Philosophies and Practices of Emancipatory Nursing

This anthology presents the philosophical and practice perspectives of nurse scholars whose works center on promoting nursing research, practice, and education within frameworks of social justice and critical theories. Social justice nursing is defined by the editors as nursing practice that is emancipatory and rests on the principle of praxis, which is practice aimed at attaining social justice goals and outcomes that improve health experiences and conditions of individuals, their communities, and society. There is a lack in the nursing discipline of resources that contain praxis approaches and there is a need for new concepts, models, and theories that could encompass scholarship and practice aimed at purposive reformation of nursing, other health professions, and health care systems. Chapters bridge critical theoretical frameworks and nursing science in ways that are understandable and useful for practicing nurses and other health professionals in clinical settings, in academia, and in research.

In this book, nurses' ideas and knowledge development efforts are not limited to problems and solutions emerging from the dominant discourse or traditions. The authors offer innovative ways to work towards establishing alternative forms of knowledge, capable of capturing both the roots and complexity of contemporary problems as distributed across a diversity of people and communities. It fills a significant gap in the literature and makes an exceptional contribution as a collection of new writings from some of the foremost nursing scholars whose works are informed by critical frameworks.

Paula N. Kagan is an associate professor at DePaul University, Chicago.

Marlaine C. Smith is Dean and Helen K. Persson Eminent Scholar at the Christine E. Lynn College of Nursing at Florida Atlantic University.

Peggy L. Chinn is the founding editor of *Advances in Nursing Science*, which since 1978 has been a premier journal publishing cutting-edge scholarship in nursing.

Routledge Studies in Health and Social Welfare

Philosophies and Practices of Emancipatory Nursing

Social Justice as Praxis

Edited by Paula N. Kagan, Marlaine C. Smith, and Peggy L. Chinn

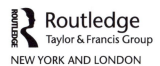

Routledge
Taylor & Francis Group

NEW YORK AND LONDON

First published 2014
by Routledge
711 Third Avenue, New York, NY 10017

and by Routledge
2 Park Square, Milton Park, Abingdon, Oxfordshire OX14 4RN

First issued in paperback 2016

Routledge is an imprint of the Taylor & Francis Group, an informa business

Library of Congress Cataloging-in-Publication Data

Philosophies and practices of emancipatory nursing : social justice as praxis /
    edited by Paula N. Kagan, Marlaine C. Smith, Peggy L. Chinn. — 1st Edition.
       pages cm. — (Routledge studies in health and social welfare ; 11)
    Includes bibliographical references and index.
   1. Social service—Research.   2. Nursing—Social aspects.   3. Social
justice.   4. Critical theory.   I. Kagan, Paula N., editor of compilation.
II. Smith, Marlaine C. (Marlaine Cappelli), editor of compilation.
III. Chinn, Peggy L., editor of compilation.
   RT86.5.P55 2014
   362.14—dc23
   2014004055

ISBN 13: 978-0-415-79340-7 (pbk)
ISBN 13: 978-0-415-65953-6 (hbk)

Typeset in Sabon
by Apex CoVantage, LLC

Contents

SECTION II
Research Methodologies and Practices:
Critical New Knowledge Development

SECTION III
Pedagogy of Praxis: Teaching for Social Justice

Acknowledgments

I offer many thanks to DePaul University for support of my scholarship in various forms including grants and paid leave. I am deeply appreciative of my colleagues, friends, and family for their encouragement and support. For their criticality, imagination, and determination I am grateful to and in awe of the authors of these chapters and the authors of chapters for which the limitations of the publication prevented their inclusion. Most importantly, I am indebted to my partners and co-editors, Marlaine and Peggy, two incredibly wonderful and visionary scholars whose continued friendship and collaboration during this journey of praxis has meant the world to me.

Paula N. Kagan

I am grateful to the authors who contributed to this volume. I learned so much from you! Editing this book with Paula and Peggy has been the quintessential experience of collegiality, and I am so grateful for their passion and patience. I acknowledge the many scholars in the fields of caring, unitary, and critical/post-structural perspectives who have influenced my thinking about social justice, participative, and emancipatory approaches to research and practice, and the uniqueness of nursing's contribution to the world. This book was in process at the time of the birth of my first grandchild, Iyla. Her arrival calls me to our purpose: the audacious hope of creating a more humane, peaceful, and just world for all our children.

Marlaine C. Smith

Working with Paula and Marlaine has been one of the most gratifying experiences of my professional career. Thank you, Paula, for your awesome leadership in this project starting with your determination to engage a publisher for this work, your sharp intellect that has been invaluable to the editing process, and your intractable yet gentle capacity to keep us all on track. Thank you, Marlaine, for your inspiring ability to "walk the talk," your gentle way of speaking truth to power, and your insights that always point to the core of nursing. You are both dear and cherished friends and colleagues. Finally, I acknowledge the immeasurable value of my family—my partner Karen and our adult children who are integral to our daily lives, and their beautiful children who are growing up in culturally diverse worlds and who will grow to adulthood in a future we can only imagine. It is the imaginations portrayed in this book that I hope will inspire a future worthy of their dreams.

Peggy L. Chinn

Foreword: Social Justice: Continuing the Dialogue

"Although we may speak the words of social justice, it is how we act that clearly demonstrates our philosophy."[1(p29)]

This book comes at a time when social justice as praxis has never been more urgent. The inequalities and inequities we are witnessing are not new. However, as we move deeper into the 21st century, wars and unrest in many parts of the world; increasing economic uncertainties locally and globally; income disparities with the widening gap between rich and poor; and perceived and actual inequities, all of which thwart life opportunities and profoundly influence health and well-being, make the enactment of social justice an urgent issue particularly in a discipline such as nursing, with its accompanying professional mandate. Bekemeier and Butterfield[2] among others remind us that progressive nurse reformers—on whose shoulders we stand—"grew indignant from witnessing the destructive health outcomes of institutionalized poverty and of gender and ethnic inequalities. These nurses harnessed their indignation to work toward the creation of progressive health policies,"[2(p153)] and so must we! In Canada, the Canadian Nurses Association's (CNA) commitment to advancing social justice has been articulated in various policy documents over the years, culminating with a policy discussion paper in 2010.[3] Yet, despite our attentiveness to social justice in policy documents and scholarly discourse over many decades, the vexing problem of injustices and inequities remain visible in some of the populations with whom we, as nurses, work. At issue is the complexity of the concept of social justice, the competing and divergent theoretical perspectives that have informed the discourse and how we see our responsibility as nurses. But regardless of the perspectives from which we come, we might be in agreement with Amartya Sen[4] that "justice cannot be indifferent to the lives that people *can* [emphasis added] actually live."[4(p18)]

Given the opportunity to contribute to this book, there are a few points—implicit in any discussion of social justice—which I would like us to consider as we embark upon reading through this very fine collection of essays. I should point out that the intent of this foreword is not to review the chapters—the editors have done this. Rather, I offer a few brief comments on issues I have observed as I have participated in nursing discourse through the years, and reflected on, and attempted to put social justice into action.

One of the issues, I believe, that has impeded our work as we strive towards the "ideal of social justice" in the discipline and profession of nursing pertains to the tension between "individual agency" and "structure"—a tension that is pervasive in many disciplines, but which is, perhaps, more poignant in disciplines such as nursing as we struggle with the complexity of these concepts and the boundaries of our responsibility as nurses. In discussions with health professionals over the years about the structures that shape the health and illness experiences of patients and their families, some (by no means all!) have seen the socioeconomic-political "structural constraints," often highlighted in such conversations, as outside of their mandate and as independent of their individual actions. Some stressed their commitment to treating *individuals equally*, an approach that is sometimes coupled with the perspective that everyone should receive the same kind of care and information, e.g., patients and their families are encouraged to engage in post-discharge planning prior to admission to hospital (for example, filling up the fridge with food prior to elective surgery, preparing and freezing meals, etc.) to facilitate the transition from hospital to home. There is often the expectation that families ought to look after their loved ones when they are ill or needing care in old age. The subtext here, I believe, is that people ought to take responsibility for their care. Although there is merit in this approach—I certainly would not quarrel with the notion that people should make adequate preparations for post-discharge prior to being admitted to hospital—the risk is that the structural constraints of economics, social inequalities, and such like may be overlooked if we are not attuned to the varied social locations of people's everyday lives. We should keep in mind that not only do some people have few social support networks, but also, there are those who have no home to return to after hospitalization.[5] Nursing scholars through the years have been reminding us to do just that, including scholars such as Drevdahl and her colleagues[1] in their article on "Reinvesting in Social Justice: A Capital Idea for Public Health Nursing?" I was struck by the trenchant insights in this excellent article. One sentence—"[a]lthough we may speak the words of social justice, it is how we act that clearly demonstrates our philosophy"[1(p29)]—the quote that appears at the beginning of this foreword—held my attention; clearly, these scholars, and others before them, are holding us to account to demonstrate socially just actions, which by their very nature would see us engage with the material context of human existence and the structural constraints that shape some lives more than others.

At the same time we should be mindful that critical discourses in nursing—at the level of discourse—often tend to privilege "*structure*" in so far as there is overriding emphasis on the structural constraints and injustices that shape the experiences of patients and their families. As I look back on my own writings, I must confess that I, too, have tended to put emphasis on structural constraints, often reifying economic and political structures as if they were "something" "out there," to be critiqued. In other words, such processes may be conceptualized as created by a "ruling elite" and independent *of our own actions.* Yet Iris Marion Young[6] reminds us that each one of us has a responsibility for social justice: " when the injustice is structural there is no clear culprit to blame and therefore no agent clearly liable for rectification. . . . [S]tructural injustice is produced and reproduced by thousands or millions of persons usually acting within institutional rules and according to practices that most people regard as morally acceptable."[6(p95)] But Young does not leave us with a feeling of helplessness. She points out that what we do matter, as do Drevdahl and her colleagues. These scholars all remind us that each one of us has a responsibility for structural inequalities; they tell us that we must find the political will to engage in conversations about social justice not only at the local level but at the global level as well. They hold us to account and marry the concept of social justice with praxis—as do the editors of this book—and, in so doing, illuminate the agency/structure dialectic.

The distinction between "treating people equally" and "treating people equitably"—the latter, a concept that grounds social justice—has consequences for our practice. Treating people equitably requires that we understand the complex context of health, illness, and suffering, including individual agency and resiliencies; the oppressive structures—often historically located—that are constraints to agency; and, that *we grapple with the dialectics of theory and action.* This, in my view, underpins what praxis means in nursing, and what is, from a critical perspective, aligned with social justice. Although praxis might be interpreted in different ways, I take it to mean translating the critical perspectives that we theorize about into action—action with the political intent of changing oppressive structures. Thus, it could be argued that working for social justice can never be from a politically "neutral" position that is unquestioning of the power structures and injustices within societies that profoundly influence health and well-being. As we have learned more about the social, political, and economic determinants of health, we have become acutely aware that although access to health care remains out of reach for many; having access, in and of itself, does not guarantee good health or recovery from illness. For instance, it became apparent to me in some of my early research with women who were balancing living with a chronic illness, minding a family, and holding down a job in the lower tiers of Canada's workforce to make ends meet, that the mediating circumstances of women's lives had a profound impact on their ability to manage their health, even when they had access to health care and worked with compassionate health care professionals whom they held in high regard. We know that the resources for managing illness and achieving health, even in societies as affluent as Canada and the United States, are inaccessible to many. Yet, theories and perspectives that do not take into account the texture of the structural constraints operating at the *intersections* of various social relations such as "race," "gender," "class," and "age," among others, put the blame squarely on the shoulders of those who are not able to live up to the ideals of "good health" even when material deprivation makes everyday survival a struggle. So, the question to be considered is whether we can speak about social justice in nursing without critically examining and questioning the *social, political, and economic structures* in which inequities that profoundly influence health, well-being, and human suffering are embedded, *and reflecting on the ways in which each one of us, by virtue of being members of a society, unwittingly maintain and reproduce the very structures we challenge and critique.*

This book robustly addresses the complex issues of agency and structure, and in so doing, provides new insights to inform "emancipatory nursing." We know from past experience that assumptions about "power" and "powerlessness"—which often deflect attention away from the structures that perpetuate social inequities—are often the subtexts for words such as "emancipatory," "empowerment," and the like.[7] Although such terms have powerful meanings when examined in the context of "constraints" to agency—which the editors have done—as we continue the dialogue on social justice into the future, we need to be vigilant not to slip into using them to imply that those who live on the margins are bereft of human agency. Instead, we need to continue to focus on *constraints* to their agency and the triumph of agency over oppressive structures. From a postcolonial perspective, one is reminded of the words of Homi Bhabha[8]: "it is from those who have suffered the sentence of history—subjugation, domination, diaspora, displacement—that we learn our most enduring lessons for living and thinking."[8(p172)] In articulating emancipatory perspectives, we have sometimes projected the notion, though unintended, that as health professionals and academics we are positioned to emancipate those whom we regard as "oppressed," or living on the margins. In other words, we may see ourselves as having the "power" to "emancipate" the "powerless" by doing "for" them that which they cannot do for themselves. But Bhabha draws our attention to the lessons to be learned from subjugated and subaltern voices—those who have been positioned on the margins *through the sentence of history*. He beckons us to recognize their human agency and capabilities to be our teachers. Through the process of critical reflexivity on the historical processes that have shaped all of our lives, and the ongoing processes through which inequities are reproduced, we come to recognize that the emancipatory process touches all of us, in ways we may not have imagined. As the editors have so eloquently described, emancipatory nursing then becomes a process of critical reflection on our own history and positionality and how others have been positioned. *The recognition of the human agency and potentialities of all of us calls for working in a partnership with, to use Bhabha's words, "those who have suffered the sentence of history."* This engagement with, and learning from one another, is emancipatory for all and holds promise for transformative social and political action.

But how can emancipatory action be sustained? Mention of a knowledge translation study on translating "critical knowledge" into practice that colleagues and I conducted some years ago seems relevant here in light of one of sections in this book on critical practice approaches. Colleagues and I conceptualized critical knowledge as "constructed through methods of critical inquiry and as fostering an understanding of historical, political, economic, and other social processes that can be drawn on as explanatory resources as we engage with patients in promoting health and ameliorating the suffering of illness. Critical knowledge is both social and reflexive in nature, prompting us to question our assumptions, the status quo, and the taken-for-granted. It is linked to praxis as the dialectical relationship among knowledge, theory, research and action. Among its outcomes are equity and critical social justice in health and health care delivery."[9(p110)]

We have argued that critical knowledge is central to a social justice agenda in nursing, as we draw upon theoretical perspectives that bring critical and political awareness into practice. This knowledge may serve to mobilize political action among nurses, not only to change the conditions under which we work but also, as a collective, to influence broader political structures to work towards addressing inequities in health and health care. Yet we have found that there are many challenges in sustaining the knowledge translation process for the integration of critical knowledge, which requires intensive engagement in clinical settings over a protracted period of time. Such initiatives may very well come to an end upon the completion of a research project, even when there is strong collaboration and solid team building in the organizations with which we work and "champions" within these organizations who wish to carry on the work. Perhaps as we think through issues of the sustainability of social justice in different organizational contexts, we might well consider models of academic/practice relations *that go beyond* building strong collaborative relationships *between* the academy and practice settings. Might we explore, for example, models in which academic nurses become the *leaders and "expert practitioners" in practice settings* to blur the division between the academy and practice settings? This would call for major organizational change in some jurisdictions, but might such a model provide the continuity within organizations that is needed for the translation of complex theoretical concepts into practice? Might it ensure sustainability over time? Clearly, this is an issue that requires ongoing conversation.

The focus on social justice as praxis in this book sets it apart as breaking new ground in nursing. The editors have assembled chapters that not only open up a discursive space to keep social justice on the agenda; the chapters provide rich conceptualizations of social justice and emancipatory nursing by drawing on research and different theoretical perspectives. Importantly, the authors *challenge us to action* not only within the universities in which some of us work, and in communities far from academia, but also in exploring interorganizational connections for sustainable social justice. The book therefore provides significant knowledge for the enactment of social justice at the level of nursing practice, within the curricula of health professionals, and within the policy domain. The essays in this book provide a foundation for continuing the dialogue on social justice as praxis well into the future.

Joan M. Anderson

REFERENCES

1. Drevdahl D, Kneipp SM, Canales MK, Dorcy KS. Reinvesting in social justice: a capital idea for public health nursing? *ANS. Advances in Nursing Science* 2001;24(2): 19–31.
2. Bekemeier B, Butterfield P. Unreconciled inconsistencies: a critical review of the concept of social justice in 3 national nursing documents. *ANS. Advances in Nursing Science* 2005;28(2): 152–162.
3. Canadian Nurses Association (CNA). Social justice . . . a means to an end, and end in itself. 2nd ed. 2010. http://www2.cna-aiic.ca/CNA/documents/pdf/publications/Social_Justice_2010_e.pdf. Accessed July 31, 2012.
4. Sen A. *The Idea of Justice*. Cambridge, MA: The Belknap Press of Harvard University Press; 2009.
5. Anderson JM. Discourse: the politics of home care: where is "home"? *Canadian Journal of Nursing Research* 2001;33(2) 5–10.
6. Young IM. *Responsibility for Justice*. New York, NY: Oxford University Press; 2011.
7. Anderson JM. Empowering patients: issues and strategies. *Social Science & Medicine* 1996;43(5): 697–705.
8. Bhabha H. *The Location of Culture*. New York, NY: Routledge; 1994.
9. Anderson JM, Browne AJ, Reimer-Kirkham S, et al. Uptake of critical knowledge in nursing practice: lessons learned from a knowledge translation study. *Canadian Journal of Nursing Research* 2010;42(3): 106–122.

Introduction

Paula N. Kagan, Marlaine C. Smith,
and Peggy L. Chinn

This anthology is a work of audacious hope and optimism. It is a collection of papers in which nurse scholars share their musings, methodologies, and actions about creating social justice through nursing practice in novel ways. The genesis of the book emerged when the three editors, joined by our friend and colleague, Richard Cowling, published *A Nursing Manifesto: An Emancipatory Call for Knowledge Development, Conscience, and Praxis* in *Nursing Philosophy* in 2009.[1] That article was inspired by our collective experiences attending the combined Nursing Knowledge Development and International Philosophy of Nursing (IPONS) Conference in Boston in 2008, whose theme was social change for the good of people and society. Our analysis of the *Nursing Manifesto*[2] specified the philosophical frameworks grounding the manifesto and our own philosophical beliefs about nursing.

A FOUNDATION OF PRAXIS

We defined *praxis* then, as now, as professional practice directed by and toward social justice goals and outcomes—which include reflexivity, action, and transformation. We conceptualize an emancipatory framework as asserting that all persons, regardless of hierarchy, status, or privilege, should have full access in sharing awareness and participating in social processes. Praxis, as conceptualized by Paulo Freire, is simultaneous reflection and action in order to transform the world.[3] Chinn, in extending Freire's idea, has maintained that the nature of the transformation that emerges from praxis alters the social conditions and power dynamics that sustain disadvantage for some and privilege for others in the direction of equality, fairness, and justice for all persons.[4] We believe that there exists a type of nursing—which we name *emancipatory nursing*—that is capable of bringing to the forefront new forms of nursing practice, research, and education that are grounded in a critical theory or philosophical awareness and intent.

Freedom is an essential concept that underpins praxis and represents the ability to choose action. Freedom is the foundational component in arriving at progressive social change, and reflects the essence of being human: freedom to think independently, live safely, in the manner of one's choosing, perhaps even well, to speak one's views, and to protect and advocate for others. Freedom, in an emancipatory context, only exists when each person shares equally in the rights and responsibilities of the culture so that no person or group is privileged or advantaged over others. Willis, Perry, LaCoursiere-Zucchero, and Grace, in their chapter titled "Facilitating Humanization: Liberating the Profession of Nursing from Institutional Confinement on Behalf of Social Justice," emphasize the necessity for nursing as a profession to be liberated from institutional confinements in order to remain grounded in the ideals of nursing's ontological, epistemological, and ethical foundations and exercise the freedom to transform health care. They state:

> liberation of the profession from institutional confinement begins with the critically reflective and creative "essential freedom" of nursing consciousness that will devise the necessary changes to expand the range of "nursing effective freedom" for social justice action. Only then will we be able to become full actors in the efforts to transform society and facilitate humanization in the fullest sense. (Willis, Perry, LaCoursiere-Zucchero, and Grace, this volume, p. 263)

From an emancipatory nursing perspective, freedom for the professional nurse is viewed as:

- emancipation from the dogma and constraints of privileged dominant health and social discourses and practices;
- emancipation from medical model and illness-cure frameworks; emancipation from prescribed interventions derived from the experiences of white, middle-class, heterosexual, and male privilege; and
- professional emancipation from society's misunderstanding and devaluing of nursing knowledge and expertise, an emancipation that fosters acknowledgment that the nurse is central in leading health policy, ethics, research, and practice from nursing science, critical, caring, and health promotion perspectives.

From our perspective as editors, this is emancipatory nursing: nursing that embraces and nurtures social justice goals and outcomes, where practice becomes praxis. It is nursing aimed at forms of knowing and doing in order to better humankind in all its variant and valued manifestations.

We hope that this anthology will inspire and guide other nurses, regardless of their area of practice, level of education, or years of experience, toward a praxis that encompasses awareness of social injustice, understanding of how social injustice is sustained, and the knowledge on which actions aimed at challenging social injustice may be based.

OVERVIEW OF AIMS AND GOALS

This anthology includes the philosophical, theoretical, and practice perspectives of nurse scholars whose work centers on frameworks of social justice and critical theories. It makes a unique contribution to the literature in that it contains original, new writings from leading nursing scholars whose works are informed by critical and/or unitary theoretical frameworks. The number of nurse scholars dedicated to non-traditional perspectives such as critical social theory, critical feminisms, intersectionality, post-colonial discourse, American Pragmatism, and unitary-transformative and caring nursing theories as underlying frameworks for practice, research, and pedagogy has increased worldwide.[5-10] However, until this volume, there has been no single collection of works such as those forwarded here.

Currently, the discipline of nursing lacks a resource focused on praxiological approaches. Nurses, nurse educators, and students have identified a need for new concepts, models, and theories encompassing scholarship and practice aimed at purposive reformation of the nursing profession specifically and health care systems and practices generally. We believe the authors of the chapters in this book provide the pathways nurses need if they are to bridge critical theoretical frameworks, nursing science, and practice in a way that is understandable and useful for all nursing to embrace the practice of emancipatory nursing.

The International Council of Nurses,[11] and other organizations and institutions, have stated that the complexity of contemporary issues facing human beings poses a broad array of questions that beg for answers; they have called for the development of suitable methods of addressing these questions. New answers need to be articulated and considered in relation to their potential for resolving the health problems of both individual persons and society as a whole. The Council further suggests that nurses' work, ideas, and knowledge development efforts should not be limited to problems and solutions emerging from the dominant discourse or tradition. It is the ethical obligation of the profession to work towards establishing alternative forms of knowledge capable of capturing both the roots and complexity of contemporary problems as distributed across a wide diversity of people and communities.

This anthology aims to address these concerns. In different ways, the authors of the works collected here advance suggestions for envisioning and enacting reformed health care services and delivery that could lead toward more equitable, sustainable, and humane models of nursing praxis. We hope this book inspires inquiry that engages participants while providing evidence of the success of novel approaches. We hope that the book prompts significant shifts in nursing education that engage and inspire learners to experience concern for social justice as central to nursing practice.

Moreover, we hope that readers will find meaningful ways to understand and practice emancipatory nursing and health care that embody a variety of social justice and critical perspectives. We anticipate that readers will revise and expand their thinking, develop frameworks, and modify their practices based on the expertise of the authors collected here, all of whom make explicit their philosophical standpoints, methods justifications, and in many cases, practical ways to "just do it." It was our goal, as editors, to offer the reader a collection that will be useful as well as inspiring and lead the reader to consider and engage in creating change for social justice.

PEDAGOGICAL APPROACHES IN NURSING AND ACROSS DISCIPLINES

In addition to appealing to nursing professionals and students, the works contained here may be helpful and informative to those from other disciplines. Educators and students in women's and gender studies, public health, social work, education, and sociology are actively seeking innovative approaches to addressing health concerns, often consulting with and collaborating with nurse scholars. We believe this anthology will be accessible to readers across disciplines for application in fields other than nursing. Nurse scholars are developing perspectives and methods that uniquely combine thought and action reflecting an ideal that is valued as praxis in many disciplines. Health professionals across disciplines are actively seeking new research processes, methodologies, and ways to resolve health disparities. The individual works collected here provide progressive ideas for addressing health problems by way of health research, education, and practice innovation.

Those disciplines and programs that are grounded in critical studies are turning their focus to health as a content area. For example, students and scholars in women's and gender studies have an increasing interest in health related to the varied way people live and identify as men and women including those of lesbian, queer, and transgender persons and communities. These researchers turn to nurse scholars for their expertise in the health, quality of life, and risks associated with such populations. Nurses have the disciplinary focus and knowledge base to guide the study of health. But without a clear commitment to issues and population health for minority and marginalized persons and communities, health knowledge alone will not adequately serve the interests of social justice in health care. Blending health knowledge with emancipatory knowledge, nurses as well as other professionals can achieve better health outcomes that respect community difference and diversity and seek methods that speak to health promotion, quality of life, and environmental sustainability. This book serves as a resource for professors and students working on health issues within critical, feminist, and/or postmodern frameworks.

EMANCIPATORY KNOWLEDGE AND PRACTICE: CONCEPTUALIZATIONS AND CHALLENGES

Within the frameworks of critical social theory, critical feminisms, intersectionality, post-colonial discourse, American Pragmatism, and unitary-transformative and caring nursing theories, we encouraged contributing authors to present their own conceptualizations and particular definitions of key terms, which, not surprisingly, they did! So, although there is a certain common theme throughout the book concerning the importance of social justice as a valued and valuable goal for nursing, there are important distinctions that bear collective reflection. These distinctions are not essentially contradictory of one another; instead, they represent the changing perspectives that emerge from envisioning a single room, depending upon where one is seated.

Quite consistently, the authors link that which is "critical" and "emancipatory" with social justice—suggesting processes and remedies that seek to address social *injustice*. Although both concepts contain elements of "knowing and doing" in their meanings, there is a clear distinction connecting "critical" as a frame of reference for seeing what might be beneath the surface. The meanings of "emancipatory" tend to be more clearly associated with frames of reference for action. Those chapters that do not explicitly define the terms focus instead on discussing scholarly work that is conducted from a critical/emancipatory perspective, and their results/conclusions are consistent with a focus on social justice and social systems that structure justice and injustice.

The purpose of our analysis was two-fold: first, to glean the richness of meaning that emerges when the content of this book is viewed as a whole and, second, to discern any contradictions or areas of tension in meanings our authors forwarded.

From a process of summary and analysis of the authors' manuscripts, four characteristic elements central to the meaning of "critical" and "emancipatory" emerged. These elements overlap, but they are also distinct. Taken together, they provide a rich description of the array of meanings related to nursing and health.

Conceptualizations of *Critical*

In this text *critical* is consistently conceptualized as having to do with social justice—becoming aware of processes and remedies that seek to address social injustice. There are four major areas of emphasis that occur around definitions of what constitutes a "critical" approach:

> **Unpacking hegemonies**—challenging what we know as truth, bringing to the surface truths that have been concealed or suppressed, and recognizing how one's own assumptions and material conditions determine what we take as "reality."

Upstream thinking—accounting for structural inequities—the "causes of causes" of health and social inequities, such as globalization of neoliberal economic and social policies, ongoing racialization of wealth and health, and the persistence of gendered inequities.

Interrogating historical/social context—examining the matrix of power relationships inherent in theories and systems—systems that privilege some knowledges and marginalize others.

Framing/anticipating transformative action—dialectic, analytic operatives of deconstruction and construction, providing a visionary inclusive framework that fosters widespread dispositions and professional habits supporting social justice.

This last characteristic reflects the inseparability of thought and action. However, it is important to note that "critical" approaches are often criticized as failing to offer constructive alternatives to that which is identified as lacking. Sally Thorne addresses this concern in her chapter titled "Nursing *as* Social Justice: A Case for Emancipatory Disciplinary Theorizing," with a particular emphasis on the imperative to remain grounded in nursing's disciplinary core. Here, she calls upon nursing's critical social scholars to "find their way back into the intrigue of nursing theorizing" so that our "our most prominent thought leaders remain aligned with nursing's disciplinary core". (Thorne, this volume, pp. 86, 87). Thorne's call for attention to nursing action provide the perfect segue for turning attention to the meanings of "emancipatory."

Conceptualizations of *Emancipatory*

In this collection the term *emancipatory* is consistently associated with actions that seek to change unjust social and political structures and to encourage a community's capacity to strive toward freedom from unjust constraints. The following four elements emerged to define characteristics of emancipatory action:

Facilitating humanization—transformative action for social justice that is grounded in the ideals of nursing's ontological, epistemological, and ethical roots.

Disrupting structural inequities—intersectional approaches to changing social structures taking into account the complexity of social life and allowing for the intersection of multiple interacting contexts.

Self-reflection—paying particular attention to the ways in which one's own experiences foster or inhibit one's ability to effectively engage in action directed at social change.

Engaging communities—building authentic relationships with communities and engaging collective action that is aimed toward political awareness, empowerment, and equitable social policy.

There are two tensions related to "emancipatory" approaches that bear particular discussion. The first tension involves the process of change itself.

The other concerns the related concepts of socio-political knowing and action and emancipatory knowing and action.

There are many complex issues surrounding change itself. There is a persistent tension around the presumption that we can "make change" on behalf of others, when at the same time we seek to respect and advocate on behalf of those with whom we work. The ethics of change involve our right to privilege our professional knowledge and insights, not *over* those we serve, but *with* them. Our responsibility to honor the choices of others or to enter into a dialogue and cooperative relationship that addresses the ethical tensions involved in making change is paramount.[12] It is generally understood, and it is our position as editors, that making change in an emancipatory context does not mean "doing for" others. However the term "emancipatory" is sometimes used in a way that implies a paternalistic intent to make change on behalf of others. Some efforts to change social conditions do hinge on making broad judgments about needed shifts in policy or practice that are eventually imposed on others without their knowledge or consent (for example, consider the social policies that have emerged with mandated seat belt use and bans on smoking in public spaces). The tensions surrounding efforts intended to create change for the better deserve ongoing dialogue and debate. Just like the social problems that emancipatory approaches seek to address, these very tensions often appear overwhelming. Gweneth Hartrick Doane, in her chapter titled "Cultivating Relational Consciousness in Social Justice Practice," provides an explanation of relational complexity and offers a notable commentary related to tensions around creating change:

> Increasing our relational complexity requires the development of a *relational consciousness*, a consciousness that involves paying close attention to how we are relating *within* situations, and inquiring into our own relational comportment—to the how, what, where, why, and when of the situation we find ourselves in. (Doane, this volume, p. 245)
>
> . . . . A relational consciousness asks: Who/what am I primarily relating to? What is dominating my attention, including my interpretations, emotions, and responses? What am I privileging? What am I *not wanting to* relate to? And how is my relational orientation shaping my experience and my action? Central to this inquiry process is *letting things be* without adding our own by-lines that result in static still shots and bounded views of people and situations. It includes noticing and exercising the skill of holding our by-lines of good/bad, right/wrong in abeyance and focusing our attention on engaging more concertedly. As we step out of the subject-object stance and relate more wholeheartedly through this inquiry process, it is possible to see beyond the dualism of letting be or change (and beyond the assumption that to 'let be' means everything stays the same). By extending ourselves to know and relate to 'what is,' we are better able to correspond within and to the situation at hand. (Doane, this volume, p. 246–247)

The second issue that is conceptually related to "emancipatory" approaches involves distinctions that can be drawn between emancipatory knowing and the concept of "socio-political" knowing. Jill White first introduced the concept of "socio-political" knowing in her insightful critique of Barbara Carper's fundamental patterns of knowing. Peggy Chinn and Maeona Kramer chose the term "emancipatory" when constructing a pattern of "emancipatory knowing" because of its link to underlying philosophies associated with critical perspectives and also because the term pointed to a desired outcome of nursing action. This is related to, but distinct from, Jill White's concept of socio-political knowing. Indeed, in her chapter for this volume, White addresses a distinction between "emancipatory" and "socio-political" knowing as follows:

> in my view socio-political knowing and emancipatory knowing are different. It may be that socio-political knowing is a necessary precursor to emancipatory knowing, but it is also a positioning and practice itself. Socio-political knowing is a broadening of the nurse's gaze to include the "wherein" or context of nursing and those who influence it. Whilst inevitably raising questions of equity and circumstance, of privilege and of invisibility, socio-political knowing does not necessitate a critical social theory or critical feminist lens. Introduction of the language of emancipation without depth of philosophical understanding can leave people with a shallow veneer of critical social theory or critical feminist theory and a rhetoric of change and emancipation without the knowledge and ability to follow through with the social challenge inherent in its philosophical stance. (White, this volume, p. 298)

The central issue, therefore, is not simply a matter of semantics but rather of the tensions between theory and action, notably the extent to which one depends upon the other, as well as the extent the two are distinct from one another.

Thus far our introduction has focused on the circumstances that led us as editors to initiate this project, our underlying intents and conceptualizations that we brought to its creation, and analysis of some of the tensions and issues inherent in the varied perspectives that constitute emancipatory nursing. We now turn to a specific description of the content that appears in this volume.

Section Overviews

This anthology is organized in sections that represent the most common domains of practice in the discipline of nursing:

- Section I—Philosophical and Theoretical Considerations: Innovative Frameworks for Health;
- Section II—Research Methodologies and Practices: Critical New Knowledge Development;

- Section III—Pedagogy of Praxis: Teaching for Social Justice; and
- Section IV—Critical Practice Approaches and Methodologies.

We offer our interpretation of the significance of each section, keeping in mind that discrete boundaries do not exist between the domains, particularly when viewed and practiced from the perspective of emancipatory praxis. We recognize a synthesis of theory, pedagogy, new knowledge acquisition, and social action in all forms of nursing praxis.

The foreword is written by Joan M. Anderson, an eminent scholar in nursing who has distinguished herself as one of the leaders in social justice research and practice. Emerita Professor of Nursing at the University of British Columbia, her record of scholarship covers almost three decades. With publications in most of the major nursing journals, Dr. Anderson's work reflects a level of productivity and critical thought that is equaled by very few. Her 1985 publication in *Advances in Nursing Science* titled "Perspectives on the Health of Immigrant Women: a Feminist Analysis" illustrated her influence in moving the discipline to a new level of discourse.[13] One of her many landmark publications in the *Canadian Journal of Nursing Research* illustrates her lasting influence: "The Conundrums of Binary Categories: Critical Inquiry through the Lens of Postcolonial Feminist Humanism."[14] In the foreword to this book, Anderson continued that trajectory emphasizing the many tensions that create challenges to emancipatory nursing, the problematic meanings of the concept *emancipatory*, and the sustainability of social justice knowledge translation as praxis.

Section I: Philosophical and Theoretical Considerations: Innovative Frameworks for Health

Social justice is embedded in nursing's ontology, epistemology, and ethic. Nursing's distinctive focus as a discipline is the study of human health and healing through caring.[15(p50)] Human-environment relationships, including physical, social, political, and economic environments, are all central to human health and healing. It follows, then, that analysis of the critical environmental interrelationships that impact health and healing fall within the discipline of nursing's domain. Social justice, as a dimension and outcome of caring, is essential to health, well-being, and human flourishing. Multiple ways of knowing are necessary to understand phenomena of concern to the discipline and to inform nursing practice. Those multiple ways of knowing have been articulated individually by Carper, White, and Chinn as empirical, aesthetic, ethical, personal, sociopolitical, and emancipatory. Emancipatory knowing has been defined at length earlier in this chapter; its foundations are rooted in critical-post-structural epistemologies that assert the influence of socio-political structures on knowledge and the purpose of reflection and action to produce transformative social change. From our earliest history nurses cared for the poor, suffering, and oppressed. Nurses have been and continue to be social activists, removing barriers, creating just systems, and working directly with communities to address what is most important to them in advancing their health. Social justice, with its emphasis on equality and equity, is part of nursing's DNA. Section I introduces readers to the philosophical and theoretical foundations of emancipatory nursing and social justice praxis.

In chapter 1, "Problematizing Social Justice Discourses in Nursing," Annette J. Browne and Sheryl Reimer-Kirkham present a critical analysis of nursing's discourse on social justice. They focus their analysis on four problematics: 1) situating social justice in the politics of difference; 2) dangers in presuming a universal epistemology of social justice; 3) the need for an ontology of social justice in the discipline and professional practice of nursing; and 4) the challenge of equity fatigue. They propose a refocused conceptualization of social justice for the discipline through a dialectic that ends in a new synthesis that can be a foundation for emancipatory praxis: 1) critiquing structures of oppression AND envisioning conditions for human flourishing; 2) understanding determinants of inequity that impact human suffering AND supporting people's resistance, self-determination, strength, and quality; 3) valuing human dignity and equity AND enacting virtues of compassion, generosity, and humility; and 4) foregrounding ideas and analysis AND focusing on goals for action.

Chapter 2, "Towards an 'Ethics of Discomfort' in Nursing: *Parrhesia* as Fearless Speech," written by Amélie Perron, Trudy Rudge, and Marilou Gagnon, is an essay about *parrhesia*, or frank speech, in nursing. The concept of parrhesia is explored from the perspectives of the Greek philosophers and Michel Foucault. The authors share their own experiences with parrhesia and assert that truth telling or speaking without fear is an emancipatory strategy that can be useful in situations of discrimination and oppression.

In chapter 3, "Compassion, Biopower, and Nursing," Jane M. Georges advances an emancipatory theory of compassion for contemporary nursing. She analyzes power, suffering, and compassion through the philosophy of Giorgio Agamben and narratives of nurses who practiced in Nazi Germany. She draws on Foucault's definition of "biopower" as "power over life" and argues that compassion is especially critical when an individual holds such power. She questions whether the current conditions of nursing practice make compassion less possible, or at times impossible, and urges nurses to speak unspeakable truths by giving voice to both the suffering and the absence of compassion they have witnessed.

Jean Watson writes about social/moral justice from a caring science cosmology and a unitary worldview. Chapter 4, "Social/Moral Justice from a Caring Science Cosmology," presents her view of social justice informed by Emmanuel Levinas' ethic of belonging and principle of universal love and nursing's disciplinary foundation in human rights. She calls for a unitary caring science, sacred science, and sacred activism that honor human unity and engender social justice that is steeped in love, connection, and belonging.

In chapter 5, "No Hiding Place: The Search for Impermeable Boundaries," Beverly Malone shares a very personal essay about the search for safety or impermeable boundaries. She recalls her experience during the horror of September 11, 2001, while working in London, and reflects on the illusions of omniscience, immortality, omnipotence, and safety and how these illusions were shattered on that day, ushering in an era of disillusionment. She concludes that although it is not possible to hide from harm, enhanced knowledge and compassion can help us to create places and spaces for healing.

In the final chapter of Section I, "Nursing *as* Social Justice: A Case for Emancipatory Disciplinary Theorizing," Sally Thorne argues that social justice is not a departure from conventional theorizing in nursing but is a natural extension of the disciplinary focus. She asserts that social justice should be within the disciplinary core and traces the historical roots of social justice in nursing. She concludes with a call to action aimed at working for social justice to permeate nursing practice.

Section II: Research Methodologies and Practices: Critical New Knowledge Development

Nursing research has been guided by several scientific paradigms. The most prominent influence on nursing research has been the traditional science or empirical-analytic paradigm. The epistemology grounding this paradigm of science is rooted in the belief that truth is "out there" waiting to be discovered; that knowledge is gained through methods that separate the influence of person and context from what we are seeking to know or understand; and that we must reduce what we are seeking to know or understand to discrete units that can be measured and compared to each other. The essence of this paradigm is radical objectivity. The human science or phenomenologic/interpretive paradigm of science is founded on the tenets that truth is subjective and value-laden, and that knowledge is cocreated through the researcher's interpretations of experiences and observations. Its essence is radical subjectivity. In the critical-post-structural or emancipatory paradigm of science truth is viewed as coconstructed through social, cultural, and political dynamics often related to power and privilege. Reflection and action are foundational to knowledge development and occur in partnership with those invested in the process and outcomes of inquiry. Critical approaches of unveiling and questioning the "truth" lead to liberating awareness and transformation. The essence is radical contextualism.[16] These paradigms of science have engendered research methodologies, methods, and practices for new knowledge development. In this section the research methods and practices within the critical-post-structural or emancipatory paradigm are described.

Chapter 7, "Community-Based Collaborative Action Research: Giving Birth to Emancipatory Knowing," written by Margaret Dexheimer Pharris and Carol Pillsbury Pavlish, focuses on community-based collaborative action research (CBCAR) as a praxis approach to engaging communities in a process of understanding their reality, addressing inequities, and advancing social justice. CBCAR is rooted in action science, the unitary-transformative and participatory paradigms, and a commitment to social justice and human rights. The authors describe the principles for and the steps in the CBCAR process.

In chapter 8, "Social Justice Nursing and Children's Rights: A Realist and Postmodern Intersectional Feminist Analysis of Nurses' Reflections on Child Risk and Protection within Domestic Violence," Nel Glass and Kierrynn Davis introduce a critical realist and postmodern intersectional feminist analysis of child protection in the context of domestic violence. Through listening to nurses' experiences of caring for children at risk for abuse and needing protection, they discovered that risk for and protection from child abuse were polarized activities, and that nurses working in this area were more focused on risk than protection. The authors argue that their analysis affords a deeper understanding of the complexities of risk and child protection within domestic violence situations.

In chapter 9, "The Identity, Research, and Health Dialogic Interview: Its Significance for Social Justice-Oriented Research," Doris M. Boutain shares her Identity, Research, and Health Dialogic Interview approach as a way to collect and interpret meaningful information about how identity relates to health and how persons with particular identities can provide insights into identity-related research findings. Born from a critical paradigm and grounded in social justice, this process transforms the intent of gathering demographic data during research from identifying static categories to engaging with participants in a process of discovering relationships between self-described identity and health. The author also provides a detailed interview guide.

Robin A. Evans-Agnew, Marie-Anne Sanon, and Doris M. Boutain offer a critical exploration of the use of Photovoice as a research method for nursing knowledge development. In chapter 10, "Critical Research Methodologies and Social Justice Issues: A Methodological Example Using Photovoice," these authors explain the process of Photovoice, provide critiques of its use, and offer two examples from a critical ethnography and critical discourse analysis, along with suggesting questions to consider when planning to use Photovoice with critical methodologies.

Section III: Pedagogy of Praxis: Teaching for Social Justice

The chapters collected in Section III focus on emancipatory pedagogy or teaching social justice within nursing. Pedagogy refers to the art and science of teaching. Emancipatory pedagogical approaches reflect the values of coparticipation of teacher and student in the process of teaching-learning; the full engagement of the teacher and student in discovery and critical thinking; and the creation of a safe environment in which the expression of diverse points of views is encouraged.

In chapter 11, "Social Justice: From Educational Mandate to Transformative Core Value," Mary K. Canales and Denise J. Drevdahl present a critical analysis of the inclusion of the concept of social justice in key literature in nursing in the United States. They reviewed the core documents that guide curriculum development in nursing education and 20 journal articles related to some aspect of social justice, and found that social justice was weakly represented or absent from the guiding documents for nursing curricula in the United States. They conclude that without our concentrated efforts, social justice may exist as mere words on the pages of mission statements and philosophies, without impact and meaning for educating the next generation of nurses and those they'll serve.

C. Susana Caxaj and Helene Berman, in chapter 12, "Anticolonial Pedagogy and Praxis: Unraveling Dilemmas and Dichotomies," describe their anticolonial approach to praxis and pedagogy evident in Caxaj's dissertation research. The authors privileged indigenous knowledge systems of the Guatemalan Mayan community as they engaged the community in activism to address the mining of their land by a Canadian company. Their emancipatory approach to can be broadly applicable within nursing education.

In chapter 13, " 'And That's Going to Help Black Women How?': Storytelling and Striving to Stay True to the Task of Liberation in the Academy," JoAnne Banks provides a deeply personal essay about her journey of reflection and discovery leading to living an authentic academic life. Storytelling is the unifying theme of her work, and she reveals how she has stayed true to this theme in the academic missions of teaching, research and service. She says, "I am an academic, a nurse scholar and a black woman, part of a group that continues to be colonized within the U.S. . . . . Survival depends of the willingness to push back." (Banks, this volume, p. 198)

Chapter 14, "Social Justice in Nursing Pedagogy: A Postcolonial Approach to American Indian Health," authored by Selina Mohammed, focuses on a postcolonial course in American Indian Health for RN-BS students. The 10-week elective course is taught using principles of emancipatory learning. Students explore how colonialism perpetuates health disparities and how decolonizing approaches are important in working with these communities.

In chapter 15, "Human Violence Interventions: Critical Discourse Analysis Praxis," Debby A. Phillips offers a synopsis of post-structural psychoanalytic discourse analysis as a way to deconstruct harmful social structures. She makes the point that unconscious judgments about normalcy are encoded unconsciously and neurobiologically and are reflected in language. Making visible the reflected meaning in language is an important consideration in both teaching and learning in nursing.

The final chapter in this section, chapter 16, "Teaching, Research, and Service Synthesized as Postcolonial Feminist Praxis" by Lucy Mkandawire-Valhmu, Patricia E. Stevens, and Peninnah M. Kako provides examples of the integration of the academic missions of teaching, research, and service into a post-colonial feminist praxis that uses emancipatory strategies to eliminate oppression and empower health. The authors sponsor a study abroad experience in East Africa for community health students, support service learning for students with nongovernmental organizations in Kenya and Malawi, and conduct their research with the communities in the region.

Section IV: Critical Practice Approaches and Methodologies

Human beings around the world daily suffer from social, political, and economic conditions that seriously compromise their health. Western systems of care delivery most often focus efforts on treatment of or rescue from illness and death, using medico-technological approaches to treat or cure. The United States has the highest per capita expenditures for health care, and yet outcomes there are less favorable than most developed countries. To improve health and well-being attention must be given to the human-environment relationships that facilitate health and well-being. This is nursing's disciplinary focus and our unique contribution to healthcare. Nurses must claim their expertise in relational caring that enhances the health and well-being of individuals, families, and communities through attention to the environment, including the social, political, and economic forces that influence health and well-being. Critical emancipatory approaches are needed to realize these goals.

The United Nations Millenium Development Goals chart a course for improved health for all citizens of the world. These eight goals are: 1) eradicating extreme poverty and hunger; 2) achieving universal primary education; 3) promoting gender equality and empowering women; 4) reducing childhood mortality; 5) improving maternal health; 6) combating diseases such as HIV/AIDS and malaria; 7) ensuring environmental sustainability; and 8) creating global systems for development. These goals can only be accomplished through advancing social justice through emancipatory practices of empowerment, equality, equity, and justice. Other countries, such as Canada, have embraced primary health care as a model to address health for all through community partnerships that address the social determinants of health, improving access to care, and focusing on disease prevention and health promotion. The Institute of Medicine/Robert Wood Johnson Foundation's report on the *Future of Nursing*[17] in the United States contains recommendations that nurses should practice to the full extent of their education, and that nurses should be prepared to lead change to advance health in full partnership with physicians and other health professionals in redesigning U.S. healthcare systems. Nurses practicing from a disciplinary perspective that considers human-environment-health interrelationships, freedom to participate fully in healthcare decisions, and health and caring relationships as primary can be instrumental in re-forming the current healthcare delivery system.

In "Cultivating Relational Consciousness in Social Justice Practice," the first chapter of the section, Gweneth Hartrick Doane provides a compelling call for nurses to cultivate a relational consciousness as they navigate toward social justice practice in the current complex healthcare environment. She offers suggestions of how to develop this relational consciousness including understanding how embracing imperfection and the dark side of human nature can lead to compassion for self and others.

Danny Willis, Donna J. Perry, Terri LaCoursiere-Zucchero, and Pamela Grace focused on humanization and authored chapter 18, "Facilitating Humanization: Liberating the Profession of Nursing from Institutional Confinement on Behalf of Social Justice." They argue that social injustice leads to dehumanization that impacts health and well-being. They link social justice to nursing ontology, epistemology, history, and ethics, and draw on Lonergan's philosophy, concluding that nursing must liberate itself from institutional confinement to realize its full potential.

In chapter 19, "Promoting Social Justice and Equity by Practicing Nursing to Address Structural Inequities and Structural Violence," Colleen Varcoe, Annette J. Browne, and Laurie M. Cender use a critical anticolonial stance and an intersectional lens to examine how structural inequities and structural violence impact health and quality of life, and they offer strategies to enhance health equity. These authors describe nine principles for health equity and social justice and identify practices to transform inequities in health care.

In chapter 20, "Military Sexual Trauma and Nursing Practice in the Veterans Administration," Ursula A. Kelly addresses the critical contemporary issue of military sexual trauma (MST). Using intersectionality as a framework she calls attention to the factors contributing to MST and presents an exemplar analysis of African-American women's experiences of MST and PTSD. Implications for social justice praxis both within and outside the VA system are detailed.

Jill White describes sociopolitical knowing in chapter 21, "Through a Socio-political Lens: The Relationship of Practice, Education, Research, and Policy to Social Justice," as an epistemological accelerant for social justice. She argues that by "shifting the gaze beyond the dyad" to the environment of care nurses can perceive the inequities driven by social-political-economic forces. She traces the roots of nursing's sociopolitical involvement to promote societal health and calls for the involvement of nurses in political action to foster new models outside of illness care within hospitals.

The final chapter, "A Passion in Nursing for Justice: Toward Global Health Equity," written by Afaf I. Meleis and Caroline G. Glickman, focuses on reclaiming nursing's mission of social justice. They describe the problem of health inequities, nursing's commitment to social justice, the uneven progress toward the Millenium Development Goals, the application of justice theories to advance health equity, and how nurses can advance health equity. The five areas that call for attention in order to advance social justice are identified as: notions of health, access to care, gender equity, maximizing potential of nurses to practice at full capacity, and breaking disciplinary silos.

The chapter sections conclude with an afterword by editor Paula N. Kagan in which she reflects on the implications for emancipatory nursing, the potential for change, and the challenges to developing nursing as a socially critical discipline.

As editors of this book, we feel privileged to have engaged with this group of nurse scholars in the completion of this important project. Each has contributed a unique and significant facet to deepen our understanding of social justice praxis leading us to new reflections, questions, and actions. We thank them for their powerful contributions, their patience and good humor through the editing process, and their willingness to share their considerable knowledge with readers.

REFERENCES

1. Kagan PN, Smith MC, Cowling WR, Chinn PL. A nursing manifesto: an emancipatory call for knowledge development, conscience, and praxis. *Nursing Philosophy* 2009;11: 67–84.
2. Cowling WR, Chinn PL, Hagedorn S. A nursing manifesto: A call to conscience and action. 2000. http://www.nursemanifest.com/manifesto_num. htm. Accessed June 12, 2013.
3. Freire P. *Pedagogy of the Oppressed*. New York, NY: The Seabury Press; 1970.
4. Chinn PL. *Peace & Power: New Directions for Building Community*. 8th ed. Burlington, MA: Jones and Bartlett Learning; 2013.
5. Chinn PL. Critical theory and emancipatory knowing. In: Butts JB, Rich KL, eds. *Philosophies and Theories for Advanced Nursing Practice*. Boston, MA: Jones & Bartlett; 2011: 143–164.
6. Kagan PN. Historical voices of resistance: crossing boundaries to praxis through documentary filmmaking for the public. ANS. *Advances in Nursing Science* 2009;32(1): 19–32.
7. Drevdahl D. Coming to voice: The power of emancipatory community interventions. ANS. *Advances In Nursing Science* 1995;18(2): 13–24.
8. Henderson DJ. Consciousness raising in participatory research: method and methodology for emancipatory nursing inquiry. ANS. *Advances in Nursing Science* 1995;17(3): 58–69.
9. Kendall J. Fighting back: promoting emancipatory nursing actions. ANS. *Advances in Nursing Science* 1992;15(2): 1–15.
10. Fontana JS. A Methodology for Critical Science in Nursing. ANS. *Advances In Nursing Science*. 2004 2004;27(2):93-101.
11. ICN. Nurses and human rights. 2011. Accessed June 12, 2013. http://www. icn.ch/images/stories/documents/publications/position_statements/E10_ Nurses_Human_Rights.pdf
12. Hess JD. The ethics of compliance: a dialectic. ANS. *Advances in Nursing Science* 1996;19(1): 18–27.

13. Anderson JM. Perspectives on the health of immigrant women: a feminist analysis. *ANS. Advances in Nursing Science* 1985;8(1): 61–76.
14. Anderson JM. The conundrums of binary categories: critical inquiry through the lens of postcolonial feminist humanism. *Canadian Journal of Nursing Research* 2004;36(4): 11–16.
15. Smith MC. Arriving at a philosophy of nursing: Discovering? Constructing? Evolving? In: Kikuchi JF, Simmons H, eds. *Developing a Philosophy of Nursing*. Thousand Oaks, CA: Sage; 1994: 43–60.
16. Smith MC. Knowledge building for the health sciences in the twenty-first century. *Journal of Sport and Exercise Psychology* 1998;20: S128–S144.
17. The future of nursing: Leading change, advancing health. 2010. http://the futureofnursing.org/sites/default/files/Future of Nursing Report_0.pdf. Accessed June 12, 2013.

Section I

Philosophical and Theoretical Considerations

Innovative Frameworks for Health

1 Problematizing Social Justice Discourses in Nursing

Annette J. Browne and Sheryl Reimer-Kirkham

INTRODUCTION

Nursing has seen a remarkable uptake of social justice discourses, a trend foundational to meeting our social mandate as a profession. The ever increasing focus on social justice in nursing discourses over the past 10 years mirrors the acceleration of social justice discourses across a variety of academic disciplines, practice fields, and policy initiatives. In Canada, the United States, and internationally, health policy statements and position papers increasingly draw on social justice in describing various public initiatives and health system interventions, for example, in relation to global health, HIV/AIDS, maternal child health, Indigenous peoples' health, and mental health. With the discourses on social justice so commonplace, we ask, is our work in promoting social justice as a concept for nursing accomplished? The pervasiveness and persistence of social gradients that result in inequities in health and health care would suggest that the ideal of social justice is far from being realized.

In earlier work, we proposed critical interpretations of social justice to guard against relativization and individualization of the social and to mobilize socially transformative efforts that shift the root causes of social and health inequities.[1] Yet critical traditions must also be held up for critique. We question whether, in the enthusiasm for the ideals represented by social justice, nurses have developed taken-for-granted assumptions and blind spots that limit how we philosophize, theorize, and enact social justice. Thus, our aims in this chapter are to explore four problematics in relation to social justice scholarship. First, we examine the consequences of grounding social justice on a politics of difference that risks "hardening" social identities by essentializing difference, oppression, and deterministically re-inscribing as "Other" those who may be disadvantaged by their social location. Second, we explore the dangers inherent in presuming a universal epistemology of social justice that imposes Western values. Third, we articulate the need to work toward an ontology of social justice enacted for nursing practice. Fourth, we consider how to respond to the "equity fatigue" that we increasingly encounter. We posit that equity fatigue often stems from paralysis at the scale of addressing health inequities or guilt about one's complicities in inequitable social relations and is not just backlash. In conclusion, we propose refocused, dialectical conceptualizations of social justice for the discipline of nursing to circumvent these problematics. To frame this discussion, we begin with an overview of the concept of health equity and comment on how social justice is taken up in the discipline of nursing.

HEALTH EQUITY AND NURSING'S COMMITMENT TO SOCIAL JUSTICE

The concept of health equity has been around for many decades but has recently gained momentum alongside social determinants of health research and health policy.[2(p86)] Health equity is defined as the absence of systematic and potentially remediable differences in one or more characteristics of health across population groups defined socially, economically, demographically, or geographically.[3,4] Implicit in the definition of health equity is the role of society in reducing the gap between those who are healthy and those who are less healthy by shifting the health and social equity gradient upward.[5] Health inequity (or health disparity as the more common term in the United States) refers to differences in health or access to health care that result from structural arrangements that are potentially remedial; in this sense, inequities can be deemed unjust.[4,6,7]

Canada was recently reprimanded by the United Nations' Special Rapporteur on the Right to Adequate Housing for failing to meet its international housing rights obligations, contributing to a national affordable housing crisis and homelessness disaster.[5,8] These structural realities intersect with and are exacerbated by poverty rates that have risen dramatically in the past decade, with Canada (along with Germany) showing the greatest increase in income inequality and poverty among the 30 member nations of Organization for Economic Cooperation and Development (OECD).[9(p221),10(p1)]

Globally, the impact of neoliberal globalization has significantly widened the income inequity gap among the richest and poorest populations around the world, and the feminization of poverty has become more and more entrenched.[11,12] Pickett and Wilkinson in their book, *The Spirit Level*,[13] argue convincingly that wide inequality is harmful for a society, and that more equal societies tend to do better on many measures of social health and wealth including: physical health, mental health, substance use, education, imprisonment, obesity, social mobility, trust and community life, violence, teenage pregnancies, and child well-being. As Dion Stout[14] reminds us, however, it is important not to define poverty only in relation to economic deprivation—and to pay due attention to the social suffering and inequities resulting from unmet human needs, displacement, grief, and loss.[14(p12)] In Canada, for example, the high rates of HIV among Indigenous women are a disturbing manifestation of embodied inequities and structural violence. This inequity cannot be attributed to cultural differences, but to issues of institutionalized poverty, racialization, and structural violence as outcomes of colonial relations. In a global era of heightened racialized tensions, sweeping neoliberal reforms, and deepening health inequities, social justice continues to hold immanent relevance. It is against this sociopolitical backdrop that we are engaging in conversations about social justice.

Nursing has a long history of concern with social justice as an integral aspect of health, health care services, and nursing praxis.[1,15] Historically, social justice aims were a central focus of public health nursing, and early leaders such as Lillian Wald, Lavinia Dock, and Margaret Sanger enacted political and social activism and advocated for broad system changes aimed at mitigating the negative health effects of widespread poverty and gendered and racialized inequities. Yet, as Lipscomb[16(p1)] points out, "social justice is, simultaneously, both an established and a renascent feature of nursing and midwifery discourse." This past decade has ushered in an unprecedented proliferation of discourses on social justice in academic, practice, and policy realms—and social justice has been taken up by professional bodies in nursing and medicine as a central focal point. In Canada, the CNA's[17(p21)] policy document, *Social Justice: A Means to an End, an End in Itself*, includes a gauge for assessing how social justice is addressed in health programs, policies, and products through the application of the following three questions: (a) Does it acknowledge that individuals and groups occupy different positions relative to one another in society?; (b) Does it acknowledge that unfair differences (inequities) exist in the opportunities and outcomes of different individuals or groups?; and (c) Does it acknowledge root causes of inequities? This landmark document signals an explicit valuing of social justice as a defining aspect of nursing's disciplinary orientation. As declared in the report, "the CNA aims to maintain its position as a strong advocate for social justice . . . and will continue to pursue greater equity in society and better health and quality of life for all by following the guiding principles of recognizing injustice and taking responsible action toward its elimination." Although this policy document focuses on health programs in the context of health services, the same questions could be applied to nursing education (e.g., nursing curricula, courses, pedagogical approaches, etc.).

The calls for nurses' involvement in social justice aims also raise concerns. Lipscomb[18] and others note that the proliferation of normative, prescriptive, and often dogmatic claims about social justice as an irrefutable "good" tend to be inadequately developed in relation to their ideological and theoretical underpinnings. Others have argued that social justice and emancipatory discourses in nursing are increasingly eroded by the prevailing ideologies of liberal individualism underpinning much of nursing's disciplinary knowledge.[19-22] The concern with individualistic readings of social justice is the emphasis placed on more proximal or downstream causes of health and social inequities. Whereas nursing's (and other health disciplines') focus on helping people to modify individual-level risk factors are beneficial in some situations, individually-based models of behavior change have been proven to be ineffective in helping people to change their behaviors or "high risk profiles" or make healthier choices.[23(p51)] Although this is shifting in nursing, individualism obscures understandings of the more distal or fundamental causes of so-called high-risk behaviors that are grounded in social, economic, and structural relations, which in turn generate nonrandom distributions of health consequences.

The question we grapple with in light of the current context of deepening inequities, and simultaneously, our commitments as a practice discipline with a social mandate is: what is nursing's role and responsibility in philosophizing, theorizing, and enacting social justice? We will do well to pause to consider the social position from which nursing is advocating for social justice; who is considered in need of social justice; the kinds of normative and often universalizing claims about social justice that are made; and our ability to enact social justice given the contexts in which we are practicing as nurses. In the next section, we summarize some key points that reflect more critical readings of social justice.

Critical Readings of Social Justice

To counter individualistic interpretations of social justice, nursing scholars have increasingly drawn on critical theoretical perspectives to better understand how peoples' health, illness, and health care experiences are shaped by historic, political, and economic conditions that exert differential effects on particular populations, groups, communities, families, and individuals. We have, for example, drawn on postcolonial feminist theory to call for the inclusion of voices and perspectives that are typically marginalized in relation to the social production of knowledge and for disrupting culturalism and the continued categorization and racialization of people according to presumed cultural characteristics.[24–27] Critical understandings of social justice take into account structural inequities—the "causes of causes"—of health and social inequities, including: globalization of neoliberal economic and social policies; the ongoing racialization of wealth and health within our societies and globally; and the persistence of gendered inequities that stem from systems of patriarchy. Framed in relation to critical readings of social justice, structural injustices can be understood as "a kind of moral wrong distinct from the wrongful action of an individual agent or the repressive policies of a state. Structural injustice occurs as a consequence of many individuals and institutions acting to pursue their particular goals and interests, for the most part within the limits of accepted rules and norms."[28(p52)] In applied health contexts such as nursing, critical perspectives on social justice are concerned with the ways that structural and social inequities shape peoples' experiences of health, illness, and health care and the role that nursing can play in responding to peoples' experiences.

However, conceptions of social justice grounded in critical perspectives must also be problematized in relation to potential blind spots. Whereas the earlier work of criticism focused on illuminating oppressions and allocating blame (what Rogoff refers to as "a vicious circle from which there is no way out"),[29(p127)] and critique examined underlying assumptions that might allow something to appear as a convincing logic, the notion of "criticality" builds on these two traditions but puts forward a self-reflexive, praxis-oriented approach to living in the present. Citing Rogoff,

> We are both fully armed with the knowledges of critique, able to analyse and unveil, while at the same time sharing and living out the very conditions which we are able to see through. As such we live out a duality that requires at the same time both an analytical mode and a demand to produce new subjectivities that acknowledge that we are what Hannah Arendt has termed "fellow sufferers" of the very conditions we are critically examining.[30]

From the stance of criticality, then, we participate in praxis toward the transformative ideals of human flourishing and social justice, seeking inclusive communities with democratic, respectful engagement. Referencing human flourishing as an ideal to complement equity offers the potential to extend both our thinking and our action (i.e., our praxis) in relation to social justice. We draw on feminists, such as Coumo,[31] who integrate the notion of human flourishing into ecological ethics as embodied, in process, and in community. Derived from the Aristolean concept of *eudemonia*, human flourishing encompasses those conditions required to foster human dignity, well-being, and agency to live in ways we find meaningful.[32(pp388,391)] In the next section, we scrutinize, in the spirit of criticality, four possible blind spots or problematics that may sabotage our social justice commitments.

FOUR PROBLEMATICS FOR CONSIDERATION

Amidst the heightened attention to social justice discourses, we wonder whether, in some cases, we are actually moving toward fostering greater health and social equity and not just toward the rhetoric of social justice. We are aware of some pitfalls that can draw us away from the ends of social justice, and in this section we discuss the problematics of: a politics of difference; a universalizing epistemology; applications to nursing practice; and equity fatigue.

(1) The Problematic of a Politics of Difference

The first problematic has to do with the consequences of nursing's proclivity for grounding conceptualizations of social justice on the politics of difference. Iris Marion Young's 1990 widely cited book *Justice and the Politics of Difference*[33] made the case to move from distributive justice to a conception of justice that recognizes that:

> typically, philosophical theories of justice have operated with a social ontology that has no room for a concept of social groups. I argue that where social group differences exist and some groups are privileged while others are oppressed, social justice requires explicitly acknowledging and attending to those group differences in order to undermine oppression.[33(p3)]

With this indictment of traditional conceptions of justice, Young set the course for critical perspectives of social justice—feminist, post-structuralist, neo-Marxist, postcolonial—that take up the politics of difference. Nancy Fraser, with her bivalent construction of social justice as redistribution and recognition[34] (and later adding participation) also took up a form of identity politics. Whereas attention to the politics of difference is integral to critical conceptualizations of social justice, as Young and Fraser have emphasized, our concerns focus on how nursing tends to articulate its assumptions about presumed cultural Others as the focus of social justice endeavors. More specifically, it is the spotlight on oppression as the object of social justice that paradoxically raises a set of cautions, those of Othering and culturalism.

(a) *Othering*. We question whether there is a tendency in our social justice discourses to exacerbate Othering (albeit unintentionally) in the identification of population groups as "vulnerable," "marginalized," or "oppressed." The politics of difference with the focus on oppression runs the risk of re-inscribing the binary opposition of oppressed/oppressor[35] with asymmetrical attention given to the oppressed as victims who become our "problem," our "mission." Critical studies (and we are speaking here from our location as scholars employing methods of critical inquiry), according to Loomba[36] foreground "Other" as their business model—with Other signifying difference, as everything that the West is not, positioning Other in a subaltern relation.

Although compelling, these calls surface tensions that can arise when considering who is assumed to be in need of social justice and who is in a position to "uncover" or redress such injustices. For example, Heron[37] argues that the rise in interest in international development work by nurses and social workers (among others) is linked to the effects of the media age in escalating our focus on the Other (but with minimal social or history analyses) who is in need of "our" help and social justice interventions. As North American nurses, policy makers, and academics, attention focused on the oppressed Other locates us as in a position of authority as we deem who is eligible for our social justice efforts. As Heron cautions, such discourse

> normalizes our centering of ourselves in relation to other people's needs, not by recognizing how we are implicated in global economic processes

of globalization that underlie these needs, but by erasing the agency of local peoples who are Othered in these processes, and by presenting "our" (read white middle-class Northern) knowledge, values, and ways of doing things as at once preferable and right, since the North, especially Canada, appears orderly, clean, and well managed in comparison. In this way, our "development' gaze . . . is constructed and directed."[37(p3)]

This type of "development gaze" was evident in a recent study with Canadian nursing students on a travel studies course in Zambia.[38] Nursing students' assumptions, shaped by media portrayals of Africa as a have-not continent, obscured their ability to see the agency and capacity of Zambians.

Othering has the effect of hardening and predetermining social identities, allowing little room for agency for the subaltern subject. The gaze (from the perspective of nursing's disciplinary center) tends toward totalizing narratives where the heterogeneity of populations groups—whether racialized, gendered, cultural, impoverished, disabled, substance using, etc.—are collapsed into a collective in need of social justice interventions. Whereas critical readings of social justice place high value on "giving voice" to marginalized perspectives, this can slip into a "speaking for" particular groups or individuals, often with presumed notions of another group's universal experiences of Other as the starting point for inquiry.[39] This is perhaps at the heart of recent calls for qualitative inquiry to necessarily be in the pursuit of "peace and social justice."[40(p29)] For example, research methodology textbooks, which are influential in nursing and other disciplines, are calling for qualitative inquiry as a means to achieving social justice aims,[40] arguing that, "the purpose of research is not to produce new knowledge, per se, but to 'uncover' and construct truths that can be used for the pursuit of peace and social justice."[40] Although these calls seem compelling, they also raise questions about the role of researchers as analysts, the criteria for rigor in scientific work, what peace and social justice may mean and for whom, and the role of generating purely descriptive knowledge that may not yet be used in the pursuit of an inherently normative direction.

(b) *Culturalism.* Related to the project of "Othering," the cultural turn of the last three decades has seen much emphasis on the social construction of identities. Whereas the first concern about social justice, as risking the collapsing of identities and inadvertently Othering, stems from the potential to operate from (and wield, albeit unwittingly) a position of power, the cultural turn has the constant pull to depoliticize social justice aims as simply a matter of exploring the difference of the discursive subject—while ignoring how global neoliberalism is resulting in deepened and racialized social (and health) inequities. Fraser[41] explains that

it is by no means clear that today's struggles for recognition are serving to complement, and deepen, struggles for egalitarian redistribution. Rather, in the context of an ascendant neoliberalism, they may be serving to displace the latter. In that case, the recent gains in our understanding of justice would be entwined with a tragic loss. Instead of arriving at a broader, richer paradigm that could encompass both redistribution and recognition, we would have traded one truncated paradigm for another—a truncated economism for a truncated culturalism. The result would be a classic case of combined and uneven development: the remarkable recent gains on the axis of recognition would coincide with stalled progress if not outright losses on the axis of distribution.[41(p2)]

In Canada, several nursing scholars and leaders recently gathered to discuss strategies for "troubling culture"[42,43] in an effort to counteract the ways that teachings on culture in nursing education have paradoxically "reinforced our complicity with imperialist practices, the exoticizing of difference, and essentialism."[42(p17)] Empirical studies continue to reveal the extent to which approaches to teaching "about culture" can inadvertently reinforce cultural stereotypes. The challenge for nursing will be to reconceptualize our pedagogical approaches to circumvent racialism and culturalism as blueprints for explaining human behavior and health issues.

(2) The Problematic of a Universal Epistemology

With the politics of difference, Heron[37] points out that the media age has had the effect of increasing and escalating Othering, with images coming with minimal social or historical analyses. As Western/Northern academics, the spotlight on the "needy and oppressed" tends to locate us as in a position of authority as we deem who is eligible for our social justice efforts. As nurses, we are inculcated with images of "doing good," replete with a gendered socialization to the "helping" imperative. With this "do-goodism" it is easy to take on an air of moral superiority—what could be more important than promoting our efforts toward fostering social justice? Add to this the presumed political neutrality and egalitarianism inherent to our profession, and as nurses and scholars it becomes increasingly difficult to be honestly and critically reflexive about where we speak from. Too often, despite our concern to disrupt Enlightenment thinking and Eurocentrism, our vantage point continues to be one firmly rooted in Western epistemology. Cautioning against a presumed universality of Western conceptualizations of social justice, Ermine,[44] a Canadian Indigenous scholar cautions:

> One of the festering irritants for Indigenous peoples, in their encounter with the West, is the brick wall of a deeply embedded belief and practice of Western universality. . . . This mono-cultural existence suggests one public sphere and one conception of justice that triumphs over all others."[44(p198)]

Ermine's observations of Western universality provide a call to step outside the dominant models to consider how social justice may be conceptualized differently in non-Western worldviews. This is particularly relevant given the predominance of White-Eurocentrically derived theorizing in nursing and Eurocentric notions of bioethical concepts such as autonomy, beneficence, maleficence, and justice. With our fervent commitment to social justice, we risk imposition in plural societies where we name Western conceptions of social justice as the "trump" ethical mandate. We, therefore, need to proceed cautiously whenever we risk passing over from a universal concern for common good and human flourishing to imperialist impositions of what have been described as the culturally specific ethical concepts of autonomy, beneficence, maleficence, and justice.[45] In other societies, differing ethical virtues may be more valued. For example, Buddhist ethics focus on virtues such as enacting nonharming, compassion, generosity, and patience in individual and relational domains, over social ethics,[46] and the wisdom of ancient prophetic Jewish writings combined justice with loving kindness (*hesed*) and humility.[47] In the European Union, the shift is to engage with concepts such as dignity, integrity, and vulnerability as a means of extending beyond conventional and North American-centric bioethical principles.[45] Ruiping Fan,[48] in the book *Reconstructionist Confucianism: Rethinking Morality after the West* lays out how Western conceptualizations of a rights-based approach to ethics (founded on views of liberal, individualist, egalitarian democracy) run counter to a virtue-based Confucian account of personhood that emphases family, honor, and ritual. Justice as a moral abstraction or ideal, he argues, is very different than lived virtue, and the modern Western notions such as justice, liberty, human rights, and egalitarianism differ vastly from Chinese moral and political concepts. In a another Eastern context, Tan-Alora and Lumitao[49(p4)] articulate how a Filipina bioethics is grounded not in views of justice and individual rights, but rather in an "embodied activity of virtue." Further, the values of personalism and caring reflect family-centered and person-oriented cultures, such that "within developing countries, abstract philosophical and political issues such as justice or fairness usually are not considered as significant as personal allegiances."[49] Indeed, in family-oriented civil societies, treating people as unequals (e.g., as in the case of nepotism) may be entirely acceptable, particularly as local communities ensure that people are loved and regarded within their families and social networks, thus ensuring everyone's collective wellbeing. With these varied examples (Indigenous, Buddhist, Jewish, European, Chinese, Filipina), the problematic of assuming a universally understood and valued conception of social justice is brought into focus.

(3) The Problematic of a Social Justice for Nursing Practice (Ontological)

The third problematic pertains to the implications of a critical reading of social justice for nursing as a practice discipline. Critical theories have been instrumental in focusing our attention on the need for structural, political, and policy change as the focus of social justice and the social justice implications of our research—but, have we undersold the ontological aspects of social justice—that is, social justice as a way of being and responding to people in the context of everyday nursing practice? As more evidence is amassed on the role of health care practices in sustaining health and health care inequities, we are increasingly concerned that nursing has not paid enough attention to "what it means" to enact social justice at the point of care. Research shows that although health care providers do not intentionally respond differentially to patients, discrimination continues to have tangible effects on health status and access to health care.[50–53] In Canada for example, despite efforts to address cultural competence and cultural safety, power relations, colonial assumptions, and negative social attitudes towards Indigenous people continue to shape health care experiences and access to services and health inequities.[54–57] Innovative strategies for fostering equity in health care organizations, and for countering marginalizing practices and policies, continue to be badly needed.[4,58] Similarly, more attention is needed in nursing education programs to teaching social justice from multiple viewpoints—so that students are exposed to various interpretations of social justice including critical theoretical and non-Western-European conceptualizations. Additionally, innovative curricular and pedagogical strategies are needed to sharpen nurses' capacities to analyze and address social justice issues in the midst of corporate-managerial drivers of efficiencies in healthcare.

The question of what it means to enact social justice in clinical contexts is further complicated by the conditions in which nurses work, characterized by pressures stemming from the corporate values of efficiency, doing more with less, and scarcity discourses.[59] Thus, there is a need to turn our social justice lens not just outward but also inward to examine the profession itself and the conditions of nursing practice and education. We see an urgent need to reconsider the social justice implications of practicing nursing in potentially unjust workplaces that often constrain the ability to practice in "socially just" ways. The concept of criticality is helpful in highlighting the dominant discourses and practices that constrain enactment of socially just responses in relation to patient care. As Varcoe and Rodney describe,

> Ideas and images of resources as scarce and unattainable abound in the day-to-day world of nursing practice. And these ideas and images in turn drive practices that emphasize certain kinds of streamlining and efficiencies. So, for example, nurses might put diapers on competent adults because they do not have time to assist them to the toilet, justifying such practice as arising out of the necessity of scarce resources."[59(p126)]

We are not suggesting that nurses are necessarily complicit with these constraints. However, efforts to preserve quality in health care will need to be restructured to align with social justice aims in relation to the care of individuals and the common good and in defiance of the dominance of corporate ideologies and practices.

(4) The Problematic of Equity Fatigue

The final problematic relates to the fatigue and frustration that we are increasingly seeing expressed in relation to terms such as oppression, emancipatory, inequity, and equity. There has been some fallout around critical theories and critical theorizing: we observe how the words "critical theorizing" can conjure up a sense of negativity, critique without end, guilt about unequal relations of power, or hopelessness about the scope of social and health inequities. There is also worry about political correctness and imposition, where only certain views are considered legitimate. Lipscomb[18] highlights impatience with how "social justice is repeatedly juxtaposed against contentious assumptions regarding market disutility"[18(p4)]; with how calls for social justice imply that nurses must adopt a particular political [leftist] position; and with the implication that nurses must distance themselves from pro-market arguments that posit that neoliberal globalization may actually "function to produce a range of personal and public moral goods including the protection and advancement of social justice."[18(p7)] The arguments that link health and social inequities to the effects of neoliberal globalization, we posit, are not intended to attribute cause exclusively to market economies. Rather, it is the ways free market economies interact with factors at the global, national, and local levels to influence inequitable outcomes that can be understood as structural injustices—because some people's options and capacities are unfairly constrained while others derive significant benefit.[28(p52)]

Nevertheless, Lipscomb's defense of the potential value of market economies in mitigating some of the negative impacts of social inequities is perhaps a reflection of the "equity and oppression fatigue" that we are seeing in our nursing classrooms at all levels. Students, when given an opportunity, often convey their frustration with hearing about neoliberalism, discrimination, racialization, gendered inequities, etc., without seeing a clear pathway for how to respond. Critical inquiry is assumed to be inherently critical to the point of being depressing and pessimistic and as focusing too much on the negatives. Rarely is critical theorizing framed as a route to garnering hopefulness and inspiration in relation to the aims of our clinical work, research, or theorizing. Despite these cautions, we are putting forward critical perspectives, and the notion of "criticality"[30] as a vehicle for engagement, action, and hopefulness. Similarly, others in nursing are framing this need for engagement and action in relation to emancipatory knowing/practice.[19,60] However, as we continue to argue, critical approaches are only successful if we can hold in tension both deconstructive and constructive motives and aims.

PHILOSOPHIZING SOCIAL JUSTICE AS DIALECTICAL

The four problematics suggest to us the need to refocus our philosophizing of social justice—to draw on dialectical conceptualizations of social justice—that operate in both complementary and contradictory ways. We put these dialectics forward not as imperatives but as fuel for further thought and dialogue. We are drawn to the notion of dialectic as more than an epistemological or methodological principle. As Kovel[61(p474)] emphasizes, more fundamentally, dialectic is "a form of praxis—consciousness, self-transformative activity." Although all of us are capable of reflexive philosophical thinking, dialectics as a domain of philosophizing occurs from our specific historical situatedness—and dialectic posits a "social relation grounded in dialog and struggle."[61] To practice dialectic well, one has to be open to contradiction and emergence, dialog and hopefulness.

As the first dialectic (see Figure 1.1), that of deconstruction and construction, we propose social justice as an interplay of critiques of oppression—"to unveil, uncover and critically re-examine"[30]—while at the same time, envisioning the conditions necessary for human flourishing. Ruger,[62] in explaining Aristotle's view, says that flourishing and health are inherent to the human condition. Amartya Sen[63] and Martha Nussbaum,[64,65] philosophers who have developed what is referred to as the "capabilities approach" in ethics, have built on Aristotle to generate a profile of capabilities that support human flourishing: life, bodily health, bodily integrity; senses, imagination, and thought; emotions; practical reason; affiliation; living in relation

Philosophizing Social Justice as Dialectical

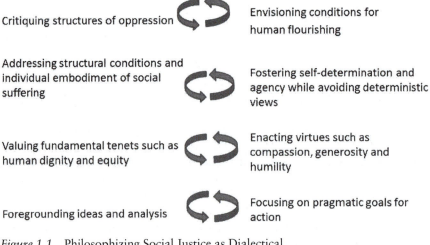

Critiquing structures of oppression ⟷ Envisioning conditions for human flourishing

Addressing structural conditions and individual embodiment of social suffering ⟷ Fostering self-determination and agency while avoiding deterministic views

Valuing fundamental tenets such as human dignity and equity ⟷ Enacting virtues such as compassion, generosity and humility

Foregrounding ideas and analysis ⟷ Focusing on pragmatic goals for action

Figure 1.1   Philosophizing Social Justice as Dialectical

to other species (animals, plants, and the world of nature); play; and control over one's environment. The capabilities approach has been criticized as individualistic in its emphasis on individual freedom (over solidarity) and as not breaking free of neoliberalism.[12,32,66] Nonetheless, our interest in featuring a capabilities approach to fostering social justice lies in its potential to offer a dialectic bridge to move between critiques of those structures that prohibit full human flourishing, and envisioning (and moving toward) those capabilities that foster human flourishing.

We are not advocating for a universalizing or "difference-blind" notion of human flourishing[67]—rather, our interest is in encouraging a form of moral humility when it comes to articulating our social justice aims precisely because we cannot assume or prescribe (in a universalist sense) exactly what human flourishing might look like for any one individual or group. This dialectic, then, creates an opening to link the projects of criticism and critique, and criticality with engagement.

As the second dialectic, that of the classic structure-agency debate, we propose social justice as a vehicle for deepening our understanding of structural forces and conditions that lead to health and social inequities and the concomitant impact on individual and collective experiences of social suffering, in dialectical exchange with the need to avoid the trap of determinism by supporting people's resistance, self-determination, strengths, and capabilities. As Young[28(p55)] points out, one of the first observations to make about social structures is that "they appear as objective, given, and constraining." She explains, "For many decades, a debate has raged among social theorists about whether conceptualizing social relations in terms of structures commits a theorist to the position that persons in a social structures are not really agents, or that that agency is something entirely independent of the structures."[28(p59)] These debates abate to some extent with the recognition that structure and agency operate in dialectical tension. Nonetheless, the challenge for nursing is to, on the one hand, bridge responsiveness to inequitable social conditions and their embodied effects on peoples' lives without presupposing that particular people or groups lack capacity (or have limited capacity) for exerting agency even in the face of extreme vulnerability, while on the other hand simultaneously working backwards, as it were, to consider how social forces and marginalizing social conditions operate to shape people's lives. Nursing's engagement with social justice will therefore need to be continually located in the often unarticulated power relations that exist between nurses and patients, relations that carry with them the very real potential of (unwittingly) undermining peoples' agency and resilience.[39]

Third, with a dialectic of principle and virtue, we propose the mapping of virtues such as compassion, generosity, patience, and humility onto our critical conceptualizations of social justice. We are not holding these out as substitutes for, or to detract from, social justice as a focus for nursing, rather, our aims are heuristic—so that we might develop more nuanced notions of what social justice may imply for our discipline and practice. This dialectic is posited as a move to decenter universalizing tendencies and to enter into an ontology of social justice at the level of clinical encounters.

At the core of this dialectic is the realization that although societies share the ideal of human flourishing, what differs is how this end is achieved. Rather than focusing on the ways in which divergent moral paradigms are incommensurable, we take up this dialectic in ways that make our efforts toward justice more compassionate, humble, generous, and infused with patience, and our person-oriented care more attuned to how people embody inequities (social suffering). The existence of divergent moral paradigms, particularly in our era of globalization, also calls forth a large degree of moral humility. Young's analysis, as cited in Clifford,[67] applied in relation to the social professions, enjoins "moral humility on individuals precisely because there is no way in which there can be absolute certainty about the knowledge that a social professional might attain."[67(p13)] This dialectic then draws us into an ontology of social justice at the level of clinical encounters. Enacting social justice in clinical interactions will simultaneously require the moral fortitude to practice in socially just ways in increasingly demoralizing workplaces—and to work collectively to transform those working conditions.

Fourth, with the dialectic of analyst-advocate—as Reimer-Kirkham and Anderson[39] have argued in relation to the tensions that must be navigated in research that aims to engage with analytic scholarship and action-oriented activism and praxis—we similarly hold that nursing needs to grapple with the advocate-analyst dialectic if it is to engage critically with the aims and subjects of social justice. As we have discussed above, advocacy for social justice needs to be understood as located in sometimes unarticulated or unrecognized power relations and problematized in relation to the very real potential of undermining agency or speaking on behalf of the other, in some cases reproducing dominant patterns of inequitable social relations. Such complexity undoubtedly requires rigorous empirical and philosophic inquiry so that our social justice efforts are based not on ideology, but rather are informed by evidence and ethics. However, the dialectic also challenges us to move beyond ideas and ideals (i.e., the "ivory tower") to engage practically and locally to affect human flourishing. Here we agree with Sen's position that focusing on the ideal of getting society's institutions and arrangements "right" can sidetrack us from very practical inroads into improving the lives of citizens: "the importance of human lives, experiences and realizations cannot be supplanted by information about institutions that exist and rules that operate."[63(p18)] As Arjona et al.[68] explain in relation to Sen's work, what is important is the ability to make decisions and engage in "justice-enhancing" responses to particular problems rather than being "paralysed into inaction" because of ideological disagreements.[63(p156)] Nursing, with its immanently practical social mandates of ameliorating illness and promoting wellness, will do well to wed rigorous analysis with thoughtful action.

In closing, to counter the four problematics we have outlined, nursing will need to delve into the tensions that arise in the midst of deconstruction and construction, structure and agency, principles and virtue, and analysis and advocacy. Entering into these dialectics will inevitably evoke tentativeness in relation to the social justice theories and frameworks we are drawn toward. The questions we have raised are held out in the spirit of evolving inquiry, toward a refocusing of social justice aims from a nursing perspective.

REFERENCES

1. Reimer-Kirkham S, Browne AJ. Toward a critical theoretical interpretation of social justice discourses in nursing. *Advances in Nursing Science* 2006;29(4): 324–339.
2. Venkatapuram S, Marmot M. Epidemiology and social justice in light of social determinants of health research. *Bioethics* 2009;23(2): 79–89.
3. World Health Organization. *The World Health Report 2008—Primary Health Care (Now More than Ever)*. Geneva, Switzerland: World Health Organization; 2008.
4. Baum FE, Bégin M, Houweling TAJ, Taylor S. Changes not for the faint-hearted: reorienting health care systems toward health equity through action on the social determinants of health. *Am J Public Health* 2009;99(11): 1967–1974.
5. Shapcott M, Blickstead R, Gardner B, Roche B. *Precarious Housing in Canada*. Toronto, ON, Canada: Wellesley Institute; 2010.
6. World Health Organization. *Closing the Gap in a Generation: Health Equity through Action on the Social Determinants of Health. Final Report of the Commission on Social Determinants of Health*. Geneva, Switzerland: World Health Organization; 2008.
7. World Health Organization. *Priorities for Research on Equity and Health: Implications for Global and National Priority Setting and the Role of WHO to take the Health Equity Research Agenda Forward*. Geneva, Switzerland: World Health Organization; 2010.
8. Shapcott M. *Universal Periodic Review—Canada—2013*. Toronto, ON, Canada: Wellesley Institute; 2012.
9. Raphael D. Mainstream media and the social determinants of health in Canada: is it time to call it a day? *Health Promotion International* June 1, 2011;26(2): 220–229.
10. OECD. *Growing Unequal? Income Distribution and Poverty in OECD Countries. Country Note: Canada*. Paris, France: OECD; 2008.
11. Hausmann R, Tyson LD, Zahidi S. *The Global Gender Gap Report 2012*. Geneva, Switzerland: World Economic Forum; 2012.
12. Jaggar A. "Saving Amina": global justice for women and intercultural dialogue. In: Follesdal A, Pogge T, eds. *Real World Justice*. Vol. 1. Dordrecht: Springer Netherlands; 2005: 37–63.
13. Pickett K, Wilkinson R. *The Spirit Level: Why Greater Equality Makes Societies Stronger*. New York, NY: Bloomsbury Publishing; 2010.
14. Dion Stout M. Ascribed health and wellness, Atikowisi miýw-āyāwin, to achieved health and wellness, Kaskitamasowin miýw-āyāwin: shifting the paradigm. *Can J Nurs Res* 2012;44(2): 11–14.
15. Falk-Rafael A, Betker C. Witnessing social injustice downstream and advocating for health equity upstream: "the trombone slide" of nursing. *Advances in Nursing Science* 2012;35(2): 98–112.

16. Lipscomb M. Social justice—special issue. *Nursing Philosophy* 2012; 13(1): 1–5.
17. Canadian Nurses Association. *Social Justice . . . A Means to an End, an End in Itself*. Ottawa, ON, Canada: Canadian Nurses Association; 2010.
18. Lipscomb M. Challenging the coherence of social justice as a shared nursing value. *Nursing Philosophy* 2011;12(1): 4–11.
19. Kagan PN, Smith MC, Cowling Iii WR, Chinn PL. A nursing manifesto: an emancipatory call for knowledge development, conscience, and praxis. *Nursing Philosophy* 2009;11(1): 67–84.
20. Daly LK. Slaves immersed in a liberal ideology. *Nursing Philosophy* 2012; 13(1): 69–77.
21. Boutain DM. Social justice in nursing: a review of the literature In: de Chesnay M, Andersen ML, eds. *Caring for the Vulnerable: Perspectives in Nursing Theory, Practice and Research*. 3rd ed. Burlington, MA: Jones and Bartlett Learning; 2012: 43–56.
22. Bekemeier B, Butterfield P. Unreconciled inconsistencies: a critical review of the concept of social justice in 3 national nursing documents. *Advances in Nursing Science* 2005;28(2): 152–162.
23. Frohlich KL, Poland B. Points of intervention in health promotion practice. In: O'Neill M, Pederson A, Dupere S, Rootman I, eds. *Health Promotions in Canada: Critical Perspectives*. 2nd ed. Toronto, ON, Canada: Canadian Scholars' Press Inc; 2007: 46–60.
24. Anderson JM, Rodney P, Reimer-Kirkham S, Browne AJ, Khan KB, Lynam JM. Inequities in health and healthcare viewed through the ethical lens of critical social justice: contextual knowledge for the global priorities ahead. *Advances in Nursing Science* 2009;32(4): 282–294.
25. Reimer-Kirkham S, Anderson JM. Postcolonial nursing scholarship: from epistemology to method. *Advances in Nursing Science* 2002;25(1): 1–17.
26. Browne AJ, Smye V, Varcoe C. Postcolonial feminist theoretical perspectives and women's health. In: Morrow M, Hankivsky O, Varcoe C, eds. *Women's Health in Canada: Critical Perspectives on Theory and Policy*. Toronto, ON, Canada: University of Toronto Press; 2007: 124–142.
27. Racine L. Implementing a postcolonial feminist perspective in nursing research related to non-Western populations. *Nurs Inq* 2003;10: 91–102.
28. Young IM. *Responsibility for Justice*. New York, NY: Oxford University Press; 2011.
29. Roseneil S. Criticality, not paranoia: a generative register for feminist social research. *NORA—Nordic Journal of Feminist and Gender Research* June 1, 2011;19(2): 124–131.
30. Rogoff I. From Criticism to Critique to Criticality. eipcp—European Institute for Progressive Cultural Policies Web site. http://eipcp.net/transversal/0806/rogoff1/en. Accessed December 21, 2012.
31. Cuomo C. *Feminism and Ecological Communities: An Ethic of Flourishing*. London, UK: Routledge; 1998.
32. Walker M. A capital or capabilities education narrative in a world of staggering inequalities? *International Journal of Educational Development* May 2012; 32(3): 384–393.
33. Young IM. *Justice and the Politics of Difference*. Princeton, NJ: Princeton University Press; 1990.
34. Fraser N. Multiculturalism and gender equity: the U.S. 'difference' debates revisited. *Constellations: An International Journal of Critical & Democratic Theory* 1996;3(1): 61.
35. Parry B. *Postcolonial Studies: A Materialist Critique*. London, UK: Routledge; 2004.

36. Loomba A. *Colonialism/Postcolonialism*. London, UK: Routledge; 2005.
37. Heron B. *Desire for Development: Whiteness, Gender, and the Helping Imperative*. Waterloo, ON: Wilfred Laurier University Press; 2007.
38. Afriyie Asenso B, Reimer-Kirkham S, & Astle B. 'In real time': Exploring nursing students' learning during an international experience. *International Journal of Nursing Education Scholarship* 2013;10(1): 1–10.
39. Reimer-Kirkham S, Anderson JM. The advocate-analyst dialectic in critical and postcolonial feminist research: reconciling tensions around scientific integrity. *Advances in Nursing Science* 2010;33(3): 196–205.
40. Denzin NK, Giardina MD. *Qualitative Inquiry and Social Justice: Toward a Politics of Hope*. Walnut Creek, CA: Left Coast Press; 2009.
41. Fraser N. Social justice in globalisation: redistribution, recognition, and participation. *Centre de Estudos Sociais (Centre for Social Studies)*. Coimbra, Portugal: Eurozine; 2003.
42. Gregory D, Harrowing J. Indigenous people's health and health-care equity: seven years later. *Canadian Journal of Nursing Research* 2012;44(2): 15–18.
43. Gregory D, Harrowing J, Lee B, Doolittle L, O'Sullivan P. Pedagogy as influencing nursing students' essentialized understanding of culture. *International Journal of Nursing Education Scholarship* 2010;7(1): 1–17.
44. Ermine W. The ethical space of engagement. *Indigenous Law Journal* 2007;6(1): 193–203.
45. Rendtorff J. Basic ethical principles in European bioethics and biolaw: autonomy, dignity, integrity and vulnerability—towards a foundation of bioethics and biolaw. *Medicine, Health Care and Philosophy* October 1, 2002;5(3): 235–44.
46. Rothberg D. *The Engaged Spiritual Life: A Buddhist Approach to Transforming Ourselves and the World*. Boston, MA: Beacon Press; 2006.
47. Forrester D. Social justice and welfare. In: Gill R, ed. *The Cambridge Companion to Christian Ethics*. Cambridge, UK: Cambridge University Press; 2012: 205–18.
48. Fan R. *Reconstructionist Confucianism: Rethinking Morality after the West*. New York, NY: Springer; 2009.
49. Tan-Alora A, Lumitao JM, eds. *Beyond a Western Bioethics: Voices from the Developing World*. Washington, DC: Georgetown University Press; 2001.
50. Agency for Healthcare Research and Quality. *National Healthcare Disparities Report 2011*. Rockville, MD: U.S. Department of Health & Human Services; 2012.
51. Canadian Institute for Health Information. *Hospitalization Disparities by Socio-Economic Status for Males and Females*. Ottawa, ON: Canadian Institute for Health Information; 2010.
52. Whitehead M, Popay J. Swimming upstream? Taking action on the social determinants of health inequalities. *Soc Sci Med* 2010;71(7): 1234–1236.
53. Institute of Medicine. *Race, Ethnicity, and Language Data: Standardization for Health Care Quality Improvement*. Washington, DC: The National Academies Press; 2009.
54. Browne AJ, Smye V, Rodney P, Tang SY, Mussell B, O'Neil JD. Access to primary care from the perspective of Aboriginal patients at an urban emergency department. *Qual Health Res* 2011;21(3): 333–348.
55. Loppie Reading C, Wien F. *Health Inequalities and Social Determinants of Aboriginal People's Health*. Prince George, BC, Canada: National Collaborating Centre for Aboriginal Health; 2009.
56. Adelson N. The embodiment of inequity: health disparities in Aboriginal Canada. *Canadian Journal of Public Health* 2005;96 (suppl 2): S45–S61.

57. Tang SY, Browne AJ. 'Race' matters: racialization and egalitarian discourses involving Aboriginal people in the Canadian health care context. *Ethn Health* 2008;13(2): 109–127.
58. Browne AJ, Varcoe CM, Wong ST, et al. Closing the health equity gap: evidence-based strategies for primary health care organizations. *International Journal for Equity in Health* 2012;11(59).
59. Varcoe CM, Rodney P. Constrained agency: the social structure of nurses' work. In: Bolaria BS, Dickinson HD, eds. *Health, Illness, and Health Care in Canada*. 4th ed. Toronto, ON, Canada: Nelson Education Ltd; 2009: 122–151.
60. Chinn PL, Kramer MK. Emancipatory knowledge development. *Integrated Theory and Knowledge Development in Nursing*. 8th ed. New York, NY: Elsevier Mosby; 2011.
61. Kovel J. Dialectic as praxis. *Science & Society* 1998;62(3): 474–482.
62. Ruger JP. Health and social justice. *The Lancet* 2004;364(9439): 1075–1080.
63. Sen A. *The Idea of Justice*. Cambridge, MA: Harvard University Press; 2009.
64. Nussbaum MC. Creating capabilities: the human development approach and its implementation. *Hypatia* 2009;24(3): 211–215.
65. Nussbaum MC. *Creating Capabilities: The Human Development Approach*. Cambridge, MA: The Belknap Press; 2011.
66. Dean H. Critiquing capabilities: The distractions of a beguiling concept. *Critical Social Policy* 2009;29(2): 261–278.
67. Clifford D. Ethics, politics and the social professions: reading Iris Marion Young. *Ethics and Social Welfare* 2013;7(1): 36–53.
68. Arjona C, Jamal AA, Menkel-Meadow C, Ramraj VV, Satiro F. Review essay. Senses of Sen: reflections of Amartya Sen's ideas of justice. *International Journal of Law in Context* 2012;8(1): 155–178.

2 Towards an "Ethics of Discomfort" in Nursing

Parrhesia as Fearless Speech

Amélie Perron, Trudy Rudge, and Marilou Gagnon

Thought is subversive and revolutionary, destructive and terrible; thought is merciless to privilege, established institutions, and comfortable habits.

—Erich Fromm

INTRODUCTION

Emancipatory practices rely on ongoing modes of critique that interrogate and challenge historic and contemporary forms of oppression that subject individuals or groups to marginalizing and disempowering mechanisms of power. Critique typically takes the shape of "critical thinking" in nursing, in that all nurses are required to question practices and policies that pose problems for patient care. Institutions themselves, including hospitals, health agencies, and universities, seem to endorse and encourage this practice, although the extent to which it is genuinely supported is open to question.

Various strategies, including advocacy, empowerment, reflective practice, and consciousness raising, have been developed in order to uphold critical reflection and provide tools for political action.[1] In health care, emancipatory strategies are usually linked to patients' and/or workers' empowerment, allowing them to identify, challenge, and transform oppressive and unethical practices. However, as we shall soon discuss, such strategies are at risk of, or have effectively been co-opted by, the very institutions and agents they target, resulting in increased containment and control of divergent opinions and actions.[2] Although the recent "integration" of emancipatory strategies officially occurs in order to address serious issues such as bullying, discrimination, and alienation, we witness in fact the consolidation and amplification of the various discourses and structures that give rise to these issues, thus leading to an ever expanding realm of government and surveillance over those who live and work in these institutions and who experience these problems.[3]

The need for critique is as relevant as ever, because issues such as discrimination, oppression, exclusion, and bullying have become so engrained and routinized (normalized) in institutional contexts of technocracy, managerialism, research orthodoxy, and corporate interests that it becomes increasingly difficult to locate and challenge them. Nurses have been called upon by professional organizations and scholars to show leadership, stand up to unethical and illegal practices, and get involved in policy. This appeal has led to numerous criticisms, namely that political involvement and professionalization constitute harmful distractions from patient care. This apparently self-serving call is often tempered by the claim that empowered nurses will better protect patient rights. This perpetuates the belief that the only valid political claim in nursing is premised on patient interests and advocacy. Indeed, for many nurses, this is the only tenable—and comfortable—political position.

In this chapter, we wish to move away from this view. We address critique, power, freedom, ethics, and political action in a way that differs from more common emancipatory practices. We discuss how Foucauldian concepts of *parrhesia* and care of the self can lead to the development of ethical and political subjectivities. To engage in this discussion however is to engage with risk, uncertainty, and vulnerability and to maintain oneself in a permanent yet ethical state of discomfort.

PARRHESIA

The Ancient Greek concept of parrhesia is essentially nonexistent in nursing or the health sciences literature. In other fields, including international relations, political theory, philosophy, literature/rhetoric, and communication, parrhesia is a widely used concept. Surprisingly, it has not been put to work in the face of concerning contemporary health issues, such as managerialism, research and best practice orthodoxy, technocracy, and medicalization.

Parrhesia refers to "frank speech" or "truth telling." It is a public articulation of one's position, a daring act that reflects one's thoughtful engagement with, and accountability to, oneself because it binds one to what one thinks and does. Parrhesia constitutes a particular discursive practice in which one speaks under specific conditions.[4] These include frankness, truth, risk, criticism, and duty.

The first condition is frankness, whereby one shares with others what one has on one's mind without resorting to artifice, without masking one's true thoughts. Frankness commands "a type of relationship between the speaker and what [s/he] says,"[4(p12)] thus rejecting rhetoric. Importantly, Foucault casts the parrhesiastic attitude in the context of relationships: "the parrhesiast primarily chooses a specific relationship to [her/himself]: [s/he] prefers [her/himself] as a truth-teller rather than as a living being who is false to [her/himself]."[4(p17)]

Parrhesia refers to truth telling because what the parrhesiast speaks is the truth, a truth acquired through certain qualities and dispositions. Truth, rather than knowledge, is central to parrhesia, and it is the second condition described by Foucault. Truth is neither the result of a reasoning process nor the product of scientific inquiry. The meaning of "truth" here departs from Foucault's earlier writing about regimes of truth. Through parrhesia, practices of truth, rather than regimes of truth, come under scrutiny. Here, Foucault argues, the parrhesiast says "what is true because [s/he] *knows* that it is true; and [s/he] *knows* that it is true because it is really true."[4(p14;emphasis in original)]

The parrhesiast possesses such truth but is also required to convey this truth to others at the risk of disrupting established practices and discourses. Risk constitutes the third condition for parrhesiastic speech. The speaker's sincerity is established because s/he speaks something that is dangerous: something that contradicts dominant thought or powerful persons. Foucault argues that the parrhesiast may risk her/his life in what he calls the "game of truth." But even if one's life is not at risk, it is easy to conceive how speaking up can damage one's social or professional life.

Speaking up entails serious consequences because it involves criticism—the fourth condition of parrhesiastic speech. Criticism is the core function of truth telling and it is conveyed in contexts where the speaker is in a position of vulnerability vis-à-vis the interlocutor. Criticism serves to point out discrepancies between their words and actions. The parrhesiast does not wish for others to act the way s/he does; rather, s/he speaks so they can see how they *could* act in ways that are consonant with what they are truly thinking, therefore taking up a new, more sincere, and more truthful relationship with themselves.

The parrhesiast speaks up but does not do so under pressure. Foucault states that s/he "is *free* to keep silent. No one forces [her/him] to speak, but [s/he] feels it is [her/his] duty to do so."[4(p19;emphasis in original)] Accordingly—and this constitutes the fifth and final condition of parrhesia—s/he feels it is her/his duty to use parrhesia: it is the only possible ethical conduct. Other courses of action, such as flattery, deceit, or silence, would leave the parrhesiast feeling that s/he is not being true to her/himself. Despite risks involved, despite the seduction of the status quo, the parrhesiast always chooses a manner of speech that is truthful, critical, and unembellished.

Foucault is less interested in what constitutes truth than what characterizes the truth teller; that is, what kind of relationship one must have to oneself in order to practice parrhesia. Parrhesia, then, focuses on the individual rather than on epistemic or power structures. And although it is concerned with the way one behaves in relation to others, it first and foremost addresses the way one behaves in relation to oneself. Parrhesia is concerned with "putting oneself first," something likely to sit uncomfortably with many, if not most, nurses.

CRITIQUE AND CARE OF THE SELF (AND CARE OF OTHERS)

Every nurse has been involved in a situation where false claims were made or the nurse was required to speak or behave in a way s/he felt conflicted about. These may be isolated events but for many such situations are alarmingly frequent. Nurses are expected to "think critically" when they occur. Here, we wish to discuss the importance of *critique* rather than critical thinking and explore the way it impacts the formation of ethical and political subjectivities.

Foucault discussed extensively how individuals are governed through techniques of power that rest on, and sustain, certain truths. As discussed earlier, speaking up through frank speech rests on continuous critique, including that of the various ever-present modes of government (understood here in the Foucauldian sense: any structure, institution, or discourse involved in shaping the conduct of individuals and populations). Critique, then, can be described as problematization aimed at generating new ways of being, acting, and thinking in relation to government: "the art of not being governed quite so much."[5(p65)]

Critique does not mean the complete dismissal of government. It is not about rejecting authority but about developing the means by which authoritative claims are evaluated and their integrity and value are judged. This opens the door to other forms of government; therefore it does not support the belief that there exists a space outside of politics, outside of power, where one is entirely free, ungoverned, and ungovernable. It does not consider that all forms of government are bad, but that they are all perilous because all may lead to imbalances of power, oppression and marginalization.[5] Not being governed "quite so much" therefore implies shifting existing relationships so as to alter established patterns of power and authority.

Therefore, Foucault sees critique as being grounded in relationships, including relationships to truth, rather than the *possession* of a particular knowledge. Parrhesia rests on dialogue between the speaker, the listener, and a community. However, its primary relationship is the self-self relationship: the relationship one has with oneself. This relationship is at the starting and end point of what Foucault calls *the care of the self.*

Care of the self is not self-care. It is a committed relationship one develops with oneself through knowledge of the self. It describes a set of embodied attitudes and practices in which the self relates to itself in a way that does not rely on prescribed biological, social, cultural, economic, or political identities and associated meanings.[6] It stands for a manner of being, a critical attitude that problematizes those discourses and rules that are mapped onto individuals and that constitute them as subjects—for example, caring, competent, or powerless nursing subjects.

Caring for oneself is concerned with "how" rather than "what" one ought to know. Foucault[7] describes three features of the care of the self: positioning oneself and behaving in relation to oneself, others, and the world; turning one's attention inward, so as to identify one's pattern of thought; and performing acts that expose one's commitment to oneself, to truth, and to freedom through practices of transformation. For Foucault, it is through a process of transformation that one has access to truth. But rather than presume what such truth might be, Foucault focuses on the kind of relationship one develops to truth. Through care of the self, one comes to know oneself, reflects on oneself, interrogates one's location in the world, judges whether one truly acts as one says and thinks, reconsiders one's attitude and behaviors, and examines how one is governed and governs others. This goes beyond the requirements of reflective practice, because it calls for changes that encompass the *entire* self, as opposed to the self specifically embodied in clinical practice. Moreover, care of the self is a practice of the self *for* the self; therefore, it does not rely on guidelines (e.g., directives, standards of practice) meant for the care of others (e.g., patients).

As discussed earlier, critique does not mean rejecting any form of governance over oneself. In fact, parrhesia rests precisely on the development of self-governance that produces an ethical subject. Self-governance comprises work over oneself (e.g., self-reflection) that leads to self-mastery. It means the ability to exercise power over oneself so that one keeps true to beliefs and ideals. Self-mastery is understood as the ability to remain *distant* and *thoughtful* in light of particular situations. This may be difficult for nurses to achieve, given the extent to which they are regulated, monitored, and governed in health care settings. Nurses are typically reacting to various demands, changes, incidents, and constraints in the "here and now," which does not provide them with the necessary space and latitude to stop and reflect properly on what these various pressures actually are, where they come from, and how they shape—and subjectivize—nurses. Critique is thus a crucial part of self-mastery because it allows one to critically reflect on what kind of subject(s) one is required to be.

Care of the self does not exclude care of others; however, one's commitment to others never supersedes one's commitment to oneself. "Care for others should not be put before the care of oneself. The care of the self is ethically prior in that the relationship with oneself is ontologically prior."[8(p30)] This may be difficult to accept for nurses, who have been socialized to perceive care of others as the only true nursing ethos. Foucault argues that care of the self is not achieved at the expense of others (e.g., patients) because, through care of the self, power is exercised over oneself that curbs one's desire to abuse others. Care of the self, then, constitutes an individualistic practice that leads to one's concern with the other. The other serves as a gauge of the degree to which self-mastery is effectively achieved.

CONTRASTING PARRHESIA WITH OTHER FORMS OF POLITICAL ACTION AND SUBJECT FORMATION

It is important to elucidate how parrhesia is similar to and varies from common critical approaches. Here we wish to explore some of the characteristics and assumptions underpinning emancipatory practices and compare these to parrhesia.

Emancipatory practices preeminently arise from critical theories associated with Marxist or neo-Marxist frameworks. Such practices suppose that structural forces and ideologies bring about oppression and a consequent inability to act freely. Emancipatory practices, explicitly or implicitly, aim for one form or another of empowerment. Power (or an understanding thereof) therefore underpins most, if not all, emancipatory practices. Power is a fundamental construct here: "having" more power (especially "formal" power) is understood as enabling a broader range of action, leading to the ability to play out a more prominent role in the realm of politics. Where parrhesia is concerned, however, power is not the driving force. Speaking out is performed neither to "gain" more power nor to give more power to others. As we shall see shortly, this allows parrhesia to escape critique often formulated against empowerment practices.

One particular assumption concerning emancipatory and social justice practices is that individuals require education to "see" how their practices or beliefs may not be in line with the "truth" of the matter. Such erroneous knowledge can be corrected by teaching how external forces shape individuals' actions and how such false consciousness leads them into error. Here, truth is construed as a relation with knowledge and social power external to, but whose beliefs are internalized by, individuals. For change to occur, dissonances and contradictory beliefs need to be confronted: first by uncovering the way they do not serve the interest of the individual/community; second, by conceiving and embodying other ways of thinking and being.

Although such contradictions may fuel the parrhesiast's reflections, assumptions about power structures are not central to the initial exploration or care of the self, although they may arise along the way. Moreover, although the parrhesiast's consciousness may be altered by her/his relation with her/himself, s/he does not seek to direct others' way of thinking and being. Rather, parrhesia constitutes a moral ideal meant to harness in others those dispositions necessary for democracy and citizenship. In comparison to consciousness raising, reflective techniques, or other forms of enlightening knowledge, parrhesia influences others only through the frankness of the parrhesiast's speech. This may lead to an educational gain and perhaps transformation conditional to the listener's own position, the parrhesiast's utterances and ethical reputation, and the associated danger, rather than expert knowledge, social influence, or status.[4]

Although power is seen to flow with knowledge in many forms of empowerment, what flows from parrhesia is increased levels of risk for the speaker.[4] For the audience no such risks exist, other than hearing something unpleasant. The risks of engaging in reflective practice, advocacy, and consciousness raising are not of the same order. Whereas risk and vulnerability are expected to diminish through these approaches, they are constant in parrhesia, inasmuch as risk is not something to be avoided or managed. Risk is an inescapable, intrinsic part of parrhesia: without risk, there is no parrhesia. In an era where risk is to be predicted, managed, and hyperrationalized, to live with risk is precisely what casts one as a parrhesiast. Risk is compounded by the fact that parrhesia is not associated with particular canons of knowledge or institutional rules. The parrhesiast does not enjoy the validation and protection afforded by a particular institution. The obligation to speak up is principally owed to oneself. One speaks only on one's own behalf and does not claim to speak for, or in defense of, anyone else, unlike those engaged in advocacy efforts for instance.

Parrhesia and care of the self are distinct forms of praxis because the parrhesiast speaks specifically to maintain a sense of identity. Therefore, unlike other practices, parrhesia does not call for a specific outcome, such as the emergence of an empowered subject, a productive subject, or a competent professional whose practice meets predetermined standards. In fact, empowerment is no longer an unproblematic concept. A critical perspective suggests instead that empowering practices can precisely perpetuate subject dependence, hierarchical relationships, objectification, marginalization, and hegemonic discourse. Because parrhesia is primarily concerned with awareness, critique, and formation of one's self, such criticism is effectively sidestepped.

With parrhesia, the outcome is unfixed, unpredictable, and shifting. For instance, unlike nurses' reflective practice, care of the self and parrhesia do not follow an organized, ritualized process whereby objectives are set (e.g., learning plan) and sanctioned by another practitioner, giving this particular activity a confessional quality.[9] Parrhesiastic self-examination leads to the willingness to learn and educate oneself for one's benefit, for a purpose that is self-determined and consistent with one's sense of ethical and political agency, rather than external norms or standards. Through care of the self and parrhesia, there can be multiple subjects formed through multiple modes of self-governance resting on multiple models of freedom, thereby circumventing the formation of a subject through disciplinary technologies and epistemic structures.

Finally, unlike advocacy work, social justice programs, or even whistleblowing, parrhesia cannot aim for large scale effects. Rather, it operates on a reduced scale and deals with the immediate circumstances of an encounter; any effect is rather limited in scope.[4] We suggest that, although Foucault did not delineate an obvious and immediate connection between parrhesia and politics, parrhesia and care of the self may be viewed as leading to a mode of political positioning, enabling a form of micro-politics that takes place in the minute details of everyday life. Consequently, we believe parrhesia can safeguard freedom and speech against the co-optation of emancipatory practices by the very structures they seek to challenge.

DISCOMFORT AS A MEANS OF EMANCIPATION

We now wish to discuss the intensifying co-optation of emancipatory strategies. In the past 50 years, management and organizational theories determined management could have happier, and hence more productive, workers by engaging in "the business of the business." Managerial theory permeated nursing through hospital missions and various management strategies, including participatory management, quality circles, case management techniques, and, more recently, team building. Such strategies are derived from empowerment experts and the concept of learning organizations. This strategy suggests a hijacking (co-optation) of emancipatory theories and techniques by management, for example in the form of so-called "emancipatory practice development."[10] Yet these strategies clearly serve organizations' interests: increased productivity, fewer complaints, decreased costs, improved efficiency, and less resistance to change, whereas accountability is shifted to individual workers.[10]

Similarly, action research methodologies informed practice changes that benefitted organizations more than nursing. Other approaches focused on human experiences were silenced, whereas randomized control trials and evidence-based medicine dominated knowledge production. Nurses wishing to get ahead readily developed numerous tools to measure nursing effort and work—many aspects of which are immeasurable. One profound deviation of traditional empowerment techniques came through the professional arm of nursing: self-regulation and reflective practice constitute powerful government techniques, with portfolios and reflective journals serving various regulatory authorities to ensure nurses are self-governing and regulated for the safety of the public. Thus a tool developed to transform nurses is now predominantly used to regulate them and their currency of practice.[9]

These instances speak to the difficulties in developing alternative forms of government—and the requirement of independent practice. The parrhesiast must remain vigilant and aware of how ideas, values, and situations may alter one's conduct. Nurses are governed by various things, namely professional bodies and workplaces. We suggest that nurses are socialized to see themselves as *extensions*—of their professional organization, their workplace, and even their patients. The values, desires, and agencies of these entities become nurses' own and this is construed as "professional" or "ethical" practice. We assert that nursing curricula do not equip nurses to problematize and challenge this arrangement, and that an overreliance on bioethics as a framework for ethical practice further conceals the intricacies of power relations that make up institutions. It is thus highly difficult for nurses to "extricate" themselves from these entities and reconnect with/ develop an agency of their own.

Nurses, like anyone else, can never be completely free. We contend, however, that they may become *a little freer* and find a space where they are no longer governed "quite so much." Extricating oneself from such compelling entities, especially when one's sense of professional self gravitates heavily around these entities, is a major undertaking. Parrhesia is a practice of truth but also a practice of freedom. To be free (or, rather, to be freer than one presently is), one needs to constitute a form of subjectivity that is not (or that is less) dependent on institutions that need regularity, predictability, and standardization to exist and perform. Critique destabilizes and disrupts this regularity. We believe that through care of the self and parrhesia, this can be effectively achieved on nurses' own terms if one is ready to engage with discomfort and vulnerability.

A WORD ON OUR OWN PARRHESIASTIC EXPERIENCES

All authors of this chapter have their own parrhesiastic experiences. Although the few examples below provide an idea of how parrhesia can be enacted in everyday contexts, they are not meant to restrict the reader's envisioning of the multiple forms of parrhesiastic speech and practices.

As nurses who have worked with vulnerable/marginalized populations, we have observed various practices that victimize patients (e.g., coercion into accepting treatment, breach of confidentiality, etc.) and nurses (e.g., mandatory overtime, bullying, threats, etc.). Parrhesia has involved confronting physicians about unfounded clinical decisions, speaking up during clinical meetings in order to advocate for patients and nurses, and denouncing bullying behaviors as they occurred. In one particular case, this led to one author becoming the next target of bullying, disparaging remarks, and harassment.

As nursing professors, we have witnessed various forms of discrimination, injustice, and bullying brought on by university policy or administrators' abuse of power that target students and academics. Parrhesia has involved speaking up in faculty meetings to denounce these processes. All authors have been subjected to unfair and violent behaviors from a senior administrator, including refusing to honor previous agreements, raising one's voice, and making covert threats. We were blamed for creating tension and conflict and for our lack of "collaboration" (understood as lack of *compliance*). Parrhesiastic practice has involved confronting the administrative person regarding dishonest and bullying practices.

Scholarly work also lends itself to parrhesia, by promoting critique in public forums (e.g., peer reviewed journals, conferences). Some of our work[11,12] has generated virulent critique because we used radical concepts, frameworks, or perspectives to shed light on policies that create problems for nurses and nursing. Some reactions have been very personal and the detractors worked to publicly undermine our work, credibility, and integrity.[13,14,15]

We have used these experiences to teach undergraduate and graduate students how nurses can become political agents. Teaching and learning enable new forms of socialization, political consciousness, and agency building. Class exchanges reveal how such situations are a daily occurrence for many nurses. Although they are aware of the need to "speak up," students and nurses often choose not to because of the anticipated discomfort and retaliation.

Discomfort takes various forms: ostracization, disparaging remarks, withholding of information, bullying, and even job loss. It also involves coming under scrutiny, as others assess the parrhesiast's own "worth." Yet, along with Foucault, we believe that care of the self and parrhesia, paradoxically perhaps, provide a sense of safety, confidence, ownership, freedom, and integrity, through consciousness, trust, anticipation, and readiness.[4] They help in identifying the words, concepts, or ideas needed to define, and practice in, the highly complex field of nursing science, without resorting to the usual restrictive and normative description of tasks, work environments, and specialty, and without giving in to the pressures of convenience, progress, speed, and efficiency.

Embodying care of the self and parrhesia also helps to move away from institutions and their discourses, which may seem comforting in the form of validation, belonging, empowerment, and protection, but they may instead induce feelings of confusion, alienation, anger, powerlessness, disengagement, and isolation. Although moral distance is needed to safeguard a sense of self, it is particularly difficult to achieve when one is overwhelmed by seductive discourses on "excellence" in patient care, "empowered workforces," "best practice," "life-saving" technologies, and "cutting-edge" scientific advances. Rather than acting as extensions of institutions' and patients' agency, nurses could regain a sense of their own agency that is robust in contexts of managerialism, technocracy, bureaucratization, research orthodoxy, health consumerism, anti-intellectualism, and the proliferation of medical-industrial-academic complexes.

Parrhesia (and care of the self) is uncharted territory in nursing. Yet as political discussions begin to flourish in our discipline and profession, we remain convinced that, because it radically links the political and the ethical, parrhesia constitutes a powerful concept that helps us (re)think emancipatory practices in nursing—practices that could be less at risk of being co-opted by the very governmental and institutional infra-structures they challenge.[2]

We expect such a stance to generate a high level of discomfort among nurses, because such framing of emancipation may seem contrary to the way nurses are socialized. Indeed, our education and self-regulation systems promote an understanding of political action limited to patient advocacy. Although such political action remains fundamental, we contend that it does not stand in opposition to the concomitant safeguarding of nurses' and nursing interests in troubling contexts of care. Care of the self and parrhesia, in fact, go beyond "critical thinking" toward *critique*. Critique fosters ones' ability and confidence to distance and extricate oneself from particular institutions and structures. One therefore develops the intellectual and moral disposition to do this successfully; parrhesia, in fact, is the public manifestation of this ethical and political disposition. However, it rests on one's (ethical) ability to tolerate discomfort rather than submit to the seemingly reassuring command of the status quo.

FINAL REMARKS

Our call for nurses to "put themselves first" is likely to elicit much discomfort among our nursing colleagues. Nurses are notorious for not caring for themselves and for focusing instead on the care of others. Care of nurses' selves (e.g., demanding fair pay, refusing to work under certain conditions or against professional expertise/standards, etc.) has been construed as being against patients' interests, unprofessional, and possibly unethical. Foucault[8] recalls that attending to oneself was long equated with egotism and vanity: negative qualities standing in stark contrast to nurses' expected attitudes of self-denial and devotion to others. However, as argued above, caring for oneself is unequivocally tied to the care of others because it provides the checks and balances needed for an exercise of power that is not abusive and unrestrained.

Vulnerability, uncertainty, and risk—in a word, discomfort—are the awkward, yet necessary, foundation for the formation of an ethical subject. They are not irritations to be avoided or overcome; instead, they provide robust grounds for ethical and political claims and actions. Valuing uncertainty and risk is difficult in a society that devalues and condemns them and whose institutions are geared towards their management and eradication—a tendency that creates individuals comfortable with relinquishing political decision-making authority and leaving it in the hands of remote institutions and so-called experts.

A radical kind of ethics must be envisioned, one that Foucault terms an "ethics of discomfort."[16] Nurses can develop a comfort zone where putting oneself first, in the form of care of the self and parrhesia, is a desirable, powerful political act that, far from distracting nurses from their professional obligations, allows them to remain true to their care ideals, their values, and their selves.

REFERENCES

1. McLaren M. *Feminism, Foucault, and Embodied Subjectivity*. Albany, NY: SUNY Press; 2002.
2. Knights D, Morgan G. Corporate strategy, organizations, and subjectivity: a critique. *Organization Studies* 1991;12: 251–273.
3. Miller P, Rose N. *Governing the Present*. Cambridge, MA: Polity; 2008.
4. Foucault M. *Fearless Speech*. Los Angeles, CA: Semiotext(e); 2001.
5. Foucault M. What is critique? In: Rabinow P, Rose N, eds. *The Essential Foucault*. New York, NY: New Press; 2003: 263–278.
6. Murray S. Care and the self: biotechnology, reproduction, and the good life. *Philos Ethics Humanit Med* 2007;2.
7. Foucault M. *The Hermeneutics of the Subject: Lectures at the College de France 1981–82*. New York, NY: Palgrave McMillan; 2005.
8. Foucault M. The ethics of the concern of the self as a practice of freedom. In: Rabinow P, Rose N, eds. *The Essential Foucault*. New York, NY: New Press; 2003: 25–42.

9. Nelson S, Purkis ME. Mandatory reflection: the Canadian reconstitution of the competent nurse. *Nurs Inq* 2004;11: 247–257.

10. Rudge T, Holmes D, Perron A. The rise of practice development with/in reformed bureaucracy: discourse, power and the government of nursing. *J Nurs Manag* 2011;19: 837–844.

11. Perron A, Rudge T, Blais AM, Holmes D. The politics of nursing knowledge and education: critical pedagogy in the face of the militarisation of nursing in the war on terror. *Adv Nurs Sci* 2010;33: 184–195.

12. Holmes D, Murray S, Perron A, Rail G. Deconstructing the evidence-based discourse in health sciences: truth, power, and fascism. *Int J Evid Based Healthc* 2006;4: 180–186.

13. Speraw S. Letter to the editor. *Adv Nurs Sci* 2011;34: 2–3.

14. Goldacre B. Archie Cochrane: "Fascist". *Bad Science*. 2006. http://www.badscience.net/2006/08/archie-cochrane-fascist/. Accessed March 27, 2013.

15. Goldacre B. Take that you pesky microfascists. . . . *Bad Science*. 2006. http://www.badscience.net/2006/12/338/. Accessed March 27, 2013.

16. Foucault M. For an ethics of discomfort. In: Faubion JD, ed. *Power: Essential Works of Foucault, 1954–1984, Volume III*. New York, NY: The New Press; 2000: 443–448.

3 Compassion, Biopower, and Nursing

Jane M. Georges

"Compassion is not religious business, it is human business, it is not luxury, it is essential for our own peace and mental stability, it is essential for human survival."

—Dalai Lama XIV[1]

This chapter synthesizes the trajectory of my work in the development of an emancipatory theory of compassion over the past decade, with implications for contemporary nursing. Although it is situated in my own perspective as a nurse scholar, this work hopefully will be helpful to anyone in a practice-based discipline that seeks to embrace compassion as an essential element of praxis. It is my belief that no true praxis—understood as reflective practice—can ever exist without an active sense of compassion. For the purposes of this chapter, *compassion* is defined as "a sympathetic consciousness of others' distress with a desire to alleviate it."[2] I use it here in the spirit of the description of compassion given by the Dalai Lama, "the wish that others be free of suffering."[3] In order to delve deeply into the roots of an emancipatory theory of compassion, I use a "local" narrative of my own expanding consciousness of the role of suffering and biopower in the development of this theory. My central thesis is that suffering and biopower are inextricably linked to the presence or absence of compassion in the practice context, and I explore these concepts as a starting point.

SUFFERING

I will never forget the moment in my life as a nursing academician when I first was struck by both the centrality—and invisibility—of suffering as a focus for nursing scholarship. In 2002, I undertook a trajectory of scholarly work into the nature of suffering in nursing. Although nursing scholars including Steeves, Kahn, and Benoliel[4] and Kahn and Steeves[5] published important initial work regarding suffering in the 1980s and 1990s, little scholarly work regarding suffering had been published in the nursing literature since that time. Nurse scholars such as John Daly[6] had undertaken analyses of suffering in the context of the Human Becoming Theory of Parse,[6] giving valuable insights into suffering as an "ineluctable aspect of life."[6(p45)] After considering this literature that explored suffering as an essentially private experience, I began to write about the contextual and political nature of suffering. I was heartened and excited by the generally positive responses to my initial publications[7,8,9] exploring the contexts in which suffering occurs. This positive feeling came crashing down when a representative from the National Institute of Nursing Research (NINR) visited my university and offered consultation for faculty planning to apply for federal research funding. I will never forget the words spoken to me by the NINR official: "Well, there's no money in suffering, you know." Actually, I didn't know. In fact, I had seen the term "suffering" positioned in central places in important nursing texts, including the ANA's Code of Ethics Preface Statement that "Nursing encompasses . . . the alleviation of suffering."[10] Instead of having discovered what I thought was a rich, relatively unstudied phenomenon on which to build a program of research, I was advised by multiple, credible nurse researchers to "forget about it." As I meditated on this advice, I remembered the axiom that "things become very powerful when people don't speak about them." Suffering, it seemed, was unspeakable for nursing science at that particular point in time. I asked the obvious question: Why? Why would a scholarly discipline so putatively invested in alleviating suffering be so uneasy about its analysis? The answer to this question took me to a place—both spiritually and intellectually—that I had never planned on going. As often happens in one's life, the intellectual and spiritual selves interweave to take us on a journey of expanded horizons. That this journey would take me to an unspeakable "shadow" side of nursing in exploring the nature of suffering and compassion in nursing was at times both painful and life changing. Suffering, then, was my entrée into what ultimately became a theory of compassion for nursing practice, but power relations would constitute the next step in my understanding.

BIOPOWER

The enormous gift of the work of Chinn,[11] Thompson,[12] and Allen[13] in rendering power *salient*—that is, visible and spoken about—to nursing scholarship is immeasurable. Although a complete summary of their work is beyond the scope of this chapter, these scholars did a Promethean task in the 1980s by foregrounding the essential role of power relations in shaping nursing practice and scholarship. "Power relations matter," I often tell my students. Prior to my PhD program in nursing science at the University of Washington, power relations had been invisible to me. I was blessed to be among the first generation of PhD students in nursing science to be given the gift of seeing nursing beyond the traditional rational-technical focus. My work in suffering quite naturally had included the salience of power relations in promoting and alleviating suffering. But something deeper was there, I felt. If so much resistance to studying suffering within academic nursing exists, the underlying power relations and social processes surrounding suffering and nursing must merit further study. Biopower, understood in its broadest sense as "power over life," can be viewed as the ultimate locus of power. By undertaking an analysis[14] of biopower, I hoped to expand my own horizons of understanding of suffering, and consequently, compassion.

AGAMBEN AND BIOPOWER

The perspectives of Italian political philosopher Giorgio Agamben (b. 1942) became useful to me in my search to understand the underlying power relations and social processes informing nursing. Agamben's principal works in the late 1990s include *Homo Sacer: Sovereign Power and Bare Life*[15] and *Remnants of Auschwitz: the Remnant and the Archive.*[16] The analysis of power relations he espouses became a useful lens for me to examine further the social processes operant in nursing that contribute to suffering and render difficult—if not impossible—the expression of compassion in many settings.

Agamben's[15,16] work is startlingly relevant to nursing. *All* power, he asserts, is by its very nature biopower. Power, or "sovereignty" as he terms it, is a socially constructed phenomenon, including the power of life and death over those being ruled. It is not difficult for me to teach graduate students in nursing about "power relations." Nurses have a keen sense of power relations understood as "who's up and who's down," having experienced the power relations operant in most health care settings. But Agamben[15] takes the idea of power relations to its ultimate conclusion: that having power over another can and does ultimately include the power of life or death. It is this critical feature of power relations that is sometimes invisible or opaque to us as nurses.

Often, my students will ask, "So you're saying that 'biopower' means that I have power over patients, like if I don't give a medication I might kill somebody?" This is, of course, true in a limited sense, but Agamben is suggesting much, much more. He asserts that any person—nurse, patient, or otherwise—who does not comply with socially constructed norms, such as maintaining employment and obeying laws, will begin to "slip down the ladder" of social status. If, for example, a person becomes homeless or a prisoner, that individual has slipped down the rungs of status to a location in which his or her very humanity is now erased. Persons in power positions may now subject that individual to violence and even death, and little or no legal protection is available. Agamben[15] terms this "non-person" status as "zoe," or "bare life." In contrast to the "zoe" classification, Agamben[15] posits that persons who possess social agency—in other words, persons considered to have a "real" person status—are termed "bios." The use of these terms is etymologically based; although both terms loosely can be used to mean "life" in classical Greek, "zoe" represents a lower rung of the "ladder" of life-forms, carrying the nuance of animalistic life[17] (hence, the English word, "zoo").

Agamben[15] asserts that in the Eurocentric narrative—meaning the shared understanding (acknowledged or not) of social processes held by Western culture—two classifications for humans exist. Either one is "bios" (possessing political agency and therefore protected by social norms) or one is "zoe" (possessing no political agency and therefore susceptible to violence and death). All cultural practices and creation of biopolitical spaces (locations where power is exerted over life—*all* locations, in fact) reflect these two classifications. Agamben's[15] work suggests that every activity in which one engages is arranged around the careful avoidance of becoming "zoe" or "bare life," from compliance with authority figures (including health care providers) to a careful maintenance of a revenue source, such as employment, in a capitalist society. Although this zoe-bios dichotomy is often opaque, it has its most visible forms in biopolitical spaces such as prisons and hospitals, where the zoe-bios divide is so prominent and all-encompassing that participants inside these locations perceive it as "natural."[16]

The implications of this dichotomous pattern in Eurocentric thought are enormous for the discipline of nursing.[14] Nurses are participants in a social process called "nursing," which on its surface espouses values such as caring and compassion. Nevertheless, nurses function in biopolitical spaces all day, every day. Using Agamben's[15,16] lens, nurses are caught up, like everyone else in Western culture, in maintaining their own "bios" status, by observing the norms of those around, above, and below them. Patients are caught up in the same zoe-bios dichotomy, but some of them have already "slipped" down the ladder to "zoe" status, according to societal norms. Perhaps they have been labeled a "non-compliant" patient or have engaged in behaviors that "nice" people (read: "bios") should not engage in, such as substance abuse. More covertly, perhaps patients are assigned a "zoe" status because of some socially constructed difference, be it ethnic, socioeconomic, or sexual orientation.[14] No one in the biopolitical space, of course, openly states this. It is "unspeakable," and understood as such by the other actors in the biopolitical space who are highly invested in maintaining their own "bios" status. If a currently "bios" person dares to point out that labeling another person as "zoe" is unethical, then that person may be viewed as being on the side of the "zoe." And once an individual sides with the "zoe," one risks being identified with that group and slipping down the social ladder oneself. And so the silence continues, resulting in the creation and maintenance of human suffering in locations ironically designed for human healing.[14]

Thus, Agamben's[15,16] work is extremely useful to me in identifying patterns of social processes that create and maintain suffering in biopolitical spaces, such as hospitals and schools of nursing. But the implications of his work for the entire discipline of nursing—including the actual *construction* of nursing knowledge run deeper and have further reaching consequences.[14] I return to my original question: what, then, underlies what I perceive as a reticence for nursing science to examine suffering in a nuanced, sociopolitical context? Why does contemporary nursing science seem "stuck" at studying suffering and compassion at the individual level of nurse-patient interaction, without regard for broader contexts in which suffering is created and maintained? On a broader note, why do many people in Western culture, including nurses, tend to avoid looking at suffering at all? I do not propose to have any answer for this question. What I can offer as a means of gaining insight is a salient exemplar case in which nurses actively participated in doing violence to patients deemed "zoe" by a fascist ideology, namely, the Nazi ideology of Germany during the Third Reich. Going deeper into this exemplar was a necessary part of my own journey of constructing an emancipatory theory of compassion, but it is not a comfortable or easy journey. It is a journey "through the looking glass" to a shadow side of nursing that bears all too many similarities to contemporary nursing in my own location.

EXEMPLAR CASE OF NURSING AND BIOPOWER

Following the publication of my initial work[7,8,9] examining the sociopolitical nature of suffering, I began working with Dr. Susan Benedict and an international research team in examining the involvement of nursing in Nazi Germany. My first response to being invited to perform discourse analysis of nurses' accounts of their participation in the Nazi agenda was disbelief. I was well aware of the highly publicized accounts of physicians in Nazism,[18] but it had never even *occurred* to me that professional nurses had been involved. This blindness on my part, an unconscious refusal to acknowledge that "my" profession had anything to do with what I considered egregious, criminal evil, was in itself an artifact of a meta-narrative shared by many in nursing. This meta-narrative, or "shared background story," says that nurses are ethical, compassionate, and embody the most positive qualities of a healer. It was an enormous, enlightening shock to read straightforward accounts of professional nurses who were mirror images of me in terms of class background and faith tradition stating that they had indeed participated in acts of murder and torture—*and had not been forced to do so.* Of course, in many instances in the Third Reich, nurses had absolutely no choice but to comply or die. But the accounts that were the most shocking to me were those of nurses who, by their own admission, did have some element of choice in their participation. They stated that they could have changed jobs, but they chose not to. Although the precise psychological dynamics driving these choices remain unknown, one can read in the narratives a certain tone of "naturalness" about their actions, a kind of "that's just the way it was." They had become true believers in the Nazi agenda, accepting of its propaganda, and were participants in its ideological belief system that certain groups (in this particular case, the mentally impaired) were not deserving of life. Like many of their contemporaries, these nurses had been socialized in societies in which anti-Semitism, homophobia, and the worthlessness of the disabled were ingrained already as part of a long-existing cultural milieu. The subsequent foregrounding of "otherness" by Nazi propaganda of the 1930s of groups such as Jews, gay/lesbian people, or mentally impaired people as "less than human" was a reinforcement of an already existing ideology. Inside this ideological belief system these nurses existed in a biopolitical space in which anything was possible, because their "patients" had been assigned a "zoe" status that removed all humanity. Of course, such ideological assignment is not unique to Nazi Germany, nor am I suggesting this. It exists here and now in contemporary U.S. culture. That is the power of this exemplar: that what happened in this exemplar case of nursing and biopower is not unique to a specific time and place, be it Nazi Germany in the 1930–40s or Abu-Ghraib in the 2000s. The assignment of "otherness" by nurses on the basis of socially constructed difference is occurring now. Nurses are participants in it every day. This exemplar was a "wake up" call for me, meaning that I also am situated in the same narrative that derides persons with disabilities, persons of color, gay/lesbian people, and other "differences." Whether consciously aware of it or not, I have been socialized in the same ideology in the contemporary United States. And it is this realization that renders this exemplar so very relevant to contemporary nursing.

Of all the work I did in collaboration with Dr. Benedict, it was a discourse analysis[19] of an account of a nurse named Luise that hit me the hardest "where I live," meaning that I recognized parts of myself in her experience. In Luise's narrative, taken from court documents obtained from the State Archive of Munich,[20,21] Luise appears neither evil nor a sociopath. She was, like me, an ostensibly well-educated and professional nurse. She had been working at a certain hospital for many years when some subtle "changes" began to be introduced. Like the metaphoric frog that jumps in a warm pan of water and eventually becomes so accustomed to the situation that it is unaware it is about to boil to death, Luise was ensconced in a slow but steady progression of institutional changes. Luise worked at a large mental health hospital, a not unusual institution in the early 1940s, both in Germany and the United States. The treatment options for severely mentally ill persons were few in that time period, and severely schizophrenic persons often required long-term hospitalization and care. Sadly, many of these patients degenerated both psychologically and physically to the point at which total nursing care was required. Luise had been working in this setting for many years and shared a collegial relationship with the physician in charge of the institution, whose opinions she valued and trusted. One day, she was approached by this physician who informed her that "incurable, sick patients were to be 'saved from their suffering' (i.e., killed) by large doses of Veronal" (a barbiturate).[20] By her own account, Luise decided that "there must be something legal"[20] allowing this or this trusted physician would not be suggesting it. She complied, and stated that, at first, it seemed like a "release" for those unfortunate patients who were in such a debilitated condition.[21] Among her patients were a variety of persons, both Jews and non-Jews, who suffered from mental conditions ranging from severe psychosis to mild depression.

The process did not end there, however. What Luise did not realize was that the institution at which she was working, the Meseritz-Obrawalde State Institution, was part of a government program instituted to "dispose of" so-called "undesirables," including what the Third Reich propaganda termed "useless eaters."[22] In the Nazi ideology, a "useless eater" was someone deemed a "non-contributing" member of society, such as a mentally or physically challenged person.[22] The ultimate goal of this "euthanasia" program was the complete emptying of all mental hospitals and facilities for persons with developmental or physical challenges. Trains full of these individuals began arriving at Luise's hospital more and more frequently during 1942 and 1943.[23]

Luise's account becomes more troubling as it continues. At times, she states, "it seemed more like killing human beings" (than at other times).[20] In many instances, she relates, the activity seemed "justifiable," particularly if patients were very physically debilitated.[20] Many of the persons arriving on the trains had been starved and left physically uncared for during the long trip, and thus the number of persons for whom killing seemed "justifiable" increased.[23] By the time the Obrawalde hospital was discovered by the advancing Russian Army in January 1945, more than 18,000 persons had been killed and buried on the grounds of the hospital.[24] Luise is estimated to have personally performed about 210 of these killings.[20] Still, she identifies herself in her account as a Christian for whom "the commandment 'Thou shall not kill' is truth for me."[21] Ultimately, she was found not guilty by a German court in 1965 on the grounds that the nurses at Obrawalde followed the orders of their superiors "without identifying themselves with the activity."[25 (p710)]

What to make of this narrative? To me, it constitutes an exemplar case of Agamben's zoe-bios dichotomy taken to its logical conclusion. Luise is part of a social context that has propagandized her into believing that her participation in the ultimate act of violence—murder—is acceptable if committed against the "zoe" on the instructions of an authority figure, approved by a larger state apparatus. Again, such social contexts are not unique to Nazi Germany. The construction of the zoe-bios dichotomy is part of the larger meta-narrative of a society in which "otherness" is assigned on the basis of some socially constructed difference, be it disability, ethnicity, or sexual orientation. Consequently, state-sanctioned violence against the socially constructed other is viewed as "natural." For example, in my own context, "legal" violence against persons crossing the border from Mexico to the United States is a daily occurrence on local television news. The subtext is that it is a "natural" outcome of the zoe-bios dichotomy.

Luise's account shows many of the patterns of the social construction of the zoe-bios dichotomy found in Eurocentric narratives.[19] There is a free-floating responsibility for the implementation of violence. Luise imagines "there must be something legal"[20] permitting the activity, and the physician hands off the commission of the actual act of violence to a nurse, thus absenting himself. Thus, no one in the situation is "really" responsible. Another discursive pattern present in the account is the distancing, both psychological and geographic, that makes the implementation of violence possible. The socially constructed "zoe" is radically different, and violence done to him or her is acceptable in special biopolitical spaces, kept carefully separated from the general public.[19] The very fact that professional nurses were the actual implementers of these ultimate acts of violence in Nazi Germany remained "hidden" and largely unreported until the 1990s. The court files regarding nursing activities at Obrawalde originally had been sealed for a period of 80 years by the West German government and were released only after a long and difficult petitioning process by Dr. Benedict.[19(p67)]

RESPONSES FROM THE NURSING COMMUNITY

What is most salient to this discussion of biopower and compassion, however, is not just the exemplar case itself of nursing's involvement in the Nazi project, but the responses I receive from the contemporary nursing community regarding this work. Imagine my surprise when confronted with this review of a manuscript I wrote concerning nursing involvement in Nazi Germany: "This is a waste of time and should not be published. These nurses were not acting like nurses when they did this. This does not belong in the nursing literature, or anywhere." The underlying message for me was stunning: "Don't go there. No 'real' nurses were involved. They were not us. So be quiet." And all I can think of is the Nazi belief in its own propaganda, and Luise situated in a biopolitical space in which anything is possible. And I cannot be quiet.

A TROUBLING PROXIMITY

The response described above is not uncommon. Not long ago, I assigned an article I had published to my students in a PhD level philosophy of science course. In this article,[26] I identify what I call a "troubling proximity" of the treatment of disadvantaged individuals within contemporary U.S. health care systems to the treatment of "undesirable" persons within Nazi Germany. The following week a student responded with open rage, berating me for "calling her a Nazi." Of course, I had never said anything of the kind. I had simply handed the students the article and said, "See you next week." The experience struck me as a sort of Rorschach test. Something in my descriptions in the article of the creation and treatment of "non persons" ("zoe") in contemporary U.S. health care had struck a raw nerve with her. Was it the same pain I had felt when confronted with Luise as a mirror image of myself? Were these parallels too close for comfort: nurses caught in the apparatus of a fascist ideology and contemporary nurses caught in a market-driven health care system in which suffering and compassion are rendered irrelevant? In the expressed rage of this student, I discovered what is truly "unspeakable" about current nursing practice. Nursing is now situated in biopolitical spaces in which compassion is rendered severely diminished to impossible. Nurses look at the worst-case exemplar of nursing in Nazi Germany, become enraged, and then deny any connection with it to their own practice. But the depth of the rage is telling. If nursing—understood as a compassionate, praxis-based discipline—is to survive, nurses must attend to the Unspeakable, inasmuch as nursing is part of a larger society of unspeakable acts and ways of being. What is meant here by "The Unspeakable" is defined in the following section.

COMPASSION AND THE UNSPEAKABLE

Compassion

As initially stated in this chapter, compassion is defined as "a sympathetic consciousness of others' distress with a desire to alleviate it."[2] I have been influenced in my thinking about compassion by the current Dalai Lama, who defines it as "the wish that others be free of suffering."[3] Note here that compassion goes beyond "having good thoughts" or "being nice." It is an *active* consciousness, a way of being that must be maintained by the cultivation of mindfulness and an honoring of other persons. Such an active consciousness cannot occur by accident. It is nourished by role modeling and practice. It is not static. Compassion grows as the individual develops the capacity for connectedness with others and is the recipient of compassion. It is a lifelong quest that begins when one begins to recognize the evil of "othering" and rejects the "radical disconnect" that makes violence possible.

The Unspeakable

The term *Unspeakable* has been used in many philosophical contexts. Tyler[27] used the term to denote patterns of discourse that appear so "natural" to the speaker that they have disappeared from his or her consciousness. Many critical/emancipatory writers have used it as a descriptor of any phenomenon so threatening to the existing power structure that no vocabulary exists for its description.[28] Thomas Merton,[29] a 20th century mystic and philosopher, used it to describe the "everyday" nature of the possibility of the total destruction of life on Earth by nuclear weapons. I honor and draw upon each of these usages to define the Unspeakable in very circumscribed manner for the purposes of this work: *the Unspeakable in nursing is the creation/maintenance of biopolitical spaces in which compassion—for oneself or one's patients—is rendered severely diminished to nearly impossible.*[30] The Unspeakable is the metaphoric "elephant in the middle of the room" for contemporary nursing. In the past decade, the biopolitical spaces in which nursing is practiced have been altered, sometimes beyond recognition, by market forces.[26,30] When I ask nurses currently working in acute care settings about changes in the "landscape" of their work, they use terms such as "mangled" and "mutated." There is not enough time or resources for praxis-based nursing. It is a "nice idea," some of my younger colleagues tell me wistfully, but it is "impossible." Constraints imposed by doing more with less, moving patients through the system faster, and coping with technology that distances the nurse from the patient have all taken their toll. In such a milieu, it is impossible to even *feel* compassion, for one's patients or oneself.[30] It is, as one young nurse said to me, "Just trying to survive, a "Hunger Game," a compassion-killer."

IMPLICATIONS FOR NURSING

Concurrent with this lived reality, nursing continues to look for answers to somehow "fix" this situation. It is asserted that if, somehow, nurses could identify what constitutes evidence of best practices, then patient "outcomes" would improve. I am supportive of this stance. But nurses run the risk of being caught up in a meta-narrative in which empirical evidence of best practices becomes a walled-off space of isolation. This space of isolation, like the biopolitical space Luise inhabited, can rapidly become a site of violence if it lacks the shared conviction that compassion is not just a sufficient but also an absolutely necessary component of nursing practice. This, then, is the substance of my emancipatory theory of compassion: that compassion is an essential element of nursing and that persons in the biopolitical spaces in which nurses practice are at an enhanced risk for increased suffering when power relations render compassion impossible.

How, then, to render compassion "possible?" That is the key question and the most pragmatic one. There are no "quick fixes" to a problem so deep and so threatening to the very integrity of nursing. I suggest a radical approach, which begins by *all* of us speaking about the Unspeakable, be it as educators, clinicians, or researchers. As Benner and co-authors[31(p167)] urge in *Educating Nurses: A Call for Radical Transformation*, nurses educators must teach for *moral imagination*. Tell the narratives of suffering you have witnessed. Broaden the moral imagination of your students and colleagues by talking about the barriers to compassion that you see every day.

Table 3.1   Guidelines for Creating a Praxis of Compassion

Compassion	The "Unspeakable"
Engages mindfully	Radically disconnects
Constructs meaning	Denies existence of meaning
Slows down in response to human needs	Speeds up to increase "productivity"
Focuses on the unique person	Renders personhood irrelevant
Listens deeply	Disregards/derides all expressions by the "Other"
Seeks understanding	Dismisses the "Other" automatically as irrelevant
Honors person as sacred	Disposes of the "Other" like trash
Seeks enlightenment	Enacts violence

As nursing faculty, freely disclose the dissonance you see between the reality of practice and the stated "missions" of institutions to alleviate suffering. Whenever possible, make the issue tangible and relevant for your specific audience: "There is no compassion in this building anymore. Because of that, patients are going to stop coming here. You are going to lose money." Be authentic and speak from your soul: "This institution was built by a faith tradition based upon compassion. Where did it go? Would you stand with me in thinking about, meditating about, praying about this?" Challenge each other: "Some of the newer nurses seem to be interacting with their patients as if they were the machine simulators they practiced on in school. What can all of us do to show more compassion for new nurses and also teach them what compassionate care looks like?" And challenge the development of new nursing knowledge: "I think the complexity of patients' experiences is far more than a single 'satisfaction score' can capture. Would you like to join me in a research study regarding patient compassion perception and identification of exemplars of compassionate care?" For the purposes of elaborating in more detail what compassionate care "looks like" in comparison with The Unspeakable, Table 3.1 contains some guidelines for creating a praxis of compassion.

CONCLUSION

The Unspeakable is a distorted, mangled form of nursing in which no compassion can or does exist. Such a distorted horror lacks the active, conscious awareness that the human beings whom nurses are privileged to touch are unique, sacred, and worthy of honor. The Unspeakable is the reduction of the transpersonal relationship to something far worse than just an "I-it" relationship. Beyond depersonalization lies the creation of biopolitical spaces in which violence—whether physical or spiritual—is not only possible but highly probable. It is a spiritual and moral void into which nursing must not be allowed to fall. To fall into that void is to allow contemporary nursing to be walled into a biopolitical space like that of our nursing colleagues in Nazi Germany. Compassion is not a luxury. It is essential for the survival of nursing. It is, ultimately, as the Dalai Lama[1] suggests, essential for human survival.

REFERENCES

1. Dalai Lama. Dalai Lama quotes. http://thinkexist.com/quotation/compassion_ is_not_religious_business-it_is_human/145362.html. Accessed May 29, 2012.
2. Merriam-Webster Online Dictionary. http://www.merriam-webster.com/dictionary/compassion. Accessed May 29, 2012.
3. Dalai Lama, Vreeland, N (ed.) *An Open Heart: Practicing Compassion in Everyday Life.* Boston, MA: Back Bay Books; 2002.
4. Steeves RH, Kahn DL, Benoliel JQ. Nurses' interpretation of the suffering of their patients. *Western Journal of Nursing Research* 1990;12(6): 715–731.
5. Kahn DL, Steeves RH. The experience of suffering: conceptual clarification and theoretical definition. *Journal of Advanced Nursing* 1986;11(6): 623–631.
6. Daly J. The view of suffering within the Human Becoming Theory. In Parse R, ed. *Illuminations: The Human Becoming Theory in Practice and Research.* Burlington, MA: Jones & Bartlett Learning; 1999: 45–59.
7. Georges, JM. An emerging contextual model of suffering. *Communicating Nursing Research* 2002;35(10): 75–77.
8. Georges, JM. Suffering: toward a contextual praxis. *Advances in Nursing Science.* 2002:25(1): 80–87.
9. Georges JM. The politics of suffering: implications for nursing science. *Advances in Nursing Science* 2004;27(4): 250–256.
10. American Nurses Association. Code of ethics for nurses with interpretive statements. http://www.nursingworld.org/MainMenuCategories/EthicsStandards/CodeofEthicsforNurses/Code-of-Ethics.pdf. Accessed May 24, 2012.
11. Chinn PL. *Peace and Power: Creative Leadership for Building Community.* 7th ed. Sudbury, MA: Jones and Bartlett; 2008.
12. Thompson JL. Practical discourse in nursing: going beyond empiricism and historicism. *Advances in Nursing Science* 1985;7(4): 59–71.
13. Allen D. Nursing research and social control: alternative models of science that emphasize understanding and emancipation. *Journal of Nursing Scholarship* 1985;17(2): 59–64.
14. Georges JM. Biopower, Agamben, and emerging nursing knowledge. *Advances in Nursing Science* 2008;31(1): 4–12.
15. Agamben G. *Homo Sacer: Sovereign Power and Bare Life* (Heller-Roazen D, Trans.). Palo Alto, CA: Stanford University Press; 1998.
16. Agamben G. *Remnants of Auschwitz: The Witness and the Archive* (Heller-Roazen D, Trans.). New York, NY: Zone Books; 1999. (D. Heller-Roazen, translator.)
17. *Lidell and Scott's Greek-English Lexicon, Abridged.* Harrogate, UK: Simon Wallenburg Press; 2007.
18. Lipton RJ. *The Nazi Doctors: Medical Killing and the Psychology of Genocide.* New York, NY: Basic Books; 2000.

19. Benedict S, Georges JM. Nurses in the Nazi "euthanasia" program: a critical feminist analysis. *Advances in Nursing Science* 2009;32(1): 63–74.
20. Statement of Luise E. Staatsarchiv Munchen, File Number 33.029/2, June 19, 1961.
21. Statement of Luise E. Staatsarchiv Munchen, File Number 33.029/2, August 23, 1961.
22. Proctor R. *Racial Hygiene.* Cambridge, MA: Harvard University Press; 1988.
23. Statement of Dr. Hilde Wernicke, December 7, 1945, File TR 10/2584, Yad Vashem, Jerusalem, Israel.
24. deMildt D. *In the Name of the People: Perpetrators of Genocide in the Reflection of their Post-War Prosecution in West Germany.* The Hague, Netherlands: Martinus Nijhoff; 1996: 65–66, 180.
25. Sagel-Grande I, Fuchs HH, Rueter CF. *Heil- und Pflegeanstalt Meseritz-Obrawalde, Justiz un NS-Verbrechen.* Vol. XX. Amsterdam, Netherlands: University Press Amsterdam; 1979: 710.
26. Georges JM, McGuire S. Deconstructing clinical pathways: mapping the landscape of health care. *Advances in Nursing Science* 2004;27(1): 2–11.
27. Tyler SA. *The Unspeakable: Discourse, Dialogue, and Rhetoric in the Postmodern World.* Madison, WI: University of Wisconsin Press; 1987.
28. Lacey N. *Unspeakable Subjects: Feminist Essays in Legal and Social Theory.* Oxford, UK: Hart Publishing; 1998.
29. Merton T. *Raids on the Unspeakable.* New York, NY: New Directions Publishing; 1964.
30. Georges JM. Evidence of the unspeakable: biopower, compassion, and nursing. *Advances in Nursing Science* 2011;34(2): 130–135.
31. Benner P, Sutphen M, Leonard V, Day L. *Educating Nurses: A Call for Radical Transformation.* San Francisco, CA: Jossey-Bass; 2010: 167.

4 Social/Moral Justice from a Caring Science Cosmology

Jean Watson

INTRODUCTION

> *Are all nations communing? [I]s there going to be but one heart to the globe? Is humanity forming en-masse?*
>
> —Walt Whitman, 1865

Social justice and human caring are not just political issues, as Al Gore noted, they are now spiritual/moral matters facing all of humanity.[1] Thus, the notion of social justice now has a new challenge to be examined within the context of a deeper ethic for survival of humanity and planet Earth at this crossroads in human history.

The "ethic of belonging" developed by Emmanuel Levinas[2] offers an evolved Caring Science Context to awaken consciousness of our shared humanity. In this evolved ethic, we acknowledge that we *belong* to the infinite field of the universe, according to Levinas, framed as universal Love, or Life Spirit, Source, consciousness—all are current and evolving terms to capture the view of One World/One Planet/One Universe of our existence that unites ALL. Each of us is a reflection of all of humanity: "I am a human being and nothing human is alien to me" (paraphrased from Maya Angelou[1]), awakens us further to this reality of oneness of ALL.

The evolved disciplinary matrix of nursing is awakening to this universal consciousness that extends, and builds upon, the vision and consciousness of Nightingale's view of global action for humanity. This consciousness and awakening shift moves nursing toward becoming more intentional about its role in serving humanity and the planet.

This evolved unitary consciousness of shared humanity requires our awareness to attend to how we are touching others and planet Earth; how we give voice and action toward human caring as perhaps a form of sacred activism[3] within a larger cosmology. Thus, moral justice, framed within a sacred unitary worldview connects human-to-human caring with deep attention to both moral and social justice, including personal/professional actions toward peace in our world.

In the 1800s, the so-called Romantics, such as Whitman and Thoreau, envisioned a future when the world would be connected by a non-physical world of electricity, leading to a unification of humankind. Electricity opened the metaphorical world to better understanding of human consciousness and evolution of humanity. This latent hope for humanity has evolved to contemporary views of energetic quantum fields, a unitary view of science, concepts of non-local consciousness, and transformative unitary paradigms, offering a new world view, if not a new cosmology.

In the 21st century turn, new dreams emerged regarding quality of life, new standards beyond hegemony of past generations, to attention to global climate change, restoring the health of biosphere, maintaining safe communities and universal access to health care, living a less materialist lifestyle, and creating communities of diversity.[4(pp546–547)] This consciousness represents a shift from the focus on self-interest of individualism to community's well-being. Perhaps it is not obvious as we experience our daily lives and politics of the time. However, underneath the outer chaos of struggles across of the globe: wars, violence, inequalities too numerous to name, there emerges an underlying pattern of the emphatic evolution of humanity. Perhaps this emergence of shared consciousness is reflected best in recent planetary disasters, floods, hurricanes, typhoons, earthquakes, and other natural and human-influenced disasters upsetting our day-to-day, taken-for-granted-reliance on Mother Earth. It is in such disasters we see the human connections and oneness of all reflected, as we are inwardly motivated to reach out and help our brothers and sisters, realizing their tragedies could be and are at some level, our shared tragedies.

"We have reached a point where we have now colonized virtually every square inch of the planet, forcing us to realize a truly global civilization connecting the human race."[4(p612)] The phenomenon of social injustice within the colonized history can be framed as a crisis in human consciousness as well as a crisis of values, which I have referred to previously as the moral failure of the patriarchy.[5] In the separatist patriarchal-control world view that is unraveling, "violence and cruelty associated (largely with white upper class mindsets) elicited injustices violating the identity and integrity or the belief system of the other-the status of his or her human dignity. These violations constitute a failure to honor the spirit-filled person. They occur in acts small and large, from humiliating a child to 'turning our face away' from others who threaten our comfort."[1(p56)]

This injustice has been developed conceptually in the field of economics by Riane Eisler[6] who indicates that the issues of social justice are excluded in our world because of a power/domination/exploitation model that ignores humanity, caring connections, and relationships and seeks to control others, as well as Mother Earth's resources, to serve a few.[1]

Eisler makes a case for 'caring economics', highlighting real circumstances in our midst facing us around the globe, when our very survival of our species and our environment is threatened. Caring ethics scholar and educator Nel Noddings asserts that the human to human caring relationships in our homes and classrooms and daily life world, are the core, the real heart of economic productivity, that can bring real social justice and caring together for world survival. Again, as Eisler framed it, it is only from the human capital of people and caring that other economic activities are possible. Thus, we see, caring, poverty, and economics and social /moral justice merge.[1(p56)]

As Rifkin put it, this is perhaps "a time for us to ask: Have we reached a turning point in the history of the human race?"[4(p612)] There seems to be at some latent, if not overt level, a universal quest for a longing and "Belonging" to the great human race across time and space and history. There remains a pull between individuation and drive for intimacy and universality. Each consciousness shift of human evolution "is an opportunity to increasingly bond the human race into a single extended family, but it needs to be continually exercised."[4(p614)]

This latent universal emergence of humanity and its timeless search for goodness, is captured by Martha Nussbaum's view of the "fragility of goodness"[7] that is, the central preoccupation of ancient Greek thought about "the human good." The ancient Greek search was for a human good and ethical philosophy that addressed the messiness of our humanity against the reliance on reason lived side by side as means to conquer all. This ancient pursuit was tarnished by human passivity against the external world of nature, which cannot be controlled, thus placing the ethic of the "fragility of human good against luck, which cannot be controlled, leading to new questions of both metaphysical and scientific-empirical questions of the human good, the beautifully human."[7]

This ancient Greek pursuit of "the beautifully human" against nature, luck, emotions, rational cognition, and the human good, perhaps now, guides humanity, in this time, toward another level of social-moral fragility. Underneath the timeless and ancient philosophical-ethical search for "the good," we witness outer manifestations of poverty, alarming mortality rates, disease, war, violence, exploitation of wealth, power, and countless human and earth suffering.

In the field of bioethics these matters often are intellectually framed as rule-driven, principle-based ethical debates—issues of race, ethnicity, control, and power. However, from a moral/ethical justice lens—a Caring Science unitary perspective—"we critique the ethic and worldview in which the other is viewed as separate—as different, often as the enemy, or as less than fully human—allowing us to reduce another human being to the moral status of an object; to separate and distance, objectify self and other. Thus, we can justify doing things to self, other, including Mother earth, as objects to control—acts we would never want to do to our true self or another, like our self."[1(p55)]

It is through an awakening to our fragile connectedness to all—the eternal now—we shift from a separatist worldview to a relational unitary worldview. Whereby we now acknowledge, have to acknowledge, that everything in the universe and all of humanity is one—one person's level of humanity reflects on the whole of humankind. This now moves us to a holographic worldview, if you will—the whole awakened oneness-consciousness is contained within a single human caring act toward self, other, our planet.

This timeless pursuit for humanity's goodness to self/other now calls us from deep inside our one-heart and one-world awakening. We cannot deny that we all depend on Mother Earth and each other for survival. Thus, why there is such a call for social/moral justice for all.

This shifting ethos of a new era takes us back to the roots within nursing as an ideal and informed moral action, exemplified by the work of Florence Nightingale. Nursing's covenant with humanity has been inspired for more than 100 years to address social policy as well as institutional, public, and community health reform. Nightingale's mandate was global, in which she envisioned a healthy world, extending her work far into the future to consider "health for all."[8] This work brought forward can be thought of as social moral action, articulating an integral worldview, a new cosmology for human-earth survival.

Across nursing's history as well as international conventions for protection of human rights, there have been universal declarations related to social justice, although not framed as such. For example, the American Nurses Association Code of Ethics declares that "the nurse in all relationships, practices with compassion, and respect for the inherent dignity, worth, and uniqueness of every individual, unrestricted by consideration of economic status, personal attributes, or the nature of health problems."[9(p207)]

These professional disciplinary action guides, consistent with United Nation writings on human rights, are imbued with ethical intent to sustain social and moral justice for all humans. Such contemporary social moral action has been referred to by Andrew Harvey and his work with the United Nations, as *sacred activism*.[3] Sacred activism and caring science as sacred science brings us to another place to consider moral criteria to guide our ethic foundation, informing our views of science. Thus, perhaps this shift introduces a moral worldview as a first principle of science.[2]

This consciousness shift reinforces the question from early theories and writing of Maslow,[10] for example. His writings underline old/new views informing our views of science.

> *But I wish to raise the more radical question: can all the sciences, all knowledge be conceptualized as a resultant of loving and caring interrelationship between knower and known? What would be the advantages to us of setting this epistemology alongside the one that now reigns in 'objective science'? . . . we can and should use both epistemologies as the situation demands. . . . enriching each other.*[10(pp108–109)]

CARING SCIENCE LENS TOWARD AN EVOLVING MORAL JUSTICE

Such earlier thinking about humanity and sciences is now congruent with emerging theories and worldviews associated with caring science, introducing a new unitary ethical and moral foundation for both science and ontological worldview shifts—consciousness shifts that can deepen the emergence of social, if not moral, justice as a new evolutionary pattern opening for humanity.

The evolution of caring science in my writings[1,11,12] (Watson, 2005, 2008, 2012) has been enhanced by the philosophy and ethic of Emmanuel Levinas.[2] Again, he asserted "Belonging before Being," that is, the ethic of belonging becomes the first principle of science, introducing a new worldview, a unitary cosmology for humankind. His ethic is that our "Belonging" (to infinite field of universal Cosmic Love) comes before our separate "Being." That is, his philosophy presupposes an ethical relation of belonging, with other human beings, with all of humanity, "Belonging" to the infinite evolution of human consciousness. This relation of belonging (to all) goes beyond comprehension on the physical plane, and touches belonging of self and humanity to the "infinite field of universal cosmic Love."[2] This line of philosophy allows for continuous evolution of human consciousness toward *infinity*. According to Levinas, to view life otherwise is to *Totalize* the other, self, humanity, and life itself.

Such an ethic for Levinas is other than knowledge, beyond clinical, not reducible to ontology or epistemology. In this sense Levinas' ethic has Kantian overtones in that there is a categorical imperative: *I should act in such a way never to treat the other person as a means to an end, but rather as an end in him or herself.*[13]

This evolving world view of unitary caring science/sacred science, philosophy, and sacred activism makes a case for "Belonging," in its deeper cosmology that acknowledges everything in the universe is connected with everything else. Levinas' notion of *originary Love, belonging, and caring* now becomes the basis for universal survival of humanity.

Brian Swimme[14] framed this evolved cosmology the fourth era of human species—"the Age of the Earth," giving the universe, the cosmos, the principal moral authority over humans. In this cosmology and moral foundation for human caring and justice where a new view of humanistic-spiritual can be reintegrated into our scientific enterprise and search for the good morally just life, Swimme invites humanity into a new cosmic story for our survival. In envisioning our larger role of the human as a dimension of the emergent universe, we realize the inadequacy of dealing with the magnitude of human concerns in relation to the Earth and larger universe in which we reside.

By asserting the universe is the principal moral authority he means we are being taught the value of the Earth as a living organism:

> "the whole universe is alive . . . culminating in the present emergent reality" . . . teaching humans the deepest reaches of wisdom. Living

in creative harmony, with mountains, oceans, stars and life forms—all tremble with the same power for our survival. We face a cosmic responsibility to cherish our Belonging and Being by developing conscience in our use of energy and power of living Earth.[14(pp170–171)]

Now this cosmological shift invites us back to basics of human-to-earth-to-universe survival and a vision for the good and health for all. To break out of the social injustices in our world, we have to create a new consciousness, a new cosmology, a new science, that enables us to honor the unity of all; to see again the simple sadness of our way of life, mistreating our most vulnerable in society, clogging our lives with pollutions and poisons, material matter as primary over unseen spirit, thinking we are separate from our Earth, our environment, our universal source for life.[4]

The result forward with the next turn hopefully leads us to a moral community, one world, one heart, Oneness universe. We are required to create a new cosmological universal story shared by humanity around the globe. A morally just story, in which we have an ethical, moral responsibility to share human-to-human, all its resources in harmony and justice for all.

The discipline of nursing within a caring science cosmology, with its "ethic of belonging" can guide a deeper approach to considering social justice, injustice, moral considerations toward awareness of Oneness of all. We are no longer separate from each other, from our world, our universe; we are no longer separate from love, infinite primordial Love as the source of the cosmos and our existence on Earth. We are in need of awakening and repatterning a world that has forgotten its Source, severed its belonging, reaching a seeming abyss or fault line with respect to sustaining humanity, justice, and planetary survival.[12(p305)]

In closing, our first and deepest responses to this cosmological awakening to One World—that is, our infinite relation/responsibility to our shared humanity, to our Earth, and to the unlimited gifts of life source from the universe—is infinite gratitude,[14] surrendering in humility with apologies to the cosmos as we return to the sacred, and sacred activism, and caring for human and Earth equally to share the resources from universal source.

Finally, when all is said and done, our individual walk on the Earth plane can be described as a sacred journey that we engage in every day in our personal/professional quest toward a . . . higher form of social/ moral action in the world-awakening to a spiritual Caritas (loving unitary consciousness) walk beginning where we are right now in any given moment.[15(p296)]

REFERENCES

1. Watson J. Social justice and human caring: a model of caring science as a hopeful paradigm for moral justice. *Creative Nursing* 2008;14(2): 54–61.
2. Levinas E. *Totality and Infinity.* Pittsburgh, PA: Duquesne University; 1979.

3. Harvey A. Sacred sctivism: The power of love and wisdom in action. 12th International IONS Conference: Consciousness in Action. The Practice of Transformation; 2007; Palm Springs, CA.

4. Rifkin J. *The Empathetic Civilization. The Race to Global Consciousness in a World in Crisis.* New York, NY: Jeremy P. Tarcher/Penguin; 2009.

5. Watson J. The moral failure of the patriarchy. *Nursing Outlook* 1990;38(2): 62–66.

6. Eisler R. *The Real Wealth of Nations: Creating a Caring Economics.* San Francisco, CA: Berrett-Koehler Publishers; 2007.

7. Nussbaum MG. *The Fragility of Goodness.* Updated ed. New York, NY: Cambridge University Press; 2001.

8. Dossey BM, Selanders LC, Beck D, Attewell A. *Florence Nightingale Today: Healing, Leadership, Global Action.* Silver Spring, MD: American Nurses Association; 2005.

9. Milton C. The ethics of human dignity. *Nursing Science Quarterly* 2008;21(2): 207–210.

10. Maslow A. *The Psychology of Science: A Renaissance.* South Bend, IN: Gateway Editions; 1966.

11. Watson J. *Caring Science as Sacred Science.* Philadelphia, PA: F.A. Davis; 2005.

12. Watson J. Caring science: belonging before being as ethical cosmology. *Nursing Science Quarterly* 2010;18(4): 304–305.

13. Critchley S, Bernasconi R, eds. *The Cambridge Companion to Levinas.* Cambridge, UK: Cambridge University Press; 2002.

14. Swimme B. *The Universe Is a Green Dragon: a Cosmic Creation Story.* Santa Fe, NM: Bear and Company; 1984.

15. Watson J. Walking pilgrimage as caritas action in the world. *J Holistic Nurs* 2006;24(4): 289–296.

5   No Hiding Place
The Search for Impermeable Boundaries

Beverly Malone

When I was a child, I was constantly looking for safe places—perhaps something with impermeable boundaries. My granny's arms were strong and caring shielding me from the world. They were long, bony arms and attached were these graceful fingers that braided my hair and planted rows of vegetables and made lye soap and homemade vanilla ice cream. She was my haven of safety when I was a little girl. I thought that, when she held me in her arms and rocked me to sleep in the old rocking chair by the coal stove, I was safe inside the boundaries that her love, body, and spirit created for me.

I grew up in Kentucky, the bluegrass state with its fast horses and pretty women. Tornadoes came through every spring. I was taught: if you see a tornado coming, find a hole, a depression in the ground, and press yourself into the safety of the boundaries of the mother earth until the storm passes over. If you're in the house, get under the bed, turn out all the lights, stay away from the windows and within the wished-for impermeable boundaries of the bed frame, pray until the storm passes over. But one cataclysmic disaster was never enough, and so, with a good Kentucky rain, the creek in our back yard rose up out of its banks and made a journey to my house, entered without knocking through the holes in the floor, and would gently wake me up, announcing that our house did not provide walls and floors that were impermeable. Our house was built of wood and sat on a creek bank and had no running water, except when the creek stood up: there was running water everywhere.

Since September 11, 2001, finding impermeable (safe) boundaries has become a legitimate global conscious pastime. But perhaps its emergence from the unconscious has startled, shocked, and dismayed North Americans more than any other group of people. Even in the ultimate civilized country of the United Kingdom, the daily risk of finding one's self in a life and death situation caused by terrorism is not a new idea. The old, and in some minds honorable, conflict between Northern Ireland and England made the blowing up of a tube station (subway) in London or one's home, in Belfast, become a strongly possible occurrence. In fact major fundraising occurred in the United States to support the patriotic or terroristic activities, depending on one's politics. This violence though was far removed from the States, as far as Boston is from Belfast or New York from London.

Yet America is no foreigner to violence within its borders. Our urban cities where children in social networks called gangs perform ritualistic violence as a way to immunize one's heart from the continuous fear of perhaps not reaching 18 years of age; or even making it alive to the glorious age of 19. Surviving the streets may be the lucky option, only to find one's self incarcerated for life or permanently disabled due to a drive-by shooting. However this violence was usually isolated within the primarily impermeable boundaries of inner cities, ghettos, minority communities, and even Native American reservations. Middle-class Americans were safe in suburban villages or behind walled communities with electronic keys and rented protection in the form of security guards to maintain the illusion of impermeability of the boundaries. On occasion, a young middle-class American would demonstrate the lack of an adequate container for the violence, and a crisis of unrelenting pain, such as a shooting in a middle-class school system, would be noted and mourned by the nation.

But on September 11, 2001, the American dream of impermeable boundaries was shattered. I remember the day. Tuesday, September 11, 2001, was my son Jelani's 25th birthday. I had placed this information in a *very* special part of my head and my heart with a commitment to call to wish him happy birthday as soon as the time zones allowed. On this same day, I was speaking in Belfast at a research conference. The conference was excellent and my air travel back to London was amazingly simple. As I left the plane, I noticed a large group of people glued to the television set in the waiting area. I momentarily slowed down and heard the news of the tragedy: a plane had accidentally struck the World Trade Center. Unable to comprehend the story, the loss of lives, I could not process the information. It made no sense. Using my defense system against incomprehensible situations developed over the years, I kept moving. At the time I did not know what would occur in the next few minutes.

By the time I arrived home in London, where I was living at the time, in an area called Pimlico, the news had changed and the story was even more extraordinary. A second plane had struck the other tower of the World Trade Center. Following closely was the attack on the Pentagon and the crash in Pennsylvania. This was no accident; it was a coordinated terrorist attack on the United States, my home, my family, my friends, and my colleagues.

I was overwhelmed by the need to contact my children, my family, and to know their whereabouts, to know that they were not in harm's way. So many people around the world who simultaneously tried to contact significant others in the States must have shared my need. The phones lines ceased to exist as far as their usefulness to me in my efforts. Fortunately, my daughter Tosha, and new son-in-law Keni, found an open phone line and called the office, assuring my office mates of their well-being. All other family members were identified as safe but devastated by the horror and worry for the fates of friends and colleagues.

I found myself mesmerized by the TV. The repetition of the explosions angered me and yet when I turned away, I felt unbearable grief and guilt for my unwillingness to share with my countrymen and women even the images of these atrocities. Tuesday night was long and unending. Sometime before midnight, U.S. time, my son Jelani called and we talked about birthdays that will never be forgotten. His birthday had always been momentous. He was born in 1976, our country's 200th birthday. The country had transformed at that time and now 225 years later a different transformation had occurred. My family and I and my country were intact but shaken and changed forever.

IMPERMEABILITY AND ILLUSION

Wednesday morning finally arrived and I eagerly journeyed past Buckingham Palace and into the center of London to assume my role as general secretary of the Royal College of Nursing. Although I yearned for home, I just wanted to be with others, others to confirm my changing reality and others with whom to grieve. At work, I learned how the American Nurses Association and specifically the NY State Nurses Association, Pennsylvania State Nurses Association, and the Virginia and District of Columbia Nurses Associations were contributing to the caring of the massive casualties. Nurses responded with the skill, compassion, and unerring healing ability that represent the best of humankind. This global catastrophe required global healing at an extraordinary level and we, as nurses, are gifted healers. What I have come to realize is that not only are we healers, we are warriors. I heard the stories that spoke to the challenges facing nurses as they tried to get to their places of work. All the areas were cordoned off; the New York subway and bus system that never stopped for anything had come to a halt in and around the World Trade Center. With dogged determination and warrior strength and fortitude, nurses climbed across barriers and walked the bridges and city streets to offer their services to those in need. As healers, we are unstoppable.

For perhaps a lifetime, I have tried to place words around my fears of permeable boundaries; with the newfound realization that these fears were systemically shared by organizations, communities and countries, . . . For example, at a recent event of the Praxis International Network, which meets in Paris, this issue of safety, wholeness, and impermeability of boundaries was discussed. First let me describe the Praxis Network. The network provides an opportunity, for one weekend each May and October, to reflect collectively in a thoroughly international setting and in a comfortable space with others from various walks of life, some familiar and some unknown, on issues at work in our professional and societal lives. French and English usually predominate in the reflections, but participants have used other languages. Thirteen countries were represented: Canada, Catalonia, England, France, Israel, Italy, Mexico, Palestine, Spain, Sweden, Trinidad, Ukraine, and the United States. The network was the brainchild of Jacqueline Ternier David who is a senior partner in Praxis. The objective is to assemble global representation and through dialogue and reflection develop opportunities for transforming the world in our own organizations, communities, and nations.

At the May 2005 meeting, David Gutmann[1] introduced his latest thinking concerning individuals, groups, and organizations. He entitled the presentation *A Dialogue of Lacks*, while highlighting that the usual phrase is *a lack of dialogue*. The thinking went along these lines: if one begins with the baby in the womb, the proposition could be that there is no lack. All needs are provided for through the placenta and the relative safety of the mother's womb. The babe and mother are one. Upon birth, there is a separation, which is both physical and psychic for both mother and baby. Mother may express the physical and psychic despair through an empty womb syndrome or postpartum depression. The baby begins a lifelong journey in search of completeness—or the illusion of completeness. Without the separation, individuation does not occur for the baby, but this initial wish of being reunited and made whole is part of the fabric of life for each human being.

In a wish for unity, fusion with the other may frequently occur rather than connection with the acknowledgement of separate identities, needs, wants, loves, and fears. This is the archaic template of the search for unity illusion. Professor Gutmann identified three other illusions derived from the original: (1) Omniscience, (2) Immortality, and (3) Omnipotence. A colleague, Dr. Bruce Irvine, added a fourth: (4) Safety.

The illusion of omniscience basically portends that only if I knew enough, had researched enough, read enough, studied enough, dialogued enough, I would be complete—I would be omniscient. If I can just have all the information, I would understand everything; I would be able to make the right decision. This reminds me strongly of nursing education pushing everything into our curriculum to develop the omniscient nurse. But this is larger than the nursing profession: it is a humankind issue. The wish for omniscience puts each of us on a quest for the unknown that has some very positive aspects. It is the underpinning for our search for knowledge; it stimulates our curiosity and fires our motivation to succeed, to acquire educational and experiential learning. However, on the opposite side, it may leave us indecisive, traveling in circles rather than growing through our connections with the other; unable to acknowledge our limited knowledge and even our understanding of the other; and therefore, unwilling to accept our limitations and transform the experience into one of connection and growth. This natural process of disillusionment should occur with all four of the illusions: omniscience, immortality, omnipotence, and safety noted above. Feeling a little omniscient, immortal, omnipotent, and safe, we progress only to be disillusioned and despairing. The learning achieved from this process leads to zigzag growth, which is, for example, growth that is three steps forward and two back; five steps up and four down; overall progressing while experiencing and frequently identifying the backward steps as disastrous, instead of simply the inevitable delays progress evolves.[1]

I offer for your consideration the idea that our country experienced itself as omniscient, immortal, omnipotent, and safe with impermeable boundaries that stretched from coast to coast, somehow including Hawaii in its secure zone. So the United States was in total disbelief that we did not have the information, the knowledge, the forewarning to have avoided such a catastrophe. Congress demanded and the public concurred: why did we not know? How could we, the omniscient United States of America not know of the terror that would occur on 9/11? The reality has stunned many Americans and disturbed our trust in good 'ole American know how. Planes are no longer safe. Foreigners represent the unknown "other" and are to be expelled. The multicultural nature of the United States is to be reassessed and the fear that even our capitalistic and militaristic walls of financial success and safety are no longer holding pervades the country. For a country that out of the '90s emerged as the only true super power, omniscient power was not an illusion, it was a solid expectation and therefore a greater loss to the American people as reality came crashing down.

Next, the illusion of immortality is filled with the desperation of a life's time clock ticking away the minutes. I sometimes think that we, as nurses, with our healing scientific minds and hands struggle to hold back death, particularly our own. Death is an inevitable stressor from the cradle to the grave. I remember being told when I was very young that once I was born I started to die. This approach can be seen as a particularly depressing approach to life. Yet there is so much life to be lived along the way. Nurses are especially aware of this opportunity to engage in life regardless of years, days, hours, or minutes. Perhaps choosing nursing is the warrior's way to engage and to accompany *the other* on life's journey.

This illusion of immortality pervades our youth allowing us a panorama of hope, aspirations, and dreams. As we age, the quest simply becomes; if I can connect, unite, create the perfect other, I will be complete, and immortality will be mine. Disillusionment is frequently ushered in through illness, sickness, loss of loved ones, and other realities that push us into reality. This poem by Dr. Benjamin Mays[2] represents the precious finite minutes of our lives:

> I have only just a minute
> Only sixty seconds in it
> Forced upon me can't refuse it,
> Didn't seek it, didn't choose it,
> But it's up to me to use it.
> I must suffer if I lose it
> Give account if I abuse it.
> It's only just a minute,
> But eternity is in it.

The extensive loss of life, of middle class life for the most part, wounded the heart of America. Yes individuals die; yes a plane goes down every now and then; yes, automobile accidents, especially without seat belt usage, is incredibly high; yes, infection rates and hospital errors are taking a heavy toll on lives, one jet plane full of passengers every day. But, no "other" can enter through our secure boundaries and infiltrate our culture and strategically destroy our people. However, the other came like the Trojan horse and our people were surprised, wounded, and sad.

The third illusion, omnipotence, is clearly the wish to be in total control. It is the totalitarian society, and for nursing it's being in charge of our practice environment and at times seeming to "own" the patient. These are "my" patients, I remember saying with authority as a new graduate. The team concept integrated with patient-centered care decries that health professionals including nursing are in charge, rather that we are servants to the healing and to those for whom we care. This illusion of omnipotence frequently damages our relatedness to the other. As nurses at times we interact badly with one another under the category of workplace bullying. I wonder if it's our lack of omnipotence, our lack of knowing, and the fear and anger of being found lacking that we are projecting onto the other; only this "other" is another nurse. With omnipotence there is no room for identities or roles that are not subjective to the individual's, organization's, or government's superior role. This illusion is perhaps supported when the star basketball player describes the basket appearing as big as the ocean and as easy to swish in the basketball—all net. The player, the leader, is in the zone. There may be momentary glimpses of this high in other pursuits, not just sports. The lawyer defending his client with ease and oratorical splendor; the innovator discovering her latest invention; or the psychiatric nurse making exquisite interventions as the words are pouring from her unconscious.

At the time in 2001, the United States had a healthy economy, a mostly well-educated population, and access (for those well employed) to good health care, clean water, and housing. The United States had an omnipotent swagger to our walk; a Texan drawl of superiority to our talk; and a condescending style of interacting with the other. These characteristics provided a breeding ground of anger, hate, and violence from the other. After 9/11, for a moment, there was less swagger to the walk, less arrogance to the talk, and more connecting with the other who had also been wounded and saddened by disillusionment.

The fourth additional illusion, safety, represents the summation of the other three illusions. If I am omniscient, all-knowing, and immortal, free of death and omnipotent, all-powerful, I will be safe, my boundaries impenetrable and my envisioned world untouchable. However, the spice of life is engagement with the other; the other who dares, as I do, to transgress one's boundaries or seeks permission to cross protected boundaries. Without the "other" it is hard to simply exist. As nurses, a part of who we are is having the ability and capacity to create safe places for others to heal. We are courageous boundary navigators and, according to the most recent Gallup poll,[3] the most trusted professional in the United States. We have access to the other that is priceless and demands a high level of accountability for safeguarding the essential boundaries that promote hope and healing, two inseparable concepts wrapped up in a term called caring.[4]

September 11 began a special era of disillusionment, a smaller, more globally accessible world with wonderful and terrifying permeable boundaries. Working within close proximity with all these illusions, nurses are the real heroes. Nurses know that the boundaries of safety are permeable, they knowingly go into danger, and they put themselves at risk every day. Perhaps this is leadership. Perhaps this is transformation, knowing the reality of lack; of incompleteness and knowingly connecting, engaging with the other to make the world and ourselves a little better. This is nursing, my beloved profession. Working with the reality of no hiding place yet with the authority that comes from the freedom to choose to make a difference in the lives of others.

With the acknowledgment of lack as related to omniscience, immortality, omnipotence, and safety, we as nurses become more powerful and agile, not waiting until impenetrable boundaries are in place but establishing "good enough" boundaries and moving with thought, deliberation, and caring to engage with the other in the healing process. We free ourselves to move into the community where the patient and family have more control than in the hospital setting. We do not wait for illness and disease to present before we initiate our health promotion activities with the family and community. We understand that health includes mind, body, and spirit; and we are committed to advancing our knowledge and contributions. We authorize ourselves to work effectively and boldly with our interprofessional colleagues in the healing and health business. Nurses work at reconciling the business of healthcare with the privilege of caring and service. We are not waiting for perfection; we are aware of our limitations and the realities of life, and we affirm the uniqueness of and differences among ideas, persons, values, and ethnicities. Nurses are transformational activists, cocreating and implementing transformative strategies with daring ingenuity.[4]

Belonging to the human family, nurses, like others, at times yearn for a hiding place, for a system with impenetrable boundaries. Emancipatory awareness makes it possible for nurses to understand that constructing illusions does not satisfy this yearning. Nor is it possible to hide from harm. But as nurses, we are so alive in the moment, so committed to joining the other and making a difference that we use our creativity and compassion and knowledge to keep moving forward. Perhaps all we have is the now—this moment, each moment. But, I would suggest that we also share time and space with the "other"—real time and real space to create healing, to strengthen the potential for health and well-being even in the face of threat, danger, and illusion. Nursing has the privilege and will always be committed to being with the other in all the moments. Moment, after moment, after moment.

REFERENCES

1. Gutmann D. *Psychoanalysis and Management: The Transformation.* New York, NY: Karnac Books; 2003.
2. Colston F. *Dr. Benjamin E. Mays Speaks: Representative Speeches of a Great American Orator.* Lanham, MD: University Press of America, Inc; 2002: 257.
3. Gallup. (2012). Honesty and ethics survey. http://www.gallup.com/poll/1654/honesty-ethicsprofessions.aspx. Accessed April 17, 2013.
4. National League for Nursing. *NLN Strategic Plan 2013–2015.* http://www.nln.org/aboutnln/corevalues.htm. Accessed April 17, 2013.

6 Nursing *as* Social Justice
A Case for Emancipatory Disciplinary Theorizing

Sally Thorne

BACKGROUND TO THE CHALLENGE

An inherent challenge of the human condition is that we are trapped within the linguistic and theoretical contexts of our times. Because we tend to forefront the advantages of the newest conceptual innovations within an intellectual tradition, recognition that these too have limitations may follow at a significant delay. Further, in what seems a somewhat unfortunate scholarly discourse habit, we tend to take pleasure in denigrating former thinking and sometimes even vilifying its proponents. This all too human nature of evolving scholarly communities can constrain their capacity to fully capitalize on the benefits of their intellectual progress.

Social justice discourses within nursing, drawing strongly upon the social sciences for inspiration, seem to exemplify this tendency. In this chapter, I counter that trend by taking the somewhat provocative stance that an aspiration toward social justice has been a dominant normative position for nursing for as long as we have been professionalized.[1] I recognize that nurses may not always practice their profession in a manner that attends to the social context in which the health of their patients is determined[2] and that spectacular exceptions have been documented[3-5] within which nurses have abandoned professionalism with regard to human dignity and justice. Moreover, I acknowledge that some nursing scholars have assumed ideological positions favoring individual free will over recognition of social determinants of health.[6] However, despite these exceptions, there seems ample evidence to suggest that nursing has been remarkably faithful to the ideal of social justice as a core disciplinary ethos superseding time and context.

Examining the underlying aims of the social justice movement within nursing, I will reflect upon whether they represent a departure from or an extension upon the profession's fundamental motivation. I take the position that a significant proportion of early nursing theorizing was decidedly emancipatory in nature and consider current claims as to the necessity for a critical-social theoretical lens in disciplinary development in that light. On this basis, I hope to make a convincing case for excising the social justice thrust from its current entanglement in social theorizing so that it can be reunited with nursing's proper disciplinary theoretical core.

HISTORICAL ROOTS OF SOCIAL JUSTICE IN NURSING

Professional nursing was founded on an ideal of providing the best for all, creating the conditions under which all could attain health regardless of individual merit or worthiness.[7,8] In the classic Aristotelian sense, nursing has always proscribed differentiated nursing responses to patients on the basis of "irrelevant" grounds such as those pertaining to financial status or social standing.[9(p150)] Prepending the qualifier "social" to the ethic of "justice" signals a departure from the assumption of sameness or complete egalitarianism as the mechanism by which justice can be achieved. It implies that, because deservingness is unrelated to access to resources and assets within society, we are obliged to attend to equitable distribution of the benefits and burdens of living together.[10,11] Thus when we invoke the term "social justice," we acknowledge those conditions of unfairness within society toward which we accept a collective responsibility.[12,13]

A review of early nursing theorizing confirms that recognition of social inequities has been a consistent feature in considerations of professional justice. Although Florence Nightingale was only one of the early thinkers to shape the profession of nursing, her work is remembered for its profound influence on escalating political action in the direction of professionalizing the practice.[14] Despite her personal position of privilege, Nightingale's most influential and sustained campaign vociferously challenged the existing infrastructure within which the poor of society lived their lives.[15] In fact, this aspect of her practice leadership set the stage for the major social justice agenda of the day. Had her "ABC's of Poor Law" reform been adopted, universal health services, a self-evident plank in any modern social justice platform, would have been realized much earlier in modern history.[16]

The careers of many other outstanding leaders also brought nursing's social justice orientation to public attention. Lillian Wald was a "critical actor in developing public health nursing;" Lavinia Dock served "at the forefront of the fight for women's suffrage;" and Margaret Sanger, was "indicted and jailed for her efforts to distribute birth control information."[17(p21)] Although these early activists has attracted considerable critique,[18] their highly visible accomplishments served to align the profession's self-image with a broader societal orientation. For example, reflecting in 1934 on the political and attitudinal advances her professional association had made, Canadian nursing leader Ethel Johns remarked that "A term like 'socialized nursing' no longer conjures up horrid visions of Stalin in command on Parliament Hill, but seems quite compatible with our Canadian system of government and with the regular changing of the Guard at Buckingham Palace."[19(p167)] These exemplary historical figures inspired their colleagues and vigorously unsettled the social conventions of their day.[20] Each advanced a nursing agenda inspired by ideals of what we would now recognize as social justice, and it is this for which they are remembered.

NURSING'S SOCIAL JUSTICE THEORIZING TRADITION

Despite the volume of theorizing nursing over recent decades that has been directed toward understanding the individual patient, theorizing social justice has also continued as a pressing and persistent concern. According to Traynor, the advancement of nursing knowledge has always suffered from an inherent disjuncture between the science and the practice of the discipline.[21] Prior to about 1950, when science exploded as a means of legitimizing health practices in the western world, nursing simply went about its business on the basis of a pragmatic and evolving knowledge set, developed through trial and error, careful observation, systematic evaluation, and passed down across generations.[17] As nurses took on the mantle of this scientific imperative, their scholarship began to evolve in ways that sometimes seemed to serve a new master. In learning to deploy an empirical-analytical model of science to measure that which could be measured, nurses may have satisfied an increasingly corporatized service delivery system, but their research yielded information of a form that was quite peripheral to the core business of nursing practice. In an attempt to reorient and redirect that science, nursing theorizing emerged as a means through which to articulate a conceptual core around which scientific activity might be usefully directed.

The body of writing we collectively refer to as "nursing theory" constituted an array of conceptual frameworks to guide nursing practice. Although today we might more rightfully describe this intellectual activity as philosophizing, the fashion of the time considered theorizing as the more important intellectual activity. Before the advent of complexity science, which justified shifting the emphasis from causal relationships to dynamic, adaptive systems, and the availability of ontological and epistemological positionings beyond conventional "truth claims," nurse scholars tended to use the term *theory* as the primary rubric capturing the full complement of deeply philosophical problems with which they were concerned.

Although much of this nursing theory work focused on conceptualizing the individual as the fundamental target of nursing's action, even the earliest theorists recognized that it was not the only target.[22] As Bertha Harmer, whose 1922 *Principles and Practice of Nursing* became the iconic text of its generation,[23] noted, "The nurse finds herself not only concerned with the care of the individual, but with the health of a people."[24(p3)] Similarly, Virginia Henderson, who shepherded subsequent generations of Harmer's text to become a leading nursing theory figure in in her own right, called on the profession to be "in the forefront of those who work for social justice, for a healthful environment, for access to adequate food, shelter, and clothing, and universal opportunities for education and employment, realizing that all of these as well as preventive and curative health care are essential to the well-being of citizens."[25(p85)]

Within the body of work that now constitutes the disciplinary history of nursing's theorizing, the individual was rarely considered the singular target of nursing action. From the 1970s onward, theorists overtly wrestled with a worldview comprised of grand conceptualizations such as "health" (which inevitably included social elements) and complex contextual factors such as "environment" (specifically the sociocultural, ideological, and material contexts within which that individual did or did not attain that health) as fundamental metaparadigm concepts.[26,27] And just as conceptualizing the individual had proven to be a mammoth challenge for the discipline, building an epistemological basis for a nursing perspective on these domains was daunting. Following on Carper's publication of four *Fundamental Patterns of Knowing in Nursing* in 1978,[28] White later added "sociopolitical knowing," representing the sociopolitical and economic context within which health and illness are enacted and nursing practice takes place as "essential to an understanding of all the others."[29(p83)] The rapidity with which this fifth way of knowing was absorbed as a moral imperative into the nursing lexicon[8] confirms that it had captured ideas already embedded in the nursing consciousness of the time, even though they had been difficult to articulate within a professional health practice that understood itself to be guided by an essentially scientific orientation.[30] By 2008, Chinn and Kramer added "emancipatory knowing" as a sixth way of knowing to nursing's core syntax.[31] Thus, rather than considering the nursing theorizing movement to have been ideologically oriented toward individualism,[32] I understand the focus on the individual as simply a developmental phase within a highly complex philosophical disciplinary evolution process.

COMPLICATIONS IN CURRENT THEORIZING

Within the flourishing body of recent nursing theorizing, arguments that might once have been framed as an "advocacy" component of professional practice now appear in the syntax of "social justice." Justifications for this kind of action agenda draw on ethical theorizing[33] as well as social theoretical movements such as critical social theorizing, feminism, post-structuralism, post-colonialism, or intersectionality for their legitimizing framework.[34–37] Although one can enthusiastically embrace the moral direction toward which these scholars are aiming, I am uneasy with the corollary argument that departure from nursing's theoretical past is a necessary condition for integrating a meaningful social justice agenda into the discipline's future. Here, I frame my concerns in terms of the unintended consequences of both false dichotomizing and borrowed theorizing.

An Attraction to the False Dichotomy

I begin by taking issue with the extent to which the arguments advancing social justice theorizing are so often positioned against claims that this phenomenon was disregarded in conventional nursing disciplinary knowledge. Although arguably not all nurses have embraced a social justice worldview, it does not logically follow that the fault lies within the mainstream theorizing of the discipline. This form of argument reflects a worrisome trend within nursing scholarship of positioning claims in the form of false dichotomies.[38]

An example of this trend is the unfortunate distinction between holistic nursing and everything else. Despite nursing's long tradition of espousing theories that incorporate the relational engagement of nursing practice into an apprehension of the person/patient as an existential and material whole, scholars with a particular affinity to this aspect have sought to differentiate "holistic" nursing practice through group membership and certification.[39] Rather than advancing the cause of holistic thinking within the discipline, this maneuver sets up a dichotomy positioning those without certification as being somehow "non-holistic." If one seeks to valorize the distinctive aspirations of those with an attachment to this particular conceptual label, the mainstream roots of the idea become an inconvenience. However, holism is arguably a hallmark of excellent nursing practice regardless of the theoretical positioning. Whether or not that terminology is used, no anti-holism position exists in nursing education or practice, and holism seems inseparable from the complex web of ideational aspirations toward which all of the original nursing theorists were motivated.

Having applied a critical philosophical lens to the study of nursing theories for much of my career, I see tremendous strength in the commitment and passion underlying what was, in some instances, an admittedly awkward expression of ideas. Those familiar with the debates will recognize a commitment to the idea of paradigmatic incommensurability espoused by a subset of theorists who position their own work as a counterpoint to what they consider the objectification and social control motivations of mainstream nurse theories.[40,41]

Because I see in these early theories an intriguing attempt to grapple with the marvelous complexity of defining the discipline, working out a logic for nursing's mandate as both patient and population oriented, and consistently striving to realize deeply held social justice convictions, I emphatically reject this argument. To illustrate, in Dorothy Johnson's early behavioral systems theorizing I see attention to the complex interaction between a person's integrity and the conditions within the external environment within which it is supported or threatened.[42] Indeed Johnson's commitment to the development of models for nursing itself was inspired by the conviction that "the professions have an obligation which goes beyond accepting the current state of affairs to shaping the reality of the future."[p4] Similarly, we see in the work of Dorothea Orem, another prominent conventional theorist, attention to the complexities of the organizational and structural environments within which an iterative interaction between self-care action and nursing action occurs.[43] Indeed, although they may have lacked the philosophical sophistication of today's scholarship, thoughtful attempts to conceptualize the social and structural barriers to attaining health were common to all of the major theorists.[44]

Thus, I worry about the implications of setting social justice theorizing against what I recognize as the deeply felt, albeit conceptually challenging, intellectual foundations of our professional discipline. Rather, my aim for the next generation of fine minds is to encourage careful attention to the philosophical tradition of their discipline so that, armed with the advantage of an evolving social justice aspiration, it stands well prepared to inform and develop it.

The Appeal of Borrowed Theory

A second discomfort with the current direction of social justice theorizing in nursing concerns the assumption that a deep grounding in social science is a necessary condition for the enactment of social justice within the discipline. This seems to derive from the problematic misperception that the discipline's theorizing has not effectively resolved the sociopolitical competencies and capacities of nursing because it cannot, and that the only remedy is to reject prior theorizing and replace it with new theoretical orientations. In contrast, I argue that the philosophical foundations for social justice are alive and well within the intellectual traditions of our discipline, albeit limited by the available conceptualizations and abstractional conventions within which our theoretical traditions evolved. To illustrate, reflecting on Nightingale's thinking, we find aspects that seem incredibly awkward and embarrassing today. Her convictions about gender roles and nursing subservience to medical authority are cases in point within what has been elegantly termed her "complex legacy." Because of those problematic elements, the study of nursing's awkward Victorian history all but vanished from nursing curricula for several generations. However, enlightened scholarship allows us to see beyond those difficult bits so that we can discover much to inspire and guide us in confronting the social justice barriers of today.

Acknowledging in 1968 that the knowledge required by nursing to enact the full scope of its mandate did not exist in any scientific or scholarly tradition such that we needed to "make do" by synthesizing findings from several fields,[45(p207)] Johnson charged the profession with ensuring it understood the limits of borrowed theory by virtue of the restrictions implied by the perspectives of the disciplines from which it was drawn. Nurses need a similarly critical interpretation of the purpose of social science within the intellectual universe so that they can appreciate the ontological and epistemological underpinnings of the ideas they are extracting from it. In that the essential nature of a social science discipline has to do with theorizing, with any applied aspects being more peripheral than fundamental, many borrowed ideas will not have relevance to an inherently applied professional discipline such as nursing. Instead, a nursing disciplinary confidence is required to ensure that ideas are not merely borrowed but, more importantly, twisted and bent to appropriately serve our distinctive social mandate.[46]

An important distinction between disciplinary entities is that social science operates in much the same manner as conventional science by orienting a program of scholarship within an explicitly delineated theoretical tradition. A scholar stakes out his or her individual territory within a recognized genealogy of theoretical advancement toward the purpose of forging a lasting position within the genetic code of the lineage. In contrast, and because of its inherently applied nature, disciplinary knowledge in nursing is far less concerned with building individual monuments and much more with informing the evolving collective consciousness toward making a difference. Although nursing's profound power in the social justice arena has always resided in the collective, socialization into the more theoretical scholarly tradition shifts the orientation toward knowledge as the property of the individual scholar. Although nurse scholars immersed too deeply or uncritically within the social theorizing traditions often focus on smaller participatory action projects as their primary locus of application, the evidence for lasting impact on the structural and attitudinal barriers to social justice deriving from that kind of work remains somewhat obscure.[47] Another unintended consequence of the seduction of social theorizing among nursing scholars can be the adoption of the theoretical discipline's epistemological ethos to the extent that commitment to theorizing detracts from the motivation meaningful collective action and translating ideas into the foundational thinking that informs nursing competencies.[46,48] Thus, although emerging nurse scholars may benefit greatly from spending time in the land of social sciences, one would hope it represents a sojourn rather than a permanent destination.

The recent explosion of social justice theorizing coincides with a historical period in which the value and purpose of nursing professional associations is under some threat.[49,50] In that the social justice concerns arising from these newer scholarship forms will demand a strong capacity for collective action, these intersecting trends reflect a complication for our disciplinary future. Willmot describes a "civic professionalism"[51] through which nursing can act quite differently on matters of social concern than can the more theoretically situated social science disciplines. According to Mahlin, "It is only through the expression of advocacy as a collective responsibility, rather than an individual nurse's duty, that nursing can advocate for the necessary social and political reforms and, thus, benefit patients."[52(p253)] As Peter reminds us, "learning to take collective action as an end result of reflection and deliberation is ultimately the most powerful aspect of moral agency."[53(p15)] For these reasons, one would hope that the critically reflective among the next generation of nurse scholars will resist the intellectual attraction of dwelling too long in the explicitly theoretical world of social science so that their contributions remain solidly situated within the public policy action orientation of our discipline.

A CALL TO ACTION

As Lipscomb has pointed out, far too many of our claims with regard to social justice have taken the form of hollow rhetoric rather than action.[2] "When responsibility for justice is assigned to an impersonal society, ideas of social justice can become a clarion call for whom no one is directly accountable."[54(p46)] Formal training in social theorizing will never be accessible in nursing beyond a small minority who choose to take it up within the context of graduate education and scholarship. Our urgent imperative is therefore to find ways to frame the useful ideas we extract from other disciplinary traditions and articulate them in a form that finds it rightful place within the foundational fabric of how we prepare nurses to practice, justify a collective professional perspective within public policy debates, and mobilize nursing to ensure effective collective advocacy. In order to maximize their usefulness to the foundational disciplinary thinking that undergirds our profession, I believe we must support the critical social scholars in our midst to find their way back into the intrigue of nursing theorizing. To counter those who would discard the discipline's theoretical traditions as irrelevant or counterproductive, we need to reposition this new generation of critical scholarship to champion the intellectually exciting and complex philosophical challenge within which nursing has been engaged throughout its ideational history.

Concurrently, we need to begin thinking of and describing ourselves as "an inherently political profession."[55(p145)] We have been so entrenched in a disempowered collective identity that we have ignored opportunities to capitalize on our numbers and our unique wisdoms in becoming a sophisticated and effective force for public policy and health care change.[56] Although we have come a long way in embedding the idea of advocacy as a nursing competency within our various standards and guidelines, we consistently run into challenges by expecting nurses to enact it meaningfully at an individual level. By upholding abstract expectations that inevitably remain unmet because they demand collective action, we perpetuate a sense of frustration and moral distress within the members of the profession.

In order to build a truly strong social justice capacity, we need to ensure that the importance of our professional associations is deeply felt at all levels, through basic education, the transition into professional practice, and throughout a nursing career. Although many of the social justice positions being put forth in our literature have potential for strategically informing such processes, it will be in the capacity of the broad spectrum of nurses to take up the call that we a difference can be realized. Although we can certainly benefit from a sector of highly sophisticated, critically and scientifically oriented scholarship to help us better understand the complexities that present themselves as part of living in a social world, the more urgent requirement for advancing the field will be to perturb, develop, and strengthen the philosophical foundations of our discipline so as to rediscover the kind of disciplinary optimism and confidence we need to ensure impact.

If action, and not just theorizing, is our ultimate aim—and I argue that it must be—then perhaps the path forward becomes much more straightforward and welcoming to the disciplinary majority if we relinquish our grasp on the coattails of our critical social theorist colleagues and revisit the notion of what a coherent *nursing* social action agenda would entail. Rather than marginalizing the social justice inspiration that has drawn so many nurses into the critical social theoretical world, I am therefore presenting a case for the more global advantage of bringing the enthusiasm, intellectual commitment, and passion back into the mainstream disciplinary intellectual fold.

Nursing needs strong theoretical work toward integrating emancipatory ideals into its core conceptual frameworks. The holistic and complex disciplinary theoretical scaffolding we rely upon to guide nursing education and justify practice competencies must fully account for the social situatedness and structural inequities that are as much a part of the human health experience as are the body, mind, and spirit. Although nurse scholars will always and inevitably find inspiration in the ideas of the wider disciplinary universe, we need to ensure that the sustained commitment of our most prominent thought leaders remains aligned with nursing's intellectual core. The kind of inter- and multidisciplinary work that is increasingly encouraged across the health and academic spectrum can add real value to our scope and credibility, as long as it serves to augment, and not detract from, core disciplinary knowledge generation.

I envision a future in which nurses regain a sense of genuine pride in their discipline's intellectual history and celebrate their profession's sustained commitment to serving as a powerful force for social justice. I find considerable merit in embedding critical perspectives into our core educational requirements, not simply as a theoretical exercise, but as an animator for informed collective professional action. The social justice mandate is sufficiently complicated and challenging that it deserves explicit recognition, not as a specialty practice or an elite form of scholarship, but as a fundamental component of our core disciplinary thinking—past, present, and future. This is the ultimate societal project toward which our intellectual ancestors were trying to steer us. We must now do all in our power to ensure that the next generation of nurse scholars can put it into action.

REFERENCES

1. Buettner-Schmidt K, Lobo ML. Social justice: a concept analysis. *J Adv Nurs* 2012;68(4): 948–958.
2. Lipscomb M. Challenging the coherence of social justice as a shared nursing value. *Nurs Philos* 2011;12: 4–11.
3. Bendict S, Georges JN. Nurses and the sterilization experiments of Auschwitz: a postmodernist perspective. *Nurs Inq* 2006;13(4): 277–288.
4. Schweikardt C. The national socialist sisterhood: an instrument of national socialist health policy *Nurs Inq* 2009;16(2): 103–110.

5. Racine-Welch T, Welch M. Listening for the sounds of silence: a nursing consideration of caring for the politically tortured. *Nurs Inq* 2000;7: 136–141.
6. Browne AJ. The influence of liberal political ideology on nursing science. *Nurs Inq* 2001;8(2): 118–120.
7. Ballou K. A historical-philosophical analysis of the professional nurse obligation to participate in sociopolitical activities. *Policy, Politics, & Nursing Practice* 2000;1(3): 172–184.
8. Falk-Raphael A. Speaking truth to power: nursing's legacy and moral imperative. *Adv Nurs Sci* 2005;28(3): 212–223.
9. Sellman D. *What Makes a Good Nurse: Why the Virtues are Important for Nurses.* London, UK: Jessica Kingsley Publishers; 2011.
10. Hussey T. Just caring. *Nurs Philos* 2012;13: 6–14.
11. Reutter L, Kushner KE. 'Health equity through action on the social determinants of health': taking up the challenge in nursing. *Nurs Inq* 2010;17(3): 269–280.
12. Sandel MJ. *Justice: What's the Right Thing to Do?* New York, NY: Farrar, Straus and Giroux; 2009.
13. Grace PJ, Willis DG. Nursing responsiblities and social justice: an analysis in support of disciplinary goals. *Nurs Outlook* 2012;60: 198–207.
14. Nelson S. The Nightingale imperative. In: Nelson S, Rafferty AM, eds. *Notes on Nightingale: The Influence and Legacy of a Nursing Icon.* Ithaca, NY: Cornell University Press; 2010: 9–27.
15. Karpf T, Ferguson JT, Swift RY. Light still shines in the darkness: decent care for all. *Journal of Holistic Nursing* 2010;28(4): 266–274.
16. McDonald L. Mythologizing and de-mythologizing. In: Nelson S, Rafferty AM, eds. *Notes on Nightingale: The Influence and Legacy of a Nursing Icon.* Ithaca, NY: Cornell University Press; 2010: 91–114.
17. Drevdahl D, Kneipp SM, Canales MK, Dorcy KS. Reinvesting in social justice: a capital idea for public health nursing? *Adv Nurs Sci* 2001;24(3): 19–31.
18. Baker JH. *Margaret Sanger: A Life of Passion.* New York, NY: Hill & Wang; 2011.
19. Street MM. *Watch-Fires on the Mountains: The Life and Writings of Ethel Johns.* Toronto, ON, Canada: University of Toronto Press; 1973.
20. Grypma SJ. Profile of a leader: unearthing Ethel Johns's "buried" commitment to racial equality, 1925. *Nurs Leadership* 2003;16(4): 39–47.
21. Traynor M. The problem of dissemination: evidence and ideology. *Nurs Inq* 1999;6: 187–197.
22. Thorne S, Canam C, Dahinten S, Hall W, Henderson A, Reimer Kirkham S. Nursing's metaparadigm concepts: disimpacting the debates. *J Adv Nurs* 1998;27: 1257–1268.
23. Boschma G, Davidson L, Bonifacio N. Bertha Harmer's 1922 textbook—the principles and practice of nursing: clinical nursing from an historical perspective. *J Clin Nurs* 2009;18: 2684–2691.
24. Harmer B. *The Principles and Practice of Nursing.* New York, NY: MacMillan; 1922.
25. Henderson VA. Countdown to 2000: a major international conference for the primary health care team, 12–12 September 1987, London. *J Adv Nurs* 1989;14: 81–85.
26. Chopoorian TJ. Reconceptualizing the environment. In: Mochia P, ed. *New Approaches to Theory Development.* New York, NY: National League for Nursing; 1986: 39–54.
27. Stevens P. A critical social reconceptualization of environment in nursing: implications for methodology. *Adv Nurs Sci* 1989;11(4): 56–68.
28. Carper B. Fundamental patterns of knowing in nursing. *Adv Nurs Sci* 1978;1(1): 13–23.

29. White J. Patterns of knowing: Review, critique, and update. *Adv Nurs Sci* 1995;17(4): 73–86.
30. Chinn PL. Looking into the crystal ball: positioning ourselves for the year 2000. *Nurs Outlook* 1991;39: 251–256.
31. Chinn PL, Kramer MK. *Integrated knowledge development in nursing.* 7th ed. St Louis, MO: Elsevier-Mosby; 2008.
32. Kirkham SR, Browne AJ. Toward a critical theoretical interpretation of social justice discourses in nursing. *Adv Nurs Science* 2006;29(4): 324–339.
33. Starzomski R, Rodney P. Nursing inquiry for the common good. In: Thorne SE, Hayes VE, eds. *Nursing Praxis: Knowledge and Action.* Thousand Oaks, CA: Sage; 1997: 219–236.
34. Woods M. Exploring the relevance of social justice within a relational nursing ethic. *Nurs Philos* 2012;13: 56–65.
35. Van Herk KA, Smith D, Andrew C. Examining our privileges and oppressions: icorporating an intersectionality paradigm into nursing. *Nurs Inq* 2011;18(1): 29–39.
36. Rogers J, Kelly UA. Feminist intersectionality: bringing social justice to health disparities research. *Nurs Ethics* 2011;18(3): 397–407.
37. Anderson JM, Rodney P, Reimer-Kirkham S, Browne AJ, Khan KB, Lynam MJ. Inequities in health and healthcare viewed through the ethical lens of critical social justice: contextual knowledge for the global priorities ahead. *Adv Nurs Sci* 2009;32(4): 282–294.
38. Thorne SE, Henderson AD, McPherson GI, Pesut BK. The problematic allure of the binary in nursing theoretical discourse. *Nurs Philos* 2004;5: 208–215.
39. Mariano C. Holistic nursing as a specialty: holistic nursing—scope and standards of practice. *Nurs Clin N Am* 2007;42: 165–188.
40. Cody WK. About all those paradigms: many in the universe, two in nursing. *Nurs Sci Q* 1995;8(4): 144–147.
41. Parse RR. *Nursing Science: Major Paradigms, Theories & Critiques.* Philadelphia, PA: W.B. Saunders Co; 1987.
42. Johnson DE. One conceptual model of nursing. Lecture given at Vanderbilt University; 1968 (unpublished). http://www.mc.vanderbilt.edu/biolib/hc/documents/conceptualmodel.pdf. Accessed June 6, 2012.
43. Banfield BE. Environment: a perspective of the self-care deficit nursing theory. *Nurs Sci Q* 2011;24(2): 96–100.
44. Kleffel D. Rethinking the environment as a domain of nursing knowledge. *Adv Nurs Sci* 1991;14(1): 40–51.
45. Johnson DE. Theory in nursing: borrowed or unique. *Nurs Res* 1968;17(3): 206–209.
46. Thorne S. Toward methodological emancipation in applied health research. *Qual Health Res* 2011;21(4): 443–453.
47. Bambra C, Gibson M, Sowden A, Wright K, Whitehead M, Petticrew M. Tackling the wider social determinants of health and health inequalities: evidence from systematic reviews. *J Epidemiol Commun H* 2010;64(4): 284–291.
48. Rolfe G. Nursing scholarship and the asymmetical professor. *Nurs Educ Pract* 2007;7: 123–127.
49. Donelan K, Buerhaus PI, DesRoches C, Burke SP. Health policy thoughtleaders' views of the health workforce in an era of health reform. *Nurs Outlook* 2010;58(4): 175–180.
50. Fyffee T. Nursing shaping and influencing health and social care policy. *J Nurs Manag* 2009;17(6): 698–706.
51. Willmot S. Social justice and the Canadian Nurses Association: justifying equity. *Nurs Philos* 2012;13: 15–26.
52. Mahlin M. Individual patient advocacy, collective responsibility and activism within professional nursing associations. *Nurs Ethics* 2010;17(2): 247–254.

53. Peter E. Fostering social justice: the possibilities of a socially connected model of moral agency. *Can J Nurs Res* 2011;43(2): 11–17.
54. Pesut B, Beswick F, Robinson CA, Bottorff JL. Philosophizing social justice in rural palliative care: Hayek's moral stone? *Nurs Philos* 2012;13: 46–55.
55. Webber J. Nurses must influence governments and policy. *Int Nurs Rev* 2011;58(2): 145–146.
56. Lewis S. So many voices, so little voice. *Can Nurs* 2010;106(8): 40.

Section II

Research Methodologies and Practices

Critical New Knowledge Development

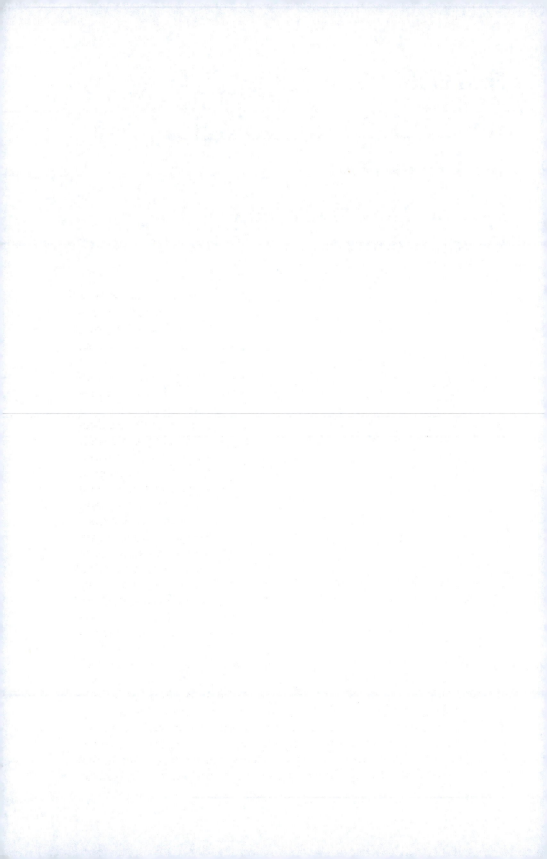

7 Community-Based Collaborative Action Research

Giving Birth to Emancipatory Knowing

Margaret Dexheimer Pharris and Carol Pillsbury Pavlish

INTRODUCTION

Emancipatory knowing sheds light on structural barriers to health and well-being, exposing the ways in which established social institutions, policies, and practices benefit some and disadvantage others.[1] We propose a community-based collaborative action research framework[2] as a process of emancipatory knowing that engages voices from across social barriers to develop new and deeper understandings of reality and uncovers actions to ameliorate inequities and produce a just social order where all life can flourish. We see this process as a form of praxis[1] that moves beyond individual reflective practice to collaborative exploration of unjust situations and collective reflection that reveals necessary actions to bring about equity and health.

The profession of nursing has arisen from, been strengthened by, and come to be known through, nurses' individual and collaborative responses to human suffering caused by structural violence—from Rfaidah bint Sa'ad in the first century dedicating her life energy to establish preventive and restorative nursing care to soldiers and the general public[3]—to Florence Nightingale who drew on her position of privilege to establish nursing care in the Crimean War and Mary Seacole, a Jamaican nurse who had extensive experience treating cholera in Central America and the Caribbean and who also set up a system of care near the Crimean War battlefield[4]—to the Henry Street Settlement nurses who responded to the physical, environmental, and social factors impacting the health of the poor in New York City—to myriad nurses around the world who are taking action to identify and address the structural determinants of poor health and the suffering experienced by patients and communities they care for. In her work on cultural safety in New Zealand, Irihapeti Ramsden[5] called nurses to be more concerned about *life chances* than *life choices* as the underlying causes of health disparities. The process of emancipatory knowing takes nurses beyond seeing *life choices* as the prevailing cause of poor health, to understanding the structural and historical factors that shape peoples' *life chances*—in which *life choices* are embedded—and responding appropriately so that health can flourish equitably for all. This process returns nurses to their roots and breaks open nurses' vision of what individuals and communities need for health to flourish, which often involves dismantling prevailing sociocultural structures.

Is it the responsibility of nurses to change unhealthy structures? Nursing innovations leader Daniel Pesut describes the complementary nature of reality, which implies that everything contains and is mutually dependent upon its opposite. A concept can be more clearly understood through defining what it is not. When speaking to groups of nurses, Pesut poses the question, "What is the opposite of nursing?" He often gets responses such as "medicine" or "self-care," but he explains that the dictionary definition of the opposite of nursing is "negligence."[6] We propose that negligence as the opposite of nursing involves not only failing to adequately care for the patients before us but also failing to address social structures that damage health or create inequitable access to appropriate, high-quality health care. In the face of health inequities, negligence in nursing involves failure to ask the four questions that Chinn and Kramer[1] identified as essential to emancipatory knowing: What is wrong in this picture? Who benefits? What are the barriers to freedom? What changes are needed? Change becomes more of a possibility if we move from an individual critique of the structural factors impacting people's health to a collective engagement representative of all who are involved in the situation—those who are suffering in the situation and those who are benefiting from it, as well as those whose efforts intentionally or unintentionally sustain the status quo, and thus perpetuate injustice by their inaction. The praxis of community-based collaborative action research (CBCAR) provides a vehicle for meaningful change that is planned in partnership between nurses and those suffering inequities to bring about a more just situation. Emancipatory knowledge arises from emancipatory processes; CBCAR is a potential birthing process for emancipatory knowing.

THE NATURE OF COMMUNITY-BASED COLLABORATIVE ACTION RESEARCH (CBCAR)

CBCAR is an emancipatory research process with roots in action-based science, the unitary-transformative and participatory paradigms, and the socio-ecological perspective. Its branches are human rights and social justice, and its fruits are equity, health, and collective flourishing. The roots of CBCAR have been nourished by a North-South dialogue on the nature of action research.

Originating in the global North with the work of Kurt Lewin in the 1940s, action research became popular across disciplines as it ruptured the pattern of researchers coming into communities to collect data and leaving without carefully listening to people most affected and ameliorating issues of concern. In the 1960s and 1970s, Brazilian educator and philosopher Paulo Freire revolutionized the means for developing knowledge by proposing active learning strategies and designing processes through which the oppressed could define and activate their own liberation. Following in the vein of Freire's teachings and in reaction to researchers from the North coming to the global South to conduct their studies only to simply leave and publish their findings to a disengaged audience in the North, a participatory action research movement rose up in Tanzania and various countries in Latin America during the 1970s.[7] In Colombia, Fals Borda[8] called researchers to move away from intellectual imperialism by aligning themselves with popular knowledge to name and change structures that cause and sustain injustices.

This North-South "dialogue" about the nature of action research has inspired many theoretical and methodological perspectives on action research, participatory action research, collaborative action research, community-based participatory research, and participatory activist research. Action research science has been enriched by indigenous and feminist movements, such as methodology of the oppressed,[9] decolonizing methodologies,[10] and feminist cultural hermeneutics.[11] To varying degrees, all of these methods acknowledge that the key to solving a group's or community's problems resides within that very group or community. Action-based research serves to unlock new insights and potential actions for meaningful change.

In our work,[2] we chose to call our action research process *community-based collaborative action research*. The concept *community-based* signifies that the research is firmly rooted within the community that is affected by the issue being studied—whether the community consists of people on a hospital unit, in a rural area, in a refugee camp, or people who are members of a group sharing a characteristic, such as people who identify as transgender. CBCAR reverses the flow of the research question from being university or institutionally defined and directed to being community defined and directed. We draw on the work of Wadsworth[12] who coined the term *critical reference group* to refer to the people whose situation the action research intends to improve—the people most adversely affected by the issue being studied. In CBCAR, the people in the critical reference group are not merely subjects or participants of the research project; they are full partners, whose lens on the subject being studied is the most important. Genet[13] encourages action research teams to privilege the critical reference group in order to discover new meanings and develop situated knowledge and theory through active collaborative engagement.

The word *collaborative* was also carefully chosen to denote equitable relationships between all who are involved in the research. Although we deeply appreciate the work of the participatory action and activist research theorists and practitioners who have honored and assured the full participation of people from the communities in which they have conducted their research, there has been a tendency in some arenas to see *participatory* as simply getting representatives from the community of interest involved as participants, often so that funding requirements can be fulfilled. We caution against falling into this trap. If there are certain pressures on members of the CBCAR team, such as grant requirements for academics or community agencies, thesis or dissertation requirements for student participants, or social and financial pressures for community participants, it is important to lay those commitments on the table at the beginning of the project so that there can be a collaborative decision on how to deal with them. When issues arise related to the pressures and commitments team members are facing, it is wise to collaboratively revisit how the team wants to deal with these dynamics. Collaborative implies deep, mutual, and respectful relationships. Collaboration across social boundaries involves bold and open dialogue that acknowledges power differentials and makes visible who is benefitting from the suffering or misfortune of people in the critical reference group.[14]

THEORETICAL UNDERPINNINGS OF CBCAR

As previously stated, CBCAR has been shaped not only by action-based science but also by practice-based theory grounded in the unitary-transformative and participatory paradigms and the nursing profession's commitment to human rights and social justice, enacted through a socio-ecological perspective. Because of this unique mix of perspectives and theoretical roots, CBCAR is a viable means for generating knowledge and change across cultures, practice settings, and community and country boundaries. Each CBCAR project unfolds uniquely because of the people involved and the sociopolitical history and environmental factors that shape the topic and community at the center of the CBCAR project's focus. Emancipatory knowing involves applying a wide socio-ecological lens to the structures that impact the situation at hand, as well as enacting a process of critical dialogue among all stakeholders and sustainers of the issue under study.

Unitary-transformative and participatory influences. The CBCAR process was heavily influenced by nurse theorist Margaret Newman,[15,16] who proposed a hermeneutic-dialectic process for knowledge development. Essential aspects of Newman's theory of health include a focus on identifying patterns of meaningful interactions and energy flow, engaging in dialogue to determine the meaning of the identified patterns, and through that dialogue, envisioning previously unseen actions; through this process, transformation of the situation being studied ensues. Newman's theory is situated within the unitary-transformative participatory paradigm, based on the premise that all of nature is one unitary, undivided whole. We are not separate, independent beings; all life on earth is intricately interwoven as one and we are evolving together in a transformative manner that cannot be predetermined or prescribed.[15,16] Knowledge is formed by our actions within the world in which we live and self-reflexive attention leads to critical conscious awareness of our presuppositions and subjective views.[17]

Newman[16(p35)] stated, "Knowledge at the unitary, transformative level includes and transcends energy transfer at the sensorial level. It is *nonenergetic, nonlocal, and present everywhere*" (emphasis in original). When we collectively and collaboratively act on our desire to create a more harmonious, healthy global community, recognizing the meaning of our current pattern of global interactions, accelerated and sudden transformation becomes a possibility. To reach this accelerated state, we must slow down and attend carefully and lovingly to that which is meaningful. Through reflective silence, quiet contemplation, and meditation, we can sense what is needed in our environment. Newman[16] pointed out that attunement and resonant receptivity are manifest in intuition and revelation—both qualities of experienced nurses who can sense what is going on within the world of the patient without objective indicators or before the objective indicators are able to be seen and measured. Newman[16(p37)] went further to state that "intellectualization breaks the field of resonance. If we analyze or evaluate an experience before we have resonated with it, the field is broken." Newman encouraged nurses to realize the whole as an active absence, drawing on the work of Bortoft[18] to give the example of actors approaching their role in a play. Skilled actors do not approach the play as an object of knowledge—lines to be memorized—but rather as an active absence which can begin to move them. They are acted upon by the play, which speaks through them. So too as the CBCAR team gathers to explore data and dialogue about the meaning of the emerging pattern of the whole, we do not approach it simply as an intellectual, analytical exercise, but rather we allow ourselves to be acted upon by the active, unseen pattern of the process.[2,16] It is in the ability to be actively absent and resonant with what we know to be an undivided whole that the process of emancipatory knowing is most powerful. As we look through the socio-ecological lens, the realization that we are an integral part of the whole and that we can resonantly be drawn into the evolving process of transformation will help us see further down the horizon of health and wholeness.

CBCAR's Socio-Ecological Lens

In the current healthcare context, the use of emancipatory research strategies embedded in praxis, such as CBCAR, becomes essential for identifying ways to change social structures. For example, as more evidence accumulates regarding social determinants of health and allostatic load factors, community-involved research and action strategies become increasingly important methods to achieve collective flourishing. Schnorpfeil and colleagues[19] described allostatic load as the stimulation of the sympathetic nervous system and the hypothalamic-pituitary-adrenal axis in response to repeated psychosocial or physical challenges, resulting in a chronic biological burden on the body. For nurses to address the chronic condition and not the underlying psychosocial and physical assaults is negligence.

CBCAR looks critically at interlocking population patterns. Informed by the questions asked in the process of emancipatory knowing,[1] CBCAR collects a broad range of structural and stakeholder data, such as information on factors that must be addressed to improve people's health, perspectives on the specific ways to make and measure those improvements, and an analysis of who is benefiting from the current situation.

CBCAR's Branches: Social Justice and Human Rights

CBCAR applies a wide ecological lens to uncover the sources of inequities and address factors impeding social justice and basic human rights. Social justice includes but reaches beyond commutative/market justice, distributive justice, retributive justice, and restorative/compensatory justice to embrace a concern for the common good of all, but most specifically for those who are suffering or on the margins of society. We see social justice and human rights as essential to a healthy society; it is us taking care of each other, particularly the most vulnerable—not as charity but as what we are morally bound to do. Social justice is the moral balance in a free market economy. Without a commitment to social justice, greed breeds gross inequities and unravels the moral fabric of society. Social justice involves analyzing who is benefiting and who is most harmed by discrimination, inequalities, oppression, and environmental exploitation, and taking action to change systems that undermine health and human flourishing.[2] Social justice involves a sense of urgency. Drevdahl, Kneipp, Canales, and Dorcy[20] questioned, "What would happen if we treated people in poverty as if they were drowning? As if they were having a myocardial infarction?"[p28]

In a comprehensive review of social justice and nursing, Boutain[21] urged nurses to adopt a multifocal approach to social justice that brings systems of advantage and disadvantage to light and dismantles them, including querying the extent to which nurses benefit from illness and suffering of others. Boutain encouraged nurses to problematize their own professionalism to determine whether, in their position of power as a professional, they are adding to the powerlessness of the person they are serving. The need to problematize professionalism extends to nurse researchers on community-based collaborative action teams. Self-reflection and critique enable nurses to resonate with patients and communities, particularly when there is an effort to enter into the world of the other without judgment or a heroic need to single-handedly *fix* a problem or impose a solution.

Farmer[22] called people into pragmatic solidarity with poor and marginalized people, which involves redressing and reversing the historic flow of resources from poor communities to wealthy communities. Farmer documents this flow as payment for professional services, benefits from low-paid human labor, exploitation of natural resources, interest payments on loans, and salaries and subsidies for government and non-governmental agency workers. In all of these instances, money and goods flow from those who have the least to those who have the most. This is an essential human rights violation. Nurses and CBCAR teams can come to a new and contextual understanding of human rights when they enter into pragmatic solidarity with those who are experiencing inequities and violations. This involves a process of listening intently. Pavlish and Ho[23] drew on Musimbi Kanyoro's[11] African perspective of feminist hermeneutics that identified *choked silence* as possessing a voice but not being heard, which increases vulnerability and marginalization. The emancipatory process of CBCAR is designed to listen intently at the margins.

THE EMANCIPATORY PROCESS OF CBCAR

CBCAR is an iterative, constructivist, and fluid process during which partners interact to make meaning of each step and plan what is to follow. Generally, the process begins as people who are interested in developing emancipatory knowledge for the purpose of improving systems and structures consider ways of working together to discover what meaningful changes are needed and best ways to create those changes. We diagram the CBCAR process circularly (see Figure 7.1), because emancipatory knowledge builds—and structural changes that equalize health opportunities and improve human flourishing perpetuate as long as passionate people partner in the constructive process.[2]

CBCAR is framed by 10 principles that serve to guide researchers through each step. First, *mutuality is a must*. Being highly relational, CBCAR focuses on creating equitable, collaborative partnerships where everyone benefits from engagement in the project. Second, *equity motivates* such that all people involved in the process consistently assess whether fair and just practices not only underlie the research process but also the research relationships. Third, *context matters*. Therefore, research data are collected and analyzed from a perspective that acknowledges the broader historical, economic, political, and social realities of those affected by the research question(s). Fourth, *inclusivity counts*. As research partners collect structural data on the systems that surround the issue being studied, they must remain alert to the emergence of new stakeholders—especially those who reside at community margins—the voices often overlooked when following traditional science that isolates and confines.

Next, *patterns connect* so researchers seek data that elicit deeper and wider understandings about interactional patterns that influence the situation being studied. Sixth, *meanings unfold* within relationships, over time, and through intentional effort. Rarely are CBCAR projects conducted rapidly or linearly; instead these partnered endeavors tend to be a circular agenda where findings and strategic action suggest subsequent research questions to explore and interventions to evaluate. Seventh, *criticality is critical* in that disruptive questions are explored, unequal power dynamics are addressed, phenomena are deconstructed, and corrective actions

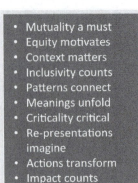

- Mutuality a must
- Equity motivates
- Context matters
- Inclusivity counts
- Patterns connect
- Meanings unfold
- Criticality critical
- Re-presentations imagine
- Actions transform
- Impact counts

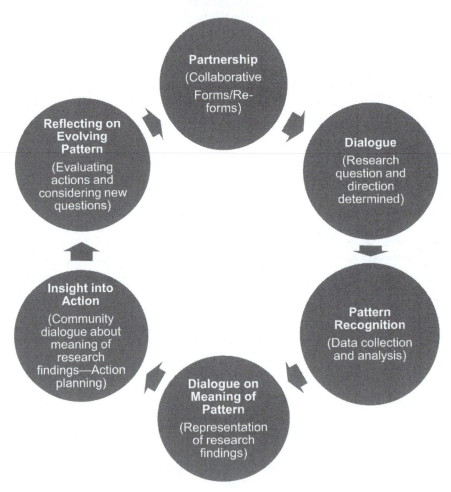

Figure 7.1 The Process of Community-Based Collaborative Action Research (CBCAR)

are sought from multiple perspectives. Eighth, *re-presentations imagine* as research partners establish creative opportunities for broadening community dialogue about preliminary findings and potential solutions. Ninth, *actions transform* so CBCAR persistently recognizes that the best ideas for health and system improvements often emerge from collaboratively studying the struggles of those most affected by the concern. Farmer[24] suggests developing solidarity and commitment to change by bearing witness to these struggles and working in solidarity to change recalcitrant systems that advantage some and disadvantage others. Tenth, *impact counts* and measuring it is both necessary and challenging. Existing measurement tools are often inadequate for evaluating the impact on underserved communities. Community members and research partners may also have to reconcile different viewpoints on desired outcomes and outcome measures. However, evaluation is important and must be included in the action planning process. Collaborations re-form as new knowledge is gained, new questions are suggested, and new people and groups are invited into the investigative and action planning process. These 10 principles merge and infuse the CBCAR process to guide action research partnerships toward health and system improvements.

CBCAR: The Process (Describing Steps in the Circle)

Seeds of thought initiate CBCAR. Whether emerging from a single, reflective moment or an intriguing conversation or silent witnessing, CBCAR takes root when a person or group experience these moments and, accompanied by a sense of collective responsibility, transition toward expressing concerns, questions, and hopes.

Step 1: Partnership—Forming the Collaboration

Any person can initiate the process by calling out their concern to others who might also be interested in pursuing the issue. As people directly affected by the issue, change makers, and researchers gather and listen attentively to one another, possibilities emerge and collaborative plans potentially ensue. A key initial step is for the partnership to determine who is most centrally affected by the issue at hand—the critical reference group. Their perspectives form the center of the partnership's work throughout the research planning, inquiry, analysis, action, and evaluation phases. For this to happen, partners must commit to a process of listening deeply to understand all perspectives and engage in relationships where deconstructing power differentials is both expected and comfortable. The process of *how* the group works together needs to be carefully and intentionally planned. The group needs to identify comfortable and meaningful ways to find and maintain its soul before going into deep analysis.[14] The key to these working partnerships is creating a healthy environment where relationships are mindful of human dignity, non-hierarchical, caringly honest and tactful, able to draw lessons from respectful conflict, and eager to address structural inequities and system ineffectiveness.[2]

Step 2: Dialogue—Planning the Process

Most collaborative efforts rely on discussion where groups volley perspectives and ideas back and forth until a suitable plan forms. In contrast, CBCAR partners intentionally create opportunities for dialogue. Bohm[25] distinguishes dialogue from discussion and suggests that people in dialogue with one another move forward more slowly, remain more alert to one another and the connectedness of ideas, suspend judgments, and become more cohesive during the planning process. Differences are acknowledged in an open, grateful manner, because people in dialogue value diversity for the chance to expand horizons, extract deep understandings, and strengthen collective planning. As a deliberate and mutual learning process, dialogue threads throughout CBCAR provide clarity to the project's meaning and direction and help identify missing or choked voices and hear them. "Critical friends"[26] are invited into the planning process to change prevailing assumptions about the research method, context, or content.

In spite of its fluidity, the CBCAR process is carefully organized. Not only do partners consider how decisions will be deliberated, communicated, and assessed but also what research questions to pursue, what research design to follow, and how to collect and analyze data. For example, partners may create research questions that suggest a traditional design such as ethnography or grounded theory or they may select research objectives that are more emergent in nature. Hesse-Biber and Leavy[27] claimed that when partners work with an emergent design, they are responsive to what direction the data suggests while still maintaining scientific and ethical integrity of the research process. They point out that emergent methods are about "methodological innovation for the purpose of enhancing knowledge building and advancing scholarly conversations."[27(p4)] Research and community partners need to be mindful of a full range of design possibilities and allow research aims and evolving dialogue to determine the best research method.

Throughout the planning and implementation process, careful record keeping ensures process integrity. For example, the partnership will benefit from clearly communicating work plans in an evolving document such as a Memorandum of Understanding which details roles, responsibilities, budget allocation, and project ownership. Additionally, careful process and content records such as an evolving Audit Trail are kept and remain accessible to all involved in the process. Clear communication, transparency, and access are critical.

Step 3: Pattern Recognition—Collecting and Analyzing the Data

Reaching deeply for authentic, individual, collective, and contextual understandings of human realities is the goal of this step. Drawing close to people's narratives of their experiences, perspectives, contexts, conditions, and interactions is an essential component, and therefore, experiential and participatory techniques are important data collection strategies to consider. As patterns emerge and deeper understandings accrue, new data such as social epidemiological data may be required. Researchers must be alert to the many data sources that deepen understandings about lived realities.

Because multiple strategies are employed in CBCAR projects, data collection is both pluralistic and triangular. Senge and Scharmer[28] described data collection as an active learning process that balances inquiry with attentive and reflective stillness within the data. Recording and sharing these inner reflections often shape emergent learning and initiate the data analysis process that, in turn, guides further data collection. This iterative movement between research questions, data collection, and expansive, reflective, and collaborative data analysis contributes to the circular and ongoing learning that occurs during CBCAR projects. Multiple voices and divergent views are treasured aspects of data collection and analysis teams. Polyvocality abandons "right" and "wrong" perspectives on data and instead explores new avenues for deeper understandings of the whole. Both methods experts (academic researchers) and content-context experts (community members) should be included and their ideas blended at this stage. As meaning emerges from systematic processing, open dialogue, and multidirectional learning, data analysis proceeds toward discovering and naming patterns of the whole that can then be brought to the community for further dialogue and even more expansive learning.

Step 4: Meaning Revealed in Pattern—Representing Research Findings
Departing from traditional ways to present data findings, CBCAR partners carefully contemplate engaging ways to share findings with the broader community such as dramatic performances, community forums, dialogue groups, artwork, video, songs, and other media or experiential forms that encourage listeners to reflect on how personal and structural factors interact to re-present people's experiences with the research phenomenon. Creating ways to transfuse data meanings and stimulating "ah-ha" moments are the goals of selecting the best media for accurately and authentically presenting research findings. This process is inherently political because social structures and arrangements are revealed and often critiqued. Building dialogue into representation design provides expanded learning opportunities that may be considered part of the evolving pattern with deeper understandings about required action.

Step 5: Action Planning—Creating Structural Changes and System Improvements
In traditional research methods, a study concludes at this point with the idea that new initiatives—be it new questions or interventions to investigate—will build on study findings. In emancipatory methods such as CBCAR, action planning directly unfolds from the findings. An action planning team that considers data findings, community responses regarding follow-up

actions, community context, and a review of the pertinent literature is well positioned to identify important actions. Creative brainstorming can be used to generate action options—always with ideal components in mind. These ideal components create a picture of human health and collective flourishing in socially just communities. The action planning team considers questions such as *why* the surfaced concerns are occurring, *what* priorities are suggested, *how* they are best addressed, *who* is in the best position to act, *who* will be affected, *where* and *when* the plan might be implemented, *what* resources are required and available, and *how* the plan could be evaluated.

As creative brainstorming and planning ensue, three principles need to be considered. First, the primary aim from an emancipatory perspective is to change systems that create the conditions impeding people's health and well-being. Multi-level strategies are generally more effective in addressing structural issues than interventions targeting only critical reference groups or other vulnerable populations.[29] Therefore, the structures that surround these groups must be included in the plan for change. Second, the team must balance community insights with best practices reported in the literature. The community provides not only creative possibilities but also valuable insights about how best practices might be contextualized; however, not all ideas from the community are sound or feasible. A full range of perspectives must be gathered as actions are considered. Third, the action planning team needs to weigh the value of available action options. In determining value, not only are the benefits deliberated but also the financial costs and potential for harm. The Institute of Medicine[30] released a framework for assessing value of community-based projects. This framework considers a full range of benefits, costs, and potential harms and provides a structure for analyzing the value of action projects.

Step 6: Evaluation—Measuring Impact and Forming New Questions

Although change cannot always be predetermined, considering impact evaluation is an important component of CBCAR. The action planning team can select from a variety of methods that range from traditional approaches to more flexible and emergent plans such as participatory[31] and empowerment[32] evaluation. Because systemic and structural changes are sought, structural impacts should be the primary outcome measures. However, changing individual and group attitudes, knowledge, and behaviors can also lead to structural change so the impact of evaluation should be multi-level and holistic with a wide range of stakeholders and structures considered, including social systems, natural resources, and the climate. Additionally, members of the critical reference group need to be included in evaluation planning, because their insights on both positive and negative consequences of the planned actions are keys to the success of any project. They can also be helpful in prioritizing and selecting critical indicators—the specific data upon which changes are tracked and measured. Although developing a timeline with intermittent monitoring periods is important—just in case the action plan needs to be adjusted because of unanticipated, negative consequences—it is also important to stay open to recognizing sudden emergent shifts in pattern and making necessary changes in the process. As impact data are collected, the action planning team analyzes its meaning and makes adjustments as needed. New questions and projects may emerge as a result, which is depicted in the circular nature of CBCAR (Figure 7.1). The research-community partnership may expand or contract as new avenues are revealed and enthusiasm for deeper learning flourishes. Moving into another cycle of CBCAR is consistent with the evolving consciousness of community potential—a manifestation of the process of emancipatory knowing.

SUMMARY

Community-based collaborative action research (CBCAR) is a circular process for developing emancipatory knowing, rooted in the socio-ecological perspective, the unitary-transformative and participatory paradigms, and action-based science. CBCAR as praxis is nourished by the efforts of inspiring nurses who embody the tenets of social justice and human rights and unleash spirited actions that change social structures. CBCAR involves a mutual partnership of people collaborating to identify issues of concern to people's health and well-being and the meaning of patterns within their community. A dialogic process that critiques and addresses power differentials, identifies and invites critical friends, and listens intently to previously unheard voices reveals what additional knowledge must be sought. That new knowledge is presented to the wider community and critiqued for its meaning, relevance, and implications for emergent knowledge. Actions are carefully crafted and potential effects are identified and measured as the actions unfold. The partnership and dialogue stay centered on emergent findings and possible new directions and evolving patterns. New questions arise and the cycle continues. The ultimate emancipatory fruits of the CBCAR process are equity, health, and collective flourishing. CBCAR is a vehicle for emancipatory knowing to take nursing back to its roots, nourishing and continually renewing its moral commitment to pragmatic solidarity with the poor and marginalized, and addressing the structural determinants of health inequalities.

REFERENCES

1. Chinn PL, Kramer MK. *Integrated Theory and Knowledge Development in Nursing.* 8th ed. St. Louis, MO: Elsevier; 2010.
2. Pavlish CP, Pharris MD. *Community-Based Collaborative Action Research: A Nursing Approach.* Sudbury, MA: Jones & Bartlett; 2012.
3. Anionwu E. A great Muslim nurse set the standard for Nightingale and Seacole. *Nurs Stand* 2006;20(38): 31.
4. Robinson J. *Mary Seacole: the Most Famous Black Woman of the Victorian Age.* New York, NY: Carroll & Graf; 2004.

5. Ramsden I. Cultural safety and nursing education in Aotearoa and Te Wal-pounamu. Unpublished doctoral dissertation. Wellington, NZ: Victoria University; 2002.

6. Pesut D. The opposite of nursing. *Gonzaga Mentor Gallery Clip*. Spokane, WA: Gonzaga University; 2007. http://www.youtube.com/watch?v=zKCnGinGDrc. Accessed February 9, 2013.

7. Hall B. Preface. In Smith SE, Willms, DG, Johnson NA, eds. *Nurtured by Knowledge: Learning to do Participatory Action-Research*. New York, NY: Apex; 1997: xiii–xv.

8. Fals Borda O. Research for social justice: some north-south convergences. Plenary Address at the Southern Sociological Society Meeting; 1995. Atlanta, GA.

9. Sandoval C. *Methodology of the Oppressed*. Minneapolis, MN: University of Minnesota Press; 2000.

10. Smith LT. *Decolonizing Methodologies: Research and Indigenous Peoples*. 2nd ed. London, UK: Zed Books; 2012.

11. Kanyoro MRA. *Introduction to Feminist Cultural Hermeneutics: A Key to African Women's Liberation Theology*. London, UK: Continuum International Publishing Group; 2002.

12. Wadsworth Y. *Everyday Evaluation on the Run*. Sydney, Australia: Allen & Unwin; 1997.

13. Genat B. Building emergent situated knowledges in participatory action research. *Action Research* 2001;7(1): 101–115.

14. Pharris MD, Pavlish CP. Critical reference group. In: Coglan D, Bryndon-Miller M, eds. *Encyclopedia of Action Research*. London, UK: Sage; 2014.

15. Newman MA. *Health as Expanding Consciousness*. 2nd ed. St. Louis, MO: Mosby; 1994.

16. Newman MA. *Transforming Presence: The Difference Nursing Makes*. Philadelphia, PA: FA Davis, 2008.

17. Heron J, Reason P. A participatory paradigm. *Qual Inq* 1997;3(3): 274–294.

18. Bortoft H. *The Wholeness of Nature: Goethe's Way toward a Science of Conscious Participation in Nature*. New York, NY: Lindisfarne; 1996.

19. Schnorpfeil P, Noll A, Schulze R, Ehlert U, Frey K, Fischer JE. Allostatic load and work conditions. *Social Science & Medicine* 2003;57: 647–656.

20. Drevdahl D, Kneipp SM, Canales MK, Dorcy KS. Reinvesting in social justice: a capital idea for public health nursing? *Adv Nurs Sci* 2001;24(2): 19–31.

21. Boutain DM. Social justice in nursing: a review of the literature. In: de Chesneay M, Anderson BA, eds. *Caring for the Vulnerable: Perspectives in Nursing Theory, Practice, and Research*. 2nd ed. Sudbury, MA: Jones and Bartlett; 2008: 152–162.

22. Farmer P. Challenging orthodoxies: the road ahead for health and human rights. *Health and Human Rights* 2008;10(1): 5–19.

23. Pavlish CP, Ho A. Pathway to social justice: research on human rights and gender-based violence in a Rwandan refugee camp. *Adv Nurs Sci* 2009;32(2): 144–157.

24. Farmer P. *Pathologies of Power: Health, Human Rights, and the New War on the Poor*. Berkeley, CA: University of California Press; 2004.

25. Bohm D. *On Dialogue*. London, UK: Routledge; 1996.

26. Sagor R. *How to Conduct Collaborative Action Research*. Alexandria, VA: Association for Supervision and Curriculum Development; 1992.

27. Hesse-Biber SN, Leavy P. *Handbook of Emergent Methods*. New York, NY; 2008.

28. Senge P, Scharmer C. Community action research: learning as a community of practitioners, consultants and researchers. In: Reason P, Bradbury H, eds. *Handbook of Action Research*. Thousand Oaks, CA: Sage; 2006: 195–206.

29. Trickett EJ. Multilevel community-based culturally situated interventions and community impact: an ecological perspective. *Am J Community Psychol* 2009;43: 257–266.

30. Institute of Medicine. *An Integrated Framework for Assessing the Value of Community-Based Prevention.* Washington, DC: The National Academies Press; 2012.

31. Suárez-Herrera JC, Springett J, Kagan C. Critical connections between participatory evaluation, organizational learning and intentional change in pluralistic organizations. *Evaluation* 2009;15(13): 321–342.

32. Fetterman D, Wandersman A. *Empowerment Evaluation Principles in Practice.* New York, NY: Guilford; 2005.

8 Social Justice Nursing and Children's Rights

A Realist and Postmodern Intersectional Feminist Analysis of Nurses' Reflections on Child Risk and Protection within Domestic Violence

Nel Glass and Kierrynn Davis

INTRODUCTION

Although all children are deserving of human rights, being treated with respect, and opportunities to reach their potential, children remain vulnerable to maltreatment and abuse and require specific protection. UNICEF's vision for children includes recognizing they are individuals as well as family and community members of a family with their own rights.[1] The Convention on the Rights of the Child explicitly advocates for their rights and identifies practices and policies to ensure protection from abuse, maltreatment, and exploitation.[1]

World governments have focused on interventions that uphold child protection, support the well-being of vulnerable children, and minimize domestic violence (DV).[2-7] Strategies with multipronged service provisions have been afforded international health, social, and legal priorities.[2,3,5] Interventions within and between diverse services have been accelerated for children exposed to DV, as exposure has been recently identified as a category of child abuse.[5,6,8] Accordingly, there are specific practice issues that need to be addressed in the management of child protection.

In this chapter, the authors present a research study grounded in critical realist and postmodern intersectional feminist theory. By using these theories, we have deeply listened to, and acknowledged the importance of, nurses' experiences in their care of children. The overall aim is to argue for social justice for children following exposure to domestic violence and acknowledge their integral human rights. This study represents emancipatory nursing as it explicitly identifies and shares nurses' challenges in assessing children exposed to risk of abuse who are in need of protection. Consistent with emancipatory nursing we propose an action care model to guide change and improve practice. The model identified from the research is a praxis example, linking theory to practice. The notion of praxis, whereby practice informs theory and theory informs practice, is clearly illuminated by linking feminist theories and philosophical standpoints.

CURRENT PRACTICE ISSUES

Co-Existence of Child Abuse and Domestic Violence

One of the most difficult practice issues is the management of co-existing child abuse and domestic violence.[5,6,9] Child abuse most commonly occurs within a context of intimate partner violence.[10] Therefore, child protection interventions remain highly problematized with a proliferation of ineffective models of practice.[6,7,11,12] Two forefront concerns are: the relationship between child abuse and maltreatment has been underacknowledged as part of the spectrum of domestic violence; and consequently, as child abuse is often hidden within DV, that child management and care is fragmented.[13–16] These concerns are the focal points for health, social service, and legal professionals, because child abuse is often concealed within DV due to a lack of a comprehensive family assessment.[9,13] A family assessment that incorporates our emancipatory philosophy is holistic in intention and guiding action. Such assessment is focused on the uniqueness of each child and family and rejects any generalizations of family violence and child abuse. Assessment includes questions and overall communication with the child and family, which are empowering and facilitative of children's rights. The child's observed behaviors and their shared experiences are acknowledged along with the interdependency of the mother-child relationship being central to the assessment. This is often in stark contrast to a traditional assessment where children's voices are minimized. The latter privileges adult voices and the experiences of medical practitioners and ignores the mother-child dyad, particularly when the assessment is framed by the bio-medical model exclusively. The inter-relatedness of child abuse within DV and the challenges associated with understanding the mother-child relationship and mandatory reporting of both child abuse and DV require nurses act skillfully and with sensitivity to recognize exposure, health risks and support children's rights.

Importance of Mother-Child Relationship

To comprehensively understand child abuse it is critical to appreciate the social context of violence and, particularly, mother-child relationships. When DV occurs, mothers are strongly aware of the increased risk of child abuse and their key concern is child protection. In DV, children are their mother's main supporters during the period of abuse in the family home, particularly in terms of attempting to ensure protection of their mothers and demonstrating behaviors to oppose the occurrence of violence.[16–18] However, actions to prevent abuse are complex as mothers tend to stay in abusive relationships for the sake of the children[17–20] yet they often leave when their children experience physical violence.

Exposure and Health Risks

Another predominant issue is related to child harm and, as such, their need for protection remains imperative. There is consistent global reporting of children and young people exposed to DV having an increased risk of harm and/or experiencing serious physical or psychological harm with either being a likely sequaelae.[4,5,9,13,14,21] Although children's reactions and responses to abuse vary, it is generally evident that witnessing and enduring family violence has detrimental effects on children. Children often live with anxiety and/or fear and some experience post-traumatic stress disorder (PTSD).[10] Therefore they have an increased health risk despite the premise that very young children could demonstrate resiliency.[22]

Mandatory Reporting of Domestic Violence

There continues to be several practical, ethical, and legal debates concerning mandatory reporting of domestic violence that result in the issue being contentious.[8,23] Mandatory reporting has not achieved its main aim: to minimize DV.[24]

Abused women may avoid health professional consultations to ensure nondisclosure of their experiences. Although mandatory reporting can increase the number of children who come to the attention of health care and service professionals[23] many issues mitigate reporting.

Mandatory Reporting of Child Abuse

As with DV, health and service professionals remain knowingly noncompliant with required legislation.[21,25,26] Complexities and privatization of abuse confound barriers to reporting.[2,4,11,23,26] The nurse's role in child protection remains fraught, and specifically role confusion, role "slippage," lack of organizational support, fear of reprisal, and increasing workload result in nonreporting.[18,24,27] The critical focus on supporting the most at risk children becomes minimized and research remains inconclusive regarding the effects of mandatory reporting.

THE STUDY

The researchers sought to explore nurses' knowledge of, and experiences with, child protection in DV through both a critical realist and postmodern intersectional feminist lens. A critical realist approach "strongly emphasizes the objective nature of reality" and is concerned with the exploration and explanation of the complexity of a social phenomena.[28(p40)] Reality is multi-layered, uses multiple approaches to inform research, and allows for a comprehensive understanding of complex social systems.

Postmodern feminism is concerned with marginalization, complexity, diversity, and plurality of perspectives based on situated knowledge.[29,30]

Postmodern feminism acknowledges an individual's mobile subjectivities and requires researchers to be empathetically engaged to reflect empowering research practices.[31,32]

Postmodern feminist intersectionality acknowledges the specificity, heterogeneity, and complexity of child abuse and protection and the forms of violence within multiple marginalized groups and contexts.[33] Thinking at the intersections is methodologically productive and allows for the critical deconstruction of binary positions. It exemplifies understanding of abuse and protection within interacting levels, types of violence, and mother and child vulnerability. This theory postulates interacting patterns of inequality, oppression, and marginalization.

In summary, the emphasis in postmodern feminism on social critique provides an emancipatory socially transformative framework for social justice, especially for marginalized and decentered individuals and groups.

Dialogical Method

Dialogue is a method that feminist researchers utilize to dismember the authoritative researcher voice, create a context for multivocality while ensuring the centrality of women's experiences.[30] The conversational process with each participant took place over 1–2 hours. This time period was critical to establish trust and rapport, encourage self-disclosure, and reciprocity.[22,34] Conversations were reciprocal as participants asked the researcher questions and experiences were willingly brought forward. In this way, researchers are facilitators rather than interrogators of the research.[18] Examples of the interview questions are outlined in Table 8.1.

Table 8.1   Example Research Questions

Researcher Questions	Participant Questions
Do you consider the witnessing of DV by a child as constituting child abuse? Explain your response?	What are your views on this issue?
What do you believe to be the role of nurses in child protection?	Did your previous research reveal nurses' frustration with child protection services?
What criteria would you use to determine if a child was at risk for abuse due to witnessing DV?	Have you used any risk assessment tools and did they help?
What are your views on mandatory reporting, by nurses, of children at risk in DV?	Do you have a view on mandatory reporting of DV?
What are your understanding and/ or experiences of the protection of children at risk in DV?	In Australia who is responsible for child protection services?

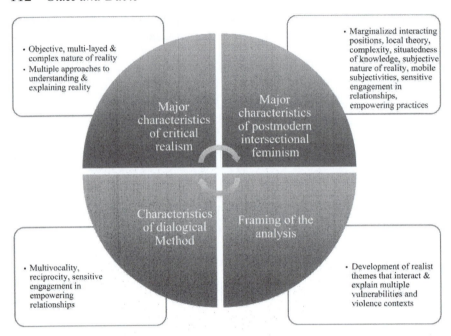

Figure 8.1 Key Characteristics of the Theoretical Framework, Methods, and Analysis

Figure 8.1 illustrates the relationships between the theoretical framing, methods, and analysis.

Participants

Four established centers of excellence or locations affiliated with well-known researchers in DV in the United States, Scotland, and Australia were the research sites. Participants were informed about the research by email and invited to participate. A total of 12 nurse and midwives consented and participated. Nurse clinicians/midwives in postgraduate nursing programs and nursing faculty at these sites were engaged in a dialogue with the researcher concerning their understanding of and/or experience with child protection in the context of family violence.

Ethical Issues

The research was approved by the relevant Human Research Ethics Committees including institutional ethics committees at each site where required. Because the sites for family violence were well known, to preserve anonymity, the data was deliberately collapsed and de-identified. The data are reported without overt site reference, by the use of pseudonyms or by grouping participants. This intentional strategy aimed to reduce the potential risk to reputation, job stability, and career.

Analytic Method

First, we completed a realist thematic analysis of the responses to the questions that guided critical conversations. Audio recordings were listened to and transcripts read to identify reoccurring words, for example "marginalized," "vulnerability," "harm," and "racism." Second, we undertook a postmodern feminist intersectional analysis to show the complex interacting factors inherent in considering child risk and protection in DV. This involved relistening to the audio recordings and rereading the transcripts to identify interacting patterns of phrases, for example, "If partner violence were the only problem," and, "taking the kids does not do any good [because] no one system needs strengthening."

Findings

The findings revealed several difficulties and dilemmas in relation to risk and protection that influence nursing practice and nursing education. Of most significance was that risk and protection were polarized and an integrated approach was absent.

Findings revealed nurses and nursing faculty were more familiar with risk than protection. Participants clearly articulated their knowledge and experience concerning children at risk in family violence. Conversely, the dialogue about protection was limited and lacked depth of knowledge and experience. These findings are related to the historical separation of responsibilities regarding violence risk and protection, confusion of terms, and/ or a lack of education and models of protection within nursing curriculum and education. Consistently, participants discussed the following dilemmas related to marginalized families.

Double Reporting

Double reporting refers to the notion that reporting DV also implicates children in the abuse and indicates a possible child risk situation. The consequence could be the removal of the child from the family.

Participants believed domestic violence threatened the integrity of the child and constituted either child abuse or neglect due to direct or indirect exposure to violence. Several participants stated there was "mandatory reporting of adult domestic violence required in some states in the US." Thus, participants thought reporting of domestic violence may become "a covert mechanism for the screening of children exposed to this violence," prompting nurses to consider whether the child is at risk of harm in the home. Courtney argued that mandatory reporting of children suspected of being at risk of DV was also considered a "covert mechanism for the surveillance/screening." The difficulty with double reporting concerns the mother-child relationship and the risk of disruption of this dyad. The relationship is interdependent particularly in isolated rural situations.[17–19]

Marginalized Families

Risk was constructed as predominately occurring in marginalized families. Marginalized families are considered to be on the edges of society, of lesser importance, or unacceptable to those in dominant social positions. Such families are seen by dominant groups to be typically characterized by poverty, unemployment, mental health problems, low levels of education, or be non-English speaking. Ethnicity was also an identified factor.

High levels of vulnerability and violence characterized these families. There were also multiple contexts within the violence and vulnerability often combined with institutional abuse such as a removal of government support payments due to illicit drug use and alcohol abuse. All of these issues impacted the families; therefore risk assessment and management by health and service providers was complex and considered difficult.

Marginalized groups came to the attention of services for two major reasons. First, there is bias within the reporting patterns of health care professionals.[35] Because health professionals tend to belong to the dominant group, a lack of critical consciousness may result in stigmatization of perceived marginalized families together with the belief that belonging to the dominant group creates immunity from violence. Second, marginalized groups come to the attention of welfare and community services more often than nonmarginalized groups. In particular, participants in both Scotland and the United States identified risk in terms of vulnerable families. These families were defined by multiple contexts of violence and social risk factors such as poverty, poor parenting skills, youth, and racialization.[36–38] Therefore, "racism and classism may function in concert with the stigmatizing nature of abuse."[38(p111)] Arguably, violence and vulnerability factors interact and are often unpredictable, ambiguous, and changing. Furthermore, although models of vulnerability may have the family at the center, service responses are often inadequate or nonexistent.[7,11]

Multiple Contexts of Violence

Participants indicated the "at risk" child in DV is exposed to violence on many levels. Violence was seen as a way of life. Alisa identified that violence for the child exists in many forms such as, "family violence . . . community violence . . . institutional violence . . . and racism." Social risk factors and the levels of violence within families varied; however, Jude suggested there were "high levels of violence" along with "chaotic families . . . aggressive parenting . . . anger management [issues] . . . mental illness, [especially] . . . a high incidence of bipolar disorder . . . substance abuse, heroin [in particular and] . . . intergeneration violence." The additive nature of the violence was recognized by three participants. Kate stated, "if partner violence were the *only* problem"; this is supported by Catriona who said, "intimate partner violence is not always top of the list." Heather raised multiple social risk factors. She said, there are "a lot of behaviors that add up to neglect."

Determining Risk

There is extensive discussion in the literature and legislation about the child at risk. Yet the strategies identified in this research and in the risk management literature remain fraught and paradoxically more difficult to protect children.[11]

In this research there were two major approaches to determining risk or identifiable harm. They varied with the three countries in relation to child protection policy, legislation, and nursing discipline or specialization. Participants identified both family centered and individual approaches. Two common themes that emerged were vulnerable families and the need for a comprehensive health assessment. In terms of the family-centered approach, participants spoke of the different ways risk was framed within their own practice. Sara implemented a "social care model" while Theresa spoke of a "communications model as an integrated approach to working with multiple agencies." Ainslee and Erin saw the importance of a health needs assessment; however, one developed from different perspectives. For vulnerable families, Ainslee saw value in a health needs assessment yet she was dependent on "intuition [as there were] no guidelines for DV screening." Erin found a "family systems approach and health needs assessment" assisted in the determination of risk of harm.

In terms of an individual approach, participants focused on their nursing specialization. Kate, a pediatric nurse found a "child behavior check list [framed within a] developmental approach" was appropriate. Inez, a mental health nurse, suggested a "legalistic-forensic nursing approach." Jacinta, a generalist nurse, utilized an "individual assessment" whereas Jude, a DV Services Coordinator, implemented a "universal screening" instrument to assess the risk of harm.

Similar to previous research, identification and acknowledgement of the complex social context of child protection is critical.[39] A "sense of unease" as an indicator of "concern" "honed by experience" and "informed by knowledge developed from specific education [informed] decision-making" was identified. Intuition acted as a "silent alarm" that caused health visitors to explore the situation more deeply and shed light on the hidden meanings in families.

Protection

Protection was described as safety planning, children's rights, advocacy, and legal obligations. Participants identified three major approaches to protection. Sara located protection within "ethical frameworks as nurses must be able to account for decisions." The rights of the child were considered a central focus by two participants. Jacinta suggested a rights-based approach, "family centered but with focus on the child." Erin explicitly stated "children's rights . . . [and] . . . advocacy" should frame protection strategies. Conversations revealed an understanding of and frustration with protective strategies. Ainslee said, "taking the kids [out of the home] does not do any good [because] no one system needs strengthening."

Four participants further articulated the problems associated with child risk and protection as the lack of resources and support by inline managers. Erin said, there is a "lack of appropriate resources to deal with the totality of the experienced violence, and the effects of parenting by children . . . there is not only a direct effect with actually experiencing the violence, but also an indirect effect, in that taking up adult roles by children in the family adds even further stress." Sara supported the idea of "lack of resources" and paradoxically this phenomenon is increased in the nonmarginalized group, such as "professional families, [where] it's non existent."

REFRAMING CHILD RISK AND PROTECTION: CRITICAL REALISM AND POSTMODERN INTERSECTIONAL FEMINISM

The framing of the research within critical methodologies and methods was an empowering praxis-orientated approach that gave voice to nurse clinicians and faculty who revealed the interacting factors contextualizing child risk. Consistent with such an approach, participants had a strong desire for a social justice advocacy framing of child protection. The following proposes a different framing of child risk assessment and protection.

Re-Designing Risk Assessments

Repeatedly participants viewed vulnerability assessment as a major focus for determining the level of risk of harm to children who are exposed to intimate partner violence. They also recognized that violence, like vulnerability, occurs on many levels and needed to be taken into account when assessing risk. Participants were aware of the intersectionality of risk factors, which revealed the complexities of risk. For example, a child experiencing racism and family violence where parental illicit drug use and mental illness is present maybe at greater risk because of these combined effects. Rose, cited in Howarth, recommends "two types of assessment to ensure a timely and proportionate response, an 'initial' assessment and then a more in-depth detailed assessment known as the 'core' assessment."[40(p1071)] Although we agree with more than one assessment, given the complexity, unpredictability, and changing nature of risk we strongly recommend regular assessment to take account of changes in the level or severity of risk.

Therefore, we propose a matrix approach for health and service professionals to utilize in risk assessments. The matrix in Table 8.2 enables a

Table 8.2   Example of an Individual Child Risk Assessment Matrix

	Multiple Contexts of Violence			
	Family Violence	Community Violence	Organizational Violence	Racism
Multiple Contexts of Vulnerability — *Type of violence*	1			1
Compromised parenting capacity	1			
Age & developmental needs of the child				
Parental illicit drug use				
Parental mental disorder/ illness				
Poverty				
Intergenerational trauma				
Chaotic families				
Parental anger management				
Marginalized group				
Number of predictors	2			1

risk predictor score to be determined. Each factor has a score value of 1; the higher the score value the greater the risk. For example, a child who experiences compromised parenting capacity, family violence, and racism would receive a predictor score of 3. Another child may experience parental mental disorder/illness, family violence, poverty, and parental illicit drug use, and these four issues would result in a predictor score of 4. The benefit of the matrix is that it can be individualized and tailored for each professional to implement irrespective of the different child risk contexts or health discipline. Although this approach does not illuminate the extent of the risk factors and does not account for the intrapersonal child characteristics, it provides a clear indicator of multiple risk factors that affect the child. The multiple assessment of risk requires organizational funding and committed inline managers to support improvements. The risk matrix provides a more dynamic and comprehensive approach to risk and protection that adds to the existing available assessment tools, such as the ecological framework proposed by Howarth[40(p1071)] that incorporates "the developmental needs of the child, parenting capacity, and family and environmental factors."

Social Justice Advocacy

The incorporation of human rights is an enactment of the political platform of critical social theory that underpins this research framing.

A rights-based framework sited within ethical principles was also revealed by participants.

Child rights fall within the broad category of human rights. Human rights discourse draws on normative ethical principles related to justice, autonomy, and dignity. It has been defined as "the basic freedoms and standards considered by most societies as belonging automatically to all people to enable them to live lives with dignity."[41(p13)] They have been enshrined in the UN Convention on the Rights of the Child (UNCRC), which upholds the notion that human rights apply to people of all ages. In the context of children's health, social justice can be considered as "doing what is best for a person" whose ability to self-advocate is compromised.[42(p192)] Child vulnerability, as shown in this research, requires a rights-based approach to child risk and protection. There are several articles within the UNCRC that relate to child risk and protection in the context of intimate partner violence, outlined in Table 8.3.

The International Council of Nurses (ICN) position statement on the Rights of Children has endorsed the UNCRC, as have other National Nursing Codes of ethics and practice.[43] However, although "professional nursing codes define social justice advocacy as an expectation of nursing practice, it is obvious from the literature, that in the practice of most nurses, this reengagement is in its infancy."[44(p66)] Health professional practice, education, and curricular has focused on individual responsibility for health and is reflected in a limited or nonexistent rights based language to explore the depth and breadth of social justice.[45] Human rights discourses in nursing are predominantly framed within Ethical Codes or strands within curricula, which, without the link to social justice, lack the socio-political framework for health practice. Nursing and health education must be framed by critical social theory and implemented by faculty who understand and articulate links to human rights and social justice. Reframing curricular and pedagogy

Table 8.3   Rights Principles within the United Nations Convention on the Rights of the Child[1,43]

Article	Principle
6	An inherent right to life, survival, and development to the maximum potential
13	Freedom of expression on all matters affecting them
18	Respect for the best interests of the child as a primary consideration
19	Protection from all forms of physical or mental violence, injury or abuse, neglect or negligence, exploitation including abuse
33	Protection from illicit drug use
34	Protection from all forms of sexual abuse and exploitation

in this way will enable nursing and health students to develop their personal critical philosophic practice guided by social justice principles where self-reflexive praxis supports sustainable socio-political thought and action.

Participants identified the importance of child centeredness and advocacy within an ethical framework. If protection is located within social justice advocacy and informed by postmodern intersectional feminist principles, outlined in Figure 8.2, an approach to child risk and protection can be formulated. Social justice advocacy combines an interest in the health of individuals as well as the social positioning of individuals within social structures and systems.[45] This new perspective takes account of the need to reframe the marginalized, considering local and individual experience, complexity, and diversity to reflect an empowering social advocacy practice for women and children. A model that frames child protection in this way aims to support and strengthen children and families rather than disempower. This supports the proactive involvement of nurses in working for broader change in structural factors within society that affect marginalized groups, such as poverty and unemployment. These main concepts are represented in Figure 8.2.

The model presented in Figure 8.3 is framed by the perspectives and practices shown in Figure 8.2 and aims to provide a teaching and practice framework for child protection. It deliberately does not provide specific guidelines to be implemented as the multiple contexts vary considerably for each child and family. The model is a framework to guide practice and is utilized with the risk assessment matrix.

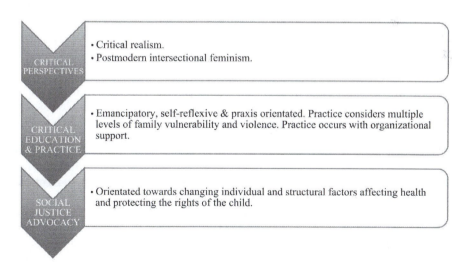

Figure 8.2 The Relationship between Critical Perspectives and Social Justice Advocacy

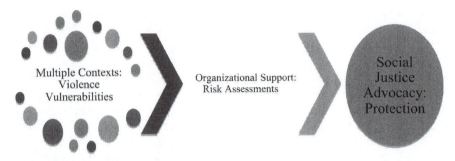

Figure 8.3   Social Justice Advocacy Framework for Child Risk and Protection

CONCLUSION

There remains a lack of clarity regarding the roles of professionals in assessing and managing the complexities of child protection.[40] Nurses have a significant role in risk assessment, notification, and care of the whole family as part of protective management. Health professionals, without an appropriate framework to conceptualize child risk and protection, often believe their role is limited. However, ongoing monitoring and care of the child remains integral to nursing practice in the community.

When critical perspectives and frameworks for analysis are incorporated, this results in emancipation "in action." The framework in Figure 8.3 opens a space for further conversation[46] and praxis orientated approaches to child protection. Social justice advocacy guided by critical perspectives aims to protect the child from further short- and long-term harm, has the child's best interest at its center, and provides a framework that will support the child to develop to their fullest potential. Social justice advocacy framing of child risk and protection is enhanced by a comprehensive assessment of interacting types of vulnerability and violence, organizational support, and the centrality of children's rights. Practice and education framed by critical perspectives and emancipatory cognitive interests advance the development of empowering, self-reflexive praxis-orientated practice that enables nurses to take up a proactive role in child protection.

REFERENCES

1. UNICEF. Convention on the Rights of the Child. http://www.unicef.org/crc/index_30160.html. Accessed April, 30, 2012.
2. Commonwealth of Australia. Protecting children is everyone's business: national framework for protecting Australia's children 2009–2020. 2009. www.coag.gov.au/sites/default/files/child_protection_framework.pdf. Accessed April, 17, 2014.
3. Commonwealth of Australia. National framework for protecting Australia's children: implementing the first three-year action plan 2009–2012. 2009.

www.dss.gov.au/our-responsibilities/families-and-children/publications-articles/national-framework-for-protecting-australias-children-implementing-the-first-three-year-action-plan-2009-2012-2009. Accessed April 17, 2014.

4. Woods Commission. Report of the special commission of inquiry into child protection services in NSW: executive summary and recommendations. Sydney, Australia; 2008.

5. Ramsay J, Carter Y, Davidson L, et al. Advocacy interventions to reduce or eliminate violence and promote the physical and psychosocial well-being of women who experience intimate partner abuse (review). *The Cochrane Library* 2009(4).

6. Rankin JM, Ornstein A. A commentary on mandatory reporting legislation in the United States, Canada, and Australia: a cross-jurisdictional review of key features, differences, and issues. *Child Maltreat* 2009;14(1): 121–123.

7. Laming H. *The protection of children in England: a progress report.* London, UK: House of Commons; 2009.

8. Mathews B, Kenny MC. Mandatory reporting legislation in the United States, Canada, and Australia: a cross-jurisdictional review of key features, differences, and issues. *Child Maltreat* 2008;13: 50–63.

9. Chan KL. Children exposed to child maltreatment and intimate partner violence: a study of co-occurrence among Hong Kong Chinese families. *Child Abuse Negl* 2011;35(7): 532–542.

10. Hester M, Pearson C, Harwin N. *Making an Impact: Children and Domestic Violence-a Reader.* 2nd ed. Philadelphia, PA: J. Kingsley Publishers; 2007.

11. Munro E. Learning to reduce risk in child protection. *British Journal of Social Work* 2010;40: 1135–1151.

12. Douglas H, Walsh T. Mothers, domestic violence, and child protection. *Violence against Women* 2010;16(5).

13. Herrenkohl TI, Sousa C, Tajima EA, Herrenkohl RC, Moylan CA. Intersection of child abuse and children's exposure to domestic violence. *Trauma Violence Abuse* 2008;9: 84–99.

14. Hill JR, Thies J. Program theory and logic model to address the co-occurrence of domestic violence and child maltreatment *Eval Program Plann* 2010;33(4): 356–364.

15. Moles K. Bridging the divide between child welfare and domestic violence services: deconstructing the change process. *Children and Youth Services Review* 2008;30: 674–688.

16. Stanley N, Miller P, Richardson Foster H, Thomson G. Children's experiences of domestic violence: developing an integrated response from police and child protection services. *J Interpers Violence* 2011;26: 2372–2391.

17. Davis K, Taylor B, Furniss D. Narrative accounts of tracking the rural domestic violence survivors' journey: a feminist approach. *Health Care Women Int* 2001;22(4): 333–347.

18. Davis K, Taylor B. Stories of resistance and healing in the process of leaving abusive relationships. *Contemp Nurse* 2006;21(2): 199–208.

19. Wendt S, Hornosty J. Understanding contexts of family violence in rural, farming communities: implications for rural women's health. *Rural Society* 2010;20(1): 51–63.

20. Hunt S, Martin A. *Pregnant Women: Violent Men-What Midwives Need to Know.* Oxford, UK: BMS; 2001.

21. de Wit K, Davis K. Nurses' knowledge and learning experiences in relation to the effects of domestic abuse on the mental health of children and adolescents. *Contemp Nurse* 2004;16(3): 214–217.

22. Elmir R, Schmied V, Jackson D, Wilkes L. Interviewing people about potentially sensitive topics. *Nurse Researcher* 2011;19(1): 12–16.

23. Cross T, Mathews B, Tonmyr L, Scott D, Ouimet C. Child welfare policy and practice on children's exposure to domestic violence. *Child Abuse Negl* 2012;36(3): 210–216.

24. Davidov D, Nadorff M, Jack S, Coben JF. Nurses home vistors' perceptions of mandatory reporting of intimate partner violence to law enforcement agencies. *J Interpers Violence* 2012;27(12): 2484–2502.

25. Francis K, Chapman Y, Sellick K, et al. The decision making processes adopted by rurally located mandated professionals when child abuse or neglect is suspected. *Contemp Nurse* 2012;41(1): 58–69.

26. Bunting L, Lazenbatt A, Wallace I. Information sharing and reporting systems in the UK and Ireland: professional barriers to reporting child maltreatment concerns. *Child Abuse Review* 2009;19(3): 187–202.

27. Fraser J, Mathews B, Walsh K, Chen L, Dunne M. Factors influencing child abuse and neglect recognition and reporting by nurses: a multivariate analysis. *Int J Nurs Stud* 2010;47(2): 146–153.

28. Alvesson M, Skoldberg K. *Reflexive Methodology: New Vistas for Qualitative Research*. Los Angeles, CA: Sage; 2009.

29. Aranda K. Postmodern feminist perspectives and nursing research: a passionately interested form of inquiry. *Nurs Inq* 2006;13(2): 135–143.

30. O'Shaughnessy S, Krogman NT. A revolution reconsidered? Examining the practice of qualitative research in feminist scholarship. *Signs* 2012;37(2): 493–520.

31. Glass N, Davis K. Reconceptualizing vulnerability: deconstruction and reconstruction as a postmodern feminist analytical research method. *Advances in Nursing Science* 2004;27(2): 82.

32. Ogle KR, Glass N. Mobile subjectivities: positioning the nonunitary self in critical feminist and postmodern research. *Advances in Nursing Science* 2006;29(2): 170.

33. Davis K, Glass N. Reframing the heteronormative constructions of lesbian partner violence: an Australian case study. In: Ristock J, ed. *Intimate Partner Violence in LGBTQ Lives*. New York, NY: Routledge Press; 2011: 13–37.

34. Dickson Swift V, James E, Kippen S, Liamputtong P. Doing sensitive research: what challenges do qualitative researchers face? *Qualitative Research* 2007;7(3): 327–353.

35. Thomas I. Against the mandatory reporting of intimate partner violence. *Virtual Mentor* 2009;11(2): 137–140.

36. Davis K, Taylor B. Voices from the margins part 1: narrative accounts of Indigenous family violence. *Contemp Nurse* 2002;14(1): 66–75.

37. Davis K, Taylor B. Voices from the margins part 2: narrative accounts of the support needs of Indigenous families experiencing violence. *Contemp Nurse* 2002;14(1): 76–85.

38. Varcoe C. Abuse obscured: an ethnographic account of emergency nursing in relation to violence against women. *Can J Nurs Res* 2001;32(4): 95–115.

39. Ling M, Luker K. Protecting children: intuition and awareness in the work of health visitors. *J Adv Nurs* 2002;32(3): 572–579.

40. Howarth J. See the practitioner, see the child: the framework for the assessment of children in need and their families ten years on. *British Journal of Social Work* 2011;41: 1070–1087.

41. Freegard H, Goddard T, Isted L. Human rights and health. In: Freegard H, ed. *Ethical Practice for Health Professionals* South Melbourne, Australia: Thomson; 2007.

42. Pacquiao D. Nursing care of vulnerable populations using a framework of cultural competence, social justice and human rights. *Contemporary Nurse* 2008;28: 189–197.

43. International Council of Nurses. Rights of children. 2008. http://www.icn.ch. Accessed May 8, 2012.
44. Paquin S. Social justice advocacy in nursing: what is it? How do we get there? *Creat Nurs* 2011;17(2): 63–67.
45. Boutain D. Social justice in nursing: a review of the literature. In: de Chesnay M, Anderson BA, eds. *Caring for the Vulnerable: Perspectives in Nursing Theory, Practice, and Research.* 3rd ed. Burlington, MA: Jones and Bartlett Learning; 2011: 43–58.
46. Jackson D, McMurray A. Recognising, responding and resisting violence: a critical challenge for nurses. *Contemp Nurse* 2006;21(2): 324–326.

9 The Identity, Research, and Health Dialogic Interview

Its Significance for Social Justice-Oriented Research

Doris M. Boutain

Sexuality, gender, racial, and class identities are well-known social constructs that inform and influence health. Yet, most research in nursing render these social constructs, or ways of thinking in society, as static demographic classifications. Thus, demographic data are ascribed as identifiers or fixed categorical labels. More attention is given to collecting categories of respondent information than understanding how identity informs health accounts and influences ways of understanding research. The limited analysis of demographic data is due, in part, to the interview design used to gather research knowledge and present that knowledge to other researchers.

Although qualitative research has both deepened and multiplied in the number of methodologies used in nursing today, the use of diverse interview methodologies have not followed suit.[1] Demographic data is frequently collected as sample, descriptive data and reported as sample categories. The notion that demographic information is identity information, social information, and health information worthy of interpretation is rare in nursing research.

The Identity, Research, and Health Dialogic Interview can offer new insights about how identity, research, and health are interrelated. This approach can reveal how people come to understand their identity, dialogue about research conundrums, and ascribe, expand, or protest meanings related to health. Current approaches to collecting identity data remain limited to collecting demographic information versus understanding demographic identity in the context of the research topic and aims. Thus, demographic data is rendered in the research report as categorical answers—even in research projects described as using a critical, social justice-oriented frameworks.

The purpose of this chapter is to describe an interview design for collecting demographic data and meaning using the Identity, Research, and Health Dialogic Interview. This approach may help researchers with critical or social justice orientations to advance their research. It has been used in research with topics such as hypertension meaning and management,[2,3] depression,[4] preconception care,[5] and asthma.[6] Methodologies used with this interview design included critical discourse analysis and critical ethnography. Using this approach, researchers and their research participants examine identity as social frames that inform health accounts and health attainment.

In this chapter, the rationale for collecting demographic data using this research interview methodology is first provided. The process of demographic interviewing follows. The suggested format for demographic interviewing is presented thereafter. The chapter is subsequently summarized. A sample worksheet and interview questions are provided as appendices. Researchers will gain another way of constructing an interview about identity, research, and health after reading this chapter.

RATIONALE FOR THE IDENTITY, RESEARCH, AND HEALTH DIALOGIC INTERVIEW

The Identity, Research, and Health Dialogic Interview was created as a way to focus on meaning production using a critical paradigm of knowledge creation or epistemology anchored by social justice. Epistemology is a way of viewing how knowledge is created in the world.[7] The critical paradigm views knowledge as social, historical, and situated in a matrix of power relationships. This paradigm acknowledges that some knowledge remains marginalized. Marginalized means the knowledge, if visible, is rendered invisible or not structured to become recognized or valued as important.

Using a social justice orientation to research, the Identity, Research, and Health Interview was created to not assume that demographic data was normative or easily assigned and understood information. Demographic data, using social justice, can be viewed as a means to understand how privilege and oppression enable contemplation and embodiment of health accounts.

Demographic data in research, using a social justice lens, are not viewed as fixed or neutral data classifications. Research participants are not simply respondents or vessels of information. Research participants are viewed as persons with historical, cultural, linguistic, and social sensibilities that influence the interview process, the data shared in the interview, and thus research generation. The researcher is also made visible as a social being sharing those same sensibilities.

This is very different from the normative idea that demographic information is sample characteristic data. That is, that demographic data are labels to describe and enumerate the research sample. Thus, it was thought that dialogue about how demographic identity influences health might best aid knowledge creation.

Significant and relevant claims are made by critical and indigenous scholars that new ways of writing in the academy can yield diversity of thought.[8] By asking research interviewees questions to open dialogue and knowledge sharing, these new understandings about health may be attained. Concurrently, a rigorous analysis of those accounts and thoughtful re-telling is also needed in research reports. Demographic data can reveal profound insights as attention is given to how and why participants come to know what they know about themselves, about health, and about research. These insights can result in re-searching topic areas—creating new interpretative spaces in research inquiry.

Despite these ideas, research in general and nursing research in particular depicts demographic data collection in written reports as a neutral process of data categorization and presentation. Few research methodologies aid researchers using a social justice orientation to imagine new strategies for building knowledge using demographic data.[9] Thus, the Identity, Research, and Health Dialogic Interview can provide another possibility for research interview design.

STEPS OF THE IDENTITY, RESEARCH, AND HEALTH DIALOGIC INTERVIEW

Three major process steps comprise the Identity, Research, and Health Dialogic Interview. First, the interview design involves a critical reflection on the purpose of the research and research aims in light of which demographic data are needed for the current research project. A sample worksheet for outlining the research purpose, aims, and necessity for demographic data is shown in Appendix A. The worksheet facilitates a detailed and explicit research-based reflection on how demographic data was used in prior research and how it will be used in the current research.

Second, the Identity, Research, and Health Dialogic Interview entails mapping and designing questions about identity, research, and health in relationship to how those questions relate to the research purposes and aims (see Appendix B). Open-ended questions are devised to elicit how participants define their identity in relation to their health and dialogue about research conundrums. For example, a participant may be asked: how does being 19 years old influence the management of hypertension? Follow-up questions may be as follows: how does being 19 years old make it easy to manage hypertension? How does being 19 years old make it difficult to manage hypertension? Thus, the age of the participant is asked in the context of research purpose of understanding hypertension management.

The third process step in the Identity, Research, and Health Dialogic Interview methodology occurs after the data are collected. It involves critical reflection and research analysis. The analysis involves researchers writing their own reflections about the process of openly asking participants about demographic information and health concerns. The researcher is to write assumptions about demographic data before the interview. Then, after the interview, the research is to write what was learned anew.

Then a re-reading of the demographic interview data is done so that the researcher takes the position of research participants. That is, the researcher reflects on how the research participants understand their identity and account for their health in light of that identity. The researcher renders an interpretation of that point of view and compares that to earlier researcher-based assumptions. In this third step, researchers may move from describing how the participants talked about their identity to analyzing how identity contextualizes health accounts. This detailed contextualization can help researchers write more thorough descriptions about possible generalizability issues. That is, how do the research findings fit with other similar contexts or research participants?

ORIENTATIONS NEEDED FOR USE OF THE IDENTITY, RESEARCH, AND HEALTH DIALOGIC INTERVIEW

The processes of designing the interview guide and flow are acts of power. Which questions researchers ask, how questions are asked, the way the questions are ordered, how responses are transcribed, how responses are coded, and the format in which results are reported are influenced by the researcher. For example, instead of asking demographic questions first, the Identity, Research, and Health Dialogic Interview focused on this as the last step in the overall research interview. This is to promote rapport building and initial trust development with less intimate questions asked earlier in the interview encounter. At the same time, it helps the research participant understand if the researcher can be trusted with more sensitive information. Overall, for critical researchers to advance inquiry—to envision new paths in knowledge development—several process orientations are outlined below to guide interviewing about demographic data differently.

PROCESS ORIENTATION I: PURPOSEFULLY ASK ABOUT DEMOGRAPHIC DATA IN THE CONTEXT OF THE RESEARCH PURPOSE AND AIMS

Sometimes demographic data may be collected that do not relate to the research aims or are not necessary to achieve the research aims. The Identity, Research, and Health Dialogic Interview insists on providing rationale for each demographic question proposed and being explicit about how it is relevant to the research aims. Often researchers ask about demographic issues that are neither significant nor noteworthy to the research topic of interest. Demographic questions are often used as normative and borrowed from study to study[10] without much thought to their relevance to the research purpose or aims. Researchers have to then link the research aims to the demographic data gathered.

An example of an interview question is needed to illustrate points previously mentioned. For example, how is being male, female, or transgender relevant to the research aims? Asking if someone is male, female, or transgender can be achieved using fixed categories. An example question may be as follows: are you male, female, transgender, or other? Relating the demographic information to the reason that makes it important for research meaning production helps detangle the normative tendency of labeling. Other examples are: how would you describe your gender? (Then wait for a reply.) Given you identify as transgender, how does being transgender influence your ability to access preconception care? The first question leaves room for four possible answers and those answers are not directly or explicitly linked by the researcher to the research aim. The second question asks for the participant's self-identification and then asks how that self-identification informs their health care access (if understanding access is the research aim).

Labeling in a social justice framework often renders assumptions more than understandings. In order to design research focusing on knowledge production, it is important to understand how demographic information and health accounts are interlaced to marginalize or privilege research data creation. Questions are created to open dialogue with research participants about how their demographic positioning (or identity) relates to their health and how persons ascribing to similar demographic positioning may be viewed in research. This technique allows participants the ability to share or protest insights about past research, about their past identity, and about how the past and present demographic issues influence their health.

PROCESS ORIENTATION II: FOCUS ON HOW DEMOGRAPHIC DATA SUPPORTS, EXPANDS, OR REFUTES PRIOR RESEARCH

Additionally, the Identity, Research, and Health Dialogic Interview has an open-ended section. Participants are asked how each demographic issue (e.g., age, gender, education) informs their health related to the research aims. This open-ended section yields data regarding participants' experiences with identity, research, and health. It places participants' health in the context of their historical, political, socioeconomic, and cultural experiences. It also can be uncomfortable for researchers to ask these questions. This discomfort can be due to uncertainty of the unknown or fear based on inexperience in asking these questions previously.

Demographic questionnaires can be designed conversationally for dialogue about the prior research findings. This allows research participants space to share a knowledge platform with researchers related to the literature. A question can be, for example, prior research on hypertension shows that persons earning low-incomes are more likely to have hypertension than persons earning higher incomes in general. However, when it comes to African-Americans as a population group specifically, hypertension is high no matter the income level. What are your thoughts on this research? Questions such as this allowed participants to express their ideas about the research on hypertension. It resulted in new directions of understanding issues about hypertension from participants' point of view. This included a focus on worry and stress and how women were positioned for additional work caring for families.[2] Through a detailed reading and re-reading of interview data, analysis can be undertaken to understand how participants engage with commonplace research findings.

PROCESS ORIENTATION III: DELIBERATELY ANALYZE DEMOGRAPHIC DATA ANEW BY LINKING QUESTIONS TO THE RESEARCH AIMS FOR CREATIVE INSIGHT DEVELOPMENT

The position of researchers shifts when using the Identity, Research, and Health Dialogic Interview. Researchers' power to neatly collect demographic data is challenged. Instead researchers witnesses how demographic issues have routed possibilities for health attainment and prior research development. The data analysis can reveal assumptions about sameness based on labeling. For example, by asking a number of participants who may use the same racial identity label (for example, White American, Native American, Multicultural, etc.) about how racial identity has influenced them, it may be easier to analyze how historical time and place variations shaped their accounts. Participants are less likely to divide themselves into demographic segmentations as they reflect on how their identity influences their health. Thus, researchers learn anew.

The imagination may be even more heightened particularly when this interview design is used with populations and communities under-represented in research. The dialogic process allows assumptions inspected and addressed to be made explicit. During an interview training session, for example, the Identity, Research, and Health Interview helped research interviewees become aware of their emotional reactions to the interview content and the research participants.[1] Imagining demographic knowledge anew and sharing that knowledge is a pathway for creative research insights.

The Identity, Research, and Health Dialogic Interview, for example, contextualizes the responses of participants and the assumptions of the researchers and creates a pathway for alternative research accounts to be told. There is a deliberate focus on analyzing how demographic data informed health. Because of the dialogic nature of the interview, researchers have information about which demographic issues most influenced participants' health accounts. These health accounts can be powerful as they are directly articulating how the demographic data is related to the research aims.

SUMMARY

Interviewing about demographic data and its influences on health versus reporting demographic data helps open new ways of researching. Research interview design is central to developing new understandings. The Identity,

Research, and Health Dialogic Interview can demystify how the research aims relate to participants' identity and how their identity influences their health and health attainment possibilities. It is also a powerful way to engage with and critique prior research. From the point of view of the researcher, it opens new thought channels while minimizing stereotypical questioning and conclusion development. This interview technique can be helpful to clarify why certain demographic data are needed and how to ask those questions to inform knowledge development. The Identity, Research, and Health Dialogic Interview promotes a process for exploring researchers' assumptions about how to collect, interpret, and re-report demographic and health data. This approach will equip researchers with another way to structure interviews to gain critical and overlooked insights about demographic data. It will also influence how participants are re-reported in research articles and presentations.

Appendix A

Identity, Research, and Health Research Analysis Worksheet

Appendix A   Identity, Research, and Health Research Analysis Worksheet

Research Purpose:

Research Aim 1:	Prior Research Studies and Demographic Information		Current Research Study Need for Demographic Information	
	What was gathered as data?	What was the rationale for gathering that data?	What will be gathered as data?	What is the rationale for gathering that data?

Research Aim 2:	Prior Research Studies and Demographic Information		Current Research Study Need for Demographic Information	
	What was gathered as data?	What was the rationale for gathering that data?	What will be gathered as data?	What is the rationale for gathering that data?

Appendix B

An Example of the Identity, Research, and Health Dialogic Interview Format

(Note: This section is the last portion of the research interview.)

Participant ID   _____

Name of Interviewer _____

Date   _____

Interview Start Time _____

Interview End Time _____

OPENING STATEMENT (THIS STATEMENT IS SPOKEN TO THE RESEARCH PARTICIPANT)

I want to understand more about you, your background, and what affects your health. I also want to discuss your thoughts about the prior research on (**state research aims of interest**). I will read some questions. Please feel free to say pass or skip if you do not want to discuss a question. At some points, the topics may become sensitive or difficult to share.

May I record this interview? (**If yes, turn the audio-recorder on now.**)
May I take notes as we talk? (**If yes, place your writing pen and pad near.**)
Now, I will begin with the questions.

(Notes to guide the development of the interview are written in parentheses.)

1. How would you describe your gender?
2. How does being a (**use the same word the person said: man, male, women, lady, girl, etc.**) influence (**state the research concept of interest using participant's term, if possible**)?
3. What is the month, day, and year of your birth?
4. What is your age today?
5. How does being (**use the same word spoken by person to re-state age**) influence (**state the research concept of interest using the participant's term, if possible**)?
6. What is your marital status? (**If more information is needed—say the words single, partnered, divorced, married, separated, etc.**)

7. How does being (use the same word spoken by person to re-state marital status) influence (state the research concept of interest using the participant's term, if possible)?

8. How many people, including yourself, live in the house with you? (If more information is needed—say the numbers 1, 2, 3, 4, 5, 6–10, 11–15, 16+)

9. How does living with (use the same word spoken by the person to re-state the number of people) influence (state the research concept of interest using the participant's terms, if possible)?

10. Of that number, how many people do you care for in that house?

11. Do you care for persons outside of that house? If so, how many?

12. So, in total, how many people do you care for overall?

13. Do you think caring for (use the same word spoken by the person to re-state the number of people) influence (state the research concept of interest using the participant's terms, if possible)?

14. What is the highest level of education you were able to complete?(If needed, say 1st, 2nd, 3rd, 4th, 5th, etc., 12th, high school, vocational school diploma, associate degree, bachelor's degree, master's degree, doctorate degree, etc.)

15. How does being (use the same word spoken by the person to re-state the educational level) influence (state the research concept of interest using the participant's terms, if possible)?

16. What was your household's total annual income last year—(state the year)? (If needed, offer a sheet for the participants to point to the numbers listed as $5, 000, $6,000, $7,000, $8,000, $9,000, $10,000 $11,000, $12,000, $13,000, etc.)

17. How does your income of (re-state the annual income) influence (state the research concept of interest using the participant's terms, if possible)?

18. How many jobs do you have? Please tell me about each one.

19. How long have you been working as a (re-state job categories sing the participant's term)? (re-state the question for each job the participant has to earn a living)

20. How does working as (re-state a job category using the participant's term) for (re-state the amount of time in months or years) influence (state the research concept of interest using the participant's terms, if possible)? (for each job re-state this question as necessary)

21. How does working (re-state the number of jobs) influence (state the research concept of interest using the participant's terms, if possible)? (If you are interviewing recent immigrants to the United States, the questions below may be useful.)

22. In which year did you come to the United States?

23. How does living in the United States since (re-state the year) influence (state the research concept of interest using the participant's terms, if possible)?

24. When you first arrived to the United States, in which state did you live?
25. How long did you live in (use the same words spoken by the person to re-state the area)?
26. How does living in the (use the same words spoken by the person to re-state the area) for (re-state the number of years) influence (state the research concept of interest using the participant's terms, if possible)?
27. How often do you return to (identify the county of origin, if appropriate for the research purpose and aims)?
28. How does returning to (re-state the country of origin) every (re-state the number) influence (state the research concept of interest using the participant's terms, if possible)?
29. Do you send goods or money to (re-state the county of origin)?
30. (If yes to the above question, say) What do you send and how often?
31. Does sending goods or money to (re-state the county of origin) every (re-state the frequency) influence (state the research concept of interest using the participant's terms, if possible)?

THOUGHTS ON THE PRIOR RESEARCH

1. In other research studies, (re-state the concept, for example, number of jobs a person has) was related to (state the research concept of interest using the participant's terms, if possible).
   a. What are your thoughts about this statement?
   b. How might those issues be related?
   c. How might those issues not be related?
   d. Have you ever heard anyone else share some thoughts about this?
2. It is not well understand in research how (state the concept of interest from prior research).
   a. What are your thoughts about this statement?
   b. What do you think might be missing from the research?
   c. Have you ever heard anyone else share some thoughts about this?

OTHER POSSIBILITIES

1. What else can we discuss which may affect your (state the research concept of interest using the participant's terms, if possible)?
2. Have you ever heard other people discuss issues that affect (state the research concept of interest using the participant's terms, if possible) that we did not discuss?

INTERVIEW IMPROVEMENT

Please help me improve this interview.

1. What can I do to make the questions easier to grasp for someone else? For example, were there any hard to understand questions?
2. Please re-state the hard to understand questions one at a time.
3. Now I wish to ask you about each one separately.
4. For (**re-state the question**), please tell me more about how you might ask that question to someone else. (**re-state the question until all difficult questions are identified and new suggestions offered.**)

CLOSING

Thank you very much for taking the time to talk with me today.
(**Turn the audio recorder off. Remember to record interview end time.**)

REFERENCES

1. Boutain D, Hitti J. Orienting multiple interviewers: the use of an interview orientation and standardized interview. *Qualitative Health Research* 2006;16(9): 1302–1309.
2. Boutain D. Worry, stress and family: critical signifiers of high blood pressure by rural dwelling African Americans. Doctoral dissertation. University of Washington School of Nursing, Seattle, WA; 2000. ProQuest: UMI Dissertations Publishing, Document ID Number 304629843.
3. Sanon M. Hypertension management among Haitian immigrant hotel housekeepers within the context of their transmigrant life. Doctoral dissertation. University of Washington School of Nursing, Seattle, WA; 2012. ProQuest: UMI Dissertations Publishing, Document ID Number 1197762361.
4. Lu L. Taiwanese older adults' and healthcare providers' views of depression and depression prevention. Doctoral dissertation. University of Washington School of Nursing, Seattle, WA; 2009. ProQuest: UMI Dissertations Publishing, Document ID Number 305016094.
5. Liu F. Exploring preconception policies and health with adult daughters, their maternal mothers and healthcare providers in rural Zhejiang Province, P.R. China. Doctoral dissertation. University of Washington School of Nursing, Seattle, WA; 2010. ProQuest: UMI Dissertations Publishing, Document ID Number 753915375.
6. Evans-Agnew R. Asthma management disparities: a critical analysis of the discourses of African American adolescent and public health stakeholders in Washington State. Doctoral dissertation. University of Washington School of Nursing, Seattle, WA; 2012. ProQuest: UMI Dissertations Publishing, Document ID Number 940892708.
7. Crotty M. *The Foundations of Social Research: Meaning and Perspective in the Research Process*. London, UK: Sage; 2003.

8. King T. *The Truth about Stories: A Native Narrative.* Minneapolis, MN: University of Minnesota Press; 2003.
9. Holstein J, Gubrium J. *Inside Interviewing: New Lens, New Concerns.* Thousand Oaks, CA: Sage; 2003.
10. Bradburn N, Sudman S, Wansink B. *Asking Questions: the Definition Guide to Questionnaire Design—For Market Research, Political Polls, and Social and Health Questionnaires.* San Francisco, CA: Jossey-Bass; 2004.

10 Critical Research Methodologies and Social Justice Issues
A Methodological Example Using Photovoice

Robin A. Evans-Agnew, Marie-Anne Sanon, and Doris M. Boutain

INTRODUCTION

New methods such as Photovoice have been increasingly utilized in nursing. Yet, as new research methods arise, many researchers succumb to the power of method over methodology. That is, methods are heralded to promote social justice, emancipation, and voice. Very little attention is given to the methodology—the philosophical orientation, strategic plan, and implementation process—underlying the choice and use of research methods.[1]

As nurse researchers engaged in social justice, our orientation to methodology and methods comes from our understanding of Paulo Friere's notion of *praxis*: "reflection and action upon the world in order to transform it."[2(p28)] In the context of our paper, praxis encourages a deeper consideration of the fit between methodology (reflection) and method (action) for social justice. Too often in research design, this close attention to praxis is ignored. With this absence comes diminished attention to improving the design, implementation, and dissemination of future nursing research studies focused on social justice.

The purpose of this chapter is to critically explore Photovoice method-use in nursing research designed to promote social justice. Firstly, a synthesis of significant critiques of the Photovoice method is presented. Secondly, two research study case examples provide a deeper exploration of how the utilization of methods in research is a social justice issue. Both studies are related in the first person of each investigator, Marie-Anne Sanon (MAS) and Robin Evans-Agnew (REA). The first example focuses on a critical ethnography of hypertension management among Haitian immigrant hotel housekeepers. The second example focuses on a critical discourse analysis of asthma management disparities among African-American adolescents. The chapter concludes with a detailed discussion of questions researchers can consider during the research design, implementation, and dissemination phases.

As a method, Photovoice was originally developed by Wang and Burris for use with rural Chinese women in 1994.[3] The original Photovoice method included the following three elements: (1) the empowerment of the voice of participants through the taking and showing of photographs, (2) the utilization of a set of structured questions to elicit texts to accompany the photographs, and (3) the presentation of these photo-texts to policy makers to inspire social action. These elements have subsequently been taken up in a variety of ways by researchers seeking to develop socially-just knowledge development and advocacy in health research.

Photovoice has been presented by some researchers as emancipatory and socially just because the method is participatory, empowering, and directed at policy change.[4,5] For example, Haque and Eng used Photovoice to promote policy change for a disadvantaged immigrant community in Canada.[5] Thus, photo-taking provides an opportunity for individual expression that can be used by nurse researchers seeking empowerment and social justice.

Carlson, Engebretson, and Chamberlain[6] described the Photovoice method as rooted in Frierian principle of *conscientização*.[2] *Conscientização* means the development of a critical consciousness; the process of developing an awareness of how one's assumptions and material conditions can determine reality and how one can choose to change or perpetuate that reality. The actions of taking, discussing, and acting on photographs as evidence, they argue, make Photovoice an emancipatory method. However nurse researchers have not explored how different methodologies would guide the use of Photovoice.

PHOTOVOICE CRITIQUED

According to Boutain,[7(p50)] social justice researchers should look to the "multiple simultaneous sites of social justice action, including awareness, amelioration, and transformation" of the oppressive structural conditions that constitute injustice. Awareness focuses on showing or making known an injustice to the public or society. Amelioration aims to limit the symptoms of injustice. Transformation is directed at understanding and addressing the root cause of injustice.

In choosing to examine such sites of social justice action and selecting an appropriate method, the researcher must pay particular attention to how such knowledge is created and disseminated. The selection of an appropriate methodology for the research aim is of paramount concern for researchers seeking such opportunities, because the methodology determines the strategy and plan of action for such knowledge discovery.[1] However, few critiques of Photovoice have explored the tensions between the research methodology and this method when used in practice. Critiques have more often been directed at ethical aspects (e.g., the risk to participant privacy in photo taking)[8,9] and participatory design issues (i.e., recruitment, involvement, analysis, and application of findings).[10,11] Other theoretical critiques of the Photovoice method have examined the implications of phenomenological[12] and anti-colonial[13] methodologies in knowledge development.

In a theoretical review of the Photovoice method, Hansen-Ketchum and Myrick[12] argued that Photovoice elicited either a relativistic or a realistic truth through the respective individual or group analysis of photos. Relativistic truths were essentially personal descriptions of photos used to construct phenomenological understandings of the lived experience of individuals. Realistic truths occurred in studies where photos were used to "represent and interpret reality"[12(p210)] by researcher and participant(s). The author's analysis made an important contribution to Photovoice design by differentiating between two data-collection objectives.

Hansen-Ketchum and Myrick[12] did not address two key issues in methodology-method praxis arising from the co-construction of data between researcher and participants, notably researcher influence on the selection, analysis, and dissemination of the photographs. Firstly, these authors did not discuss critical methodologies. Secondly, these authors did not discuss how to account for researcher influence on policy change.

Racine and Petrucka[13] described the use of critical methodologies in their application of Photovoice. With the goal of "developing transformative knowledge and achieving social justice by correcting health inequities,"[13(p16)] the authors suggested that a Photovoice method used within a critical methodological approach becomes socially just through the provision of voice(s) for the disenfranchised. These authors emphasized consideration of power relations and participant trust in method design. However, they did not critique the consequences arising from utilizing Photovoice in such a design.

CASE EXAMPLE ONE: CRITICAL ETHNOGRAPHY AND PHOTOVOICE

In this first exemplar I (MAS) describe how the Photovoice method was used in a critical ethnography study. I interviewed 31 Haitian immigrant hotel housekeepers (27 women and 4 men) to determine how they defined and managed hypertension within the context of their transmigrant life and work. "Transmigrant life" refers to the life that enables immigrants to maintain political, cultural, and socioeconomic networks and to behaviors that transcend the geographical borders of their country of residence and native country.[14]

Critical ethnography aims to understand cultural beliefs and culturally based behaviors while uncovering systemic and individual forces that may or may not be hidden from participants.[15] In this study my goal was to identify aspects of the life of Haitian immigrants that influenced their hypertension management. The methodology emphasized the co-creation of knowledge between participants and researcher as influenced by their sociocultural and work contexts. In this exemplar, the Photovoice method was emancipatory when I used it to enable participants to select and critically appraise specific contextual aspects of their life influencing their hypertension management.

For this research study, I interviewed each participant twice. I made the taking of photographs an optional activity. For those that agreed to take photos, I explained how to use a disposable camera, and asked participants to take pictures at work or at home of "any objects and/or individuals that you believe play a role in your hypertension management." During the subsequent interview of those who took photos I used three of the standard photo-text elicitation questions: (1) Why did you take this picture? (2) What is happening in this picture? and (3) How does this picture relate to how being a hotel housekeeper influences your hypertension management? I asked participants to identify pictures that best: (1) defined hypertension, (2) showed how they managed hypertension, and (3) showed their life influences on the way they managed hypertension. I addressed the ethical risks to privacy presented by photo-taking in three ways: (1) I made Photovoice an optional activity for participants, (2) I encouraged participants to seek permission from individuals they might want to take photos of, and (3) I promised not to publish any photo that identified a business or an individual.

I used a reflexive note-taking strategy to monitor power relations by asking myself the following questions: (1) how is my education influencing my interaction with the participants and the way I am collecting, analyzing, and representing the data and (2) how is my position as a researcher influencing my interaction with the participants? For example when I asked participants what they thought of hypertension, they automatically reverted the question to me saying that I needed to tell them what hypertension is because I was the nurse. This increased my awareness that participants perceived me as an individual with the power of expert "western-knowledge." I had to further underscore the importance of their expert knowledge in the management of hypertension.

Expected Consequences of Using the Photovoice Method with Critical Ethnography

I found that Photovoice enabled participants to take pictures of influences on hypertension management. For example, one participant took a picture of a pharmacy. This picture elicited a conversation between the research participant and me about the lack of health insurance, trust in the Western-biomedical system, and money to pay for medication. In contrast to previous studies that reported a positive influence of transmigrant life on health outcomes and disease management,[16] I found that these photos elicited critical reflections in the participants on the increased financial strain of a transmigrant life.

The use of a critical ethnography methodology and the Photovoice method provided me with emancipatory moment (in other words, of enlightenment or critical consciousness) during my discussions of the photos with participants. In these moments, we were able to critically examine the power relations between participants and myself. For example, the initial interviews elicited stories about what they thought *I wanted* to hear (e.g., using medication prescribed by a doctor), whereas the Photovoice interviews elicited what *they wanted* to show me (e.g., herbs used for hypertension management). When asked about the differences between the first and second interviews, participants discussed that they were not sure what I would think because of my background as a nurse. With regards to the power relation between myself as researcher and the participants, although participants informed me about their experience with hypertension and provided me with pictures to support that information, it remained up to me to decide how I was going to present that information. To address this issue I had to show the pictures along with their associated text in addition to my explanation. This ensured participants' power over data presentation and interpretation

Unexpected Consequences of Using Photovoice in a Critical Ethnography Study

The technical limitations of using a disposable camera (limited number of images, no immediate review by the photographer, and lack of an adequate viewfinder) reduced the ability of participants to express themselves through photos. Overall, 5 of the 12 participants had difficulties using the camera properly. All 12 said that they were not sure what pictures to take. For one participant, only 2 out of 24 images from the camera were discernible and therefore useful for discussion. They reported that they used the camera as they were taught and were unsure why the images were unclear. This lack of image clarity could also have been due to time constraints, as they were rushing to take the pictures, because participants had to take pictures amidst their busy schedules. I did not anticipate this as an issue because during recruitment individuals declined to participate in the study because they did not have time. Therefore I anticipated that those who opted to participate considered the time issue.

Only 12 participants out of 31 (38%) agreed to the Photovoice interview. The justification for not participating in the Photovoice interview included: lack of time ($n = 13$), not interested ($n = 5$), and fear of being fired for using a camera at work ($n = 2$). As this study explored transmigrant life in the context of the workplace I was especially concerned that Photovoice not threaten participant ability to maintain employment. Two persons from the original sample declined to participate in the Photovoice part of the study, claiming fear of reprisals from supervisors for taking pictures at their workplaces. Clearly these participants did not regard the opportunity to participate in Photovoice as emancipatory, and they had no reason to think these photos would help them improve their circumstances.

Moreover, Photovoice can be a burden to the researcher because of the researcher's responsibility towards data presentation and dissemination. Although the participants are the ones taking the photos and creating the associated texts, the interpretations attributed the photo-texts can vary. For example, in my study, when participants took photos of imported herbal medicines, they described them as replacement (14 photos) or complementary (11 photos) to the Western medicines. In presenting and disseminating my findings, I have a responsibility to provide the context (e.g., their transmigrant life) for these photo-texts. At the same time, the audience may not believe, hear, or acknowledge the interpretation of the participants and may develop their own interpretations of the photo-texts.

For my study, Photovoice became an emancipatory method when participants and I were able to critique the power relations between us that were affecting the construction of knowledge. My use of reflexivity throughout the research process provided additional appraisals of these power relations. Thus, Photovoice and reflexive practice enhanced knowledge creation between participants and me.

Future critical ethnographers who are considering methods for emancipatory action should evaluate how well the Photovoice method aligns with their methodological aims. Photovoice provided an emancipatory moment for my participants to critically appraise the power relations in data collection (i.e., saying that they took prescribed medication and yet providing me with pictures of herbal medicines), and yet the burdens of such an opportunity sometimes conflicted with my methodological intent. Through reflexivity I was able to begin to appraise power relations and become aware of the responsibility I would have in disseminating the data. Future researchers must be cautious to present not only the photo-text data but also the contextual influences (including power relations between researcher and participants and societal influences) on such data.

CASE EXAMPLE TWO: CRITICAL DISCOURSE ANALYSIS AND PHOTOVOICE

In this research exemplar my (REA) aims were to describe and compare the discourses of asthma management disparities that were introduced, promoted, or minimized by public health policy leaders and African-American adolescents with asthma. My study premise was that these discourses would be co-constructed between participants and me. I used linguistic and contextual approaches to Critical Discourse Analysis (CDA),[17] and chose the Photovoice method for collecting data from 20 adolescents (15–18 years old) and 13 policy leaders (35–70 years old) from Seattle.

Critical discourse analysis (CDA) provides nurse-researchers with opportunities to describe social problems in order to reconfigure power relations. Discourses are patterned and linked systems of text, talk, and action located in social structures.[18,19] A critical analysis of these discourses can describe the way certain discourses are introduced, promoted, or minimized and acknowledges that all knowledge is co-constructed between people. This methodology offers opportunities to develop socially-just knowledge.

Photovoice was used in this study as a photo-elicitation and an emancipatory tool for generating textual data on asthma management disparities from participants. For the purposes of photo-elicitation I first trained the adolescents to take photos to answer the following questions: (1) What is life with asthma like? (2) What makes it harder when you are not managing asthma well? (3) What may make it harder for you to manage asthma compared to others? and (4) How could your school/family help others manage asthma? Second, I conducted discussions of participant photos in focus groups. Lastly, I helped adolescents develop photo-texts for a gallery showing to public health policy leaders. I intended this method to be emancipatory through both the discovery of similarities in asthma management disparity experience amongst adolescents and the opportunity for these adolescents to influence the decisions being made by policy leaders regarding such disparities.

To address ethical concerns relating to privacy, and in consultation with the University of Washington's Institutional Review Board, I trained participants to evaluate whether a photo identified a private versus a public setting and whether persons would be identifiable or non-identifiable. I promised not to use any photo that simultaneously included both a private setting and an identifiable individual.[20]

To maintain my reflexivity throughout the data collection period I kept a daily journal. I answered a set of four questions aimed at understanding the power relations emerging in the data collection process: (1) How well am I balancing the need for critical distance and engagement? (2) How could my privilege be affecting my perspective? (3) How could I improve on protecting participants? and (4) Am I observing what I set out to observe? I then sent my comments electronically to a separate researcher for feedback.

Expected Consequences of Using Photovoice in a Critical Discourse Analysis

A key feature of a CDA methodology is an orientation to social justice.[17] The photos taken and shared by adolescent stakeholders elicited the co-construction of both textual and contextual data surrounding asthma management injustices. For example, participants used photographs of school lunches to elicit conversations both about how nutrition was an important determinant of asthma management *and* that they believed their (predominantly African-American) schools had fewer nutritional options compared to White schools. In this way, Photovoice helped shed light on specific power relations that may be propagating asthma management disparities.

Photos provided an important way to provide adolescent participants' with a *voice* in locating their identity in relation to asthma and their opinions about managing asthma.[21] Adolescents used a variety of techniques to take photos such as studio ($n = 2$), outdoor ($n = 8$), and staged shots ($n = 12$). The focus groups and gallery-showing provided participants with opportunities to discuss and *reflect* on the influence of their environment on asthma management disparities.

In the final data collection event in the study, adolescents presented their photo-texts at an event called a "Gallery Showing" to public health policy leaders. Through group discussion, parents and public health policy leaders shared how impressed they were with the leadership and creativity of the adolescents. The event empowered participating adolescents and their parents in challenging dominant discourses and asserting their own discourses on asthma management disparities. These exchanges became emancipatory through both the acknowledged leadership of the adolescents and the realization of shared discourses between participants.

Unexpected Consequences of Using Photovoice in a Critical Discourse Analysis

Texts accompanying the photographs may not have been read or may have been only read after the viewer made their own interpretation. During the gallery showing I observed that the photos generated new, observer-based texts independent of what was displayed. For example a photo of tobacco smoke prompted a discussion by gallery observers on the disparities involved in indoor environments. This discussion was in marked contrast to my focus-group observation that this photo-text was related to a racial disadvantage of being exposed to tobacco smoke. Thus, not only should researchers make consideration of the need to frame such a gallery event for an audience with the parameters for how to view the photo-texts (for example as participatory research or policy statements), but researchers could also consider such events as additional data-gathering opportunities. In this example, my research aims included the ability to critically analyze my observations of such discussions between event attendees and identify discourses that were shared/not shared between adolescents and public health leaders.

I found that my focus group questioning strategy may have been too abstract for participants. For example, in a discussion about a photograph of school stairs (and the difficulty participants found in using them and getting to class on time when the stairs triggered their asthma), I found myself continuing to contextualize the question (Figure 10.1) in order to pursue an emancipatory moment.

"PI:	Why does this asthma situation concern or strength, exist?
Participant 1:	Hmm?
PI:	Why does this asthma situation concern or strength exist?
Participant 1:	Can you break the question down?
PI:	Well, is it a concern, right? I don't know whether it's necessarily a strength... this one (pause) we've all been talking about a concern, but, what I was kind of getting with that, with that question about... why do they build schools like this if they know it's difficult for teenagers with asthma to climb up the stairs?
Participant 1:	They don't think about that.
Participant 2:	It just isn't on their mind."

Figure 10.1   Example of How I Adjusted My Focus Group Questioning Strategy

This example shows the co-construction of emancipatory reflection and action: That is, "If school builders do not consider adolescents with asthma when they design buildings with stairs, we must act to tell policy makers about this situation." My choice of a critical methodology assumed a co-construction of reality using these questions and thus fit the questioning method that I used. It was however hard to perceive from this adjustment in questioning whether I adequately balanced power between the participants and myself. In reframing the question I used my power as group leader to present an argument for inequality (in the built environment), which the adolescents responded to. Greater consideration is needed in the preparation of a socially just and emancipatory questioning strategy (one that elicits enlightenment or *conscientização*) that balances the simultaneous interests in scientific inquiry and advocacy.

The use of photos from a Photovoice project in future dissemination projects has social justice implications. In this example, the public health policy makers who had attended the gallery showing went on to publish a policy document. The document contained an inset reference (and portrait of an adolescent stakeholder holding his photo of stairs) to the gallery event together with a photo-text about disparities in adolescent and family exposure to stairs, but no mention was made of the discourse of disadvantaged urban environments.[22] Researchers may be tempted to use photos that are attractive to them for intentions not anchored in the intentions of the research participants. This is the crux, perhaps, of emancipatory nursing research: how well does the data presented through emancipatory research aims, such as in this exemplar, advance ideas about oppression and injustice for African-American adolescents managing asthma in our schools, without compromising the potency of the voice of the adolescents that articulated these ideas?

This experience has further prompted me to be cautious about use of photo-texts in my presentations to the specific social justice actions evident in my data. To underscore the argument about the potency of photographs, I decided to not use photo-texts within this exemplar. As more journals consider publishing Photovoice studies, reviewers should consider how publishing photo-texts preserves the social justice intent of the research study.

Extreme care must be taken to consider the pragmatic consequences of using the Critical Discourse Analysis (CDA) methodology (social change) to guide the Photovoice method (emancipation). The power of photographs to persuade the viewer that they are observing reality can be abrogated by those groups more powerful than others within a project such as this and utilized for their own personal gain. These issues are not new to those considering the persuasive power of photographs[23,24] and their influence on power relations.

QUESTIONS TO CONSIDER WHEN USING CRITICAL METHODOLOGIES AND THE PHOTOVOICE METHOD

When discussing study participant reactions to the photographs and photo-texts in the above exemplars, something new arises for researchers. The Photovoice method raised concerns about researcher responsibilities to research participants in (1) balancing power and (2) ensuring that the participants' intended interpretations of the photographs were communicated. Because the photographs are disseminated as research data, responsibility rests with the researcher to plan for and address power relations related to photographic interpretations. The researcher is also responsible for presenting the participants' interpretation of the photographs clearly enough to ensure that audience members acknowledge participants' interpretations. This does not mean that the audience will agree with those interpretations, however. Thus, balance of power—which may assume equal power—does not fully capture what happens as the photographs and photo-texts are disseminated. In our experience it is the researcher who controls the opportunities for dissemination. The researcher also stages and engages in the interpretative (with an acknowledgement of the primacy of the participants interpretation) moments that arise during the discussions of the photographs, such as the gallery event that happened in the second exemplar.

For these reasons, several questions arise that are important for evaluating the intentional and unintentional consequences of using critical methodologies to guide the Photovoice method. These questions can be divided into issues to plan for during the research design, implementation, and dissemination phases of the study. Important questions for the researcher to consider are offered in Table 10.1 below.

Critical methodologies are informed by social justice concerns that interrogate power relations, assert that all knowledge is socially constructed and political, and attend to social justice issues in the processes of research.[25] The issues described in this chapter illustrate that Photovoice, if used appropriately with critical methodologies, can yield complex reflections that may or may not promote socially-just knowledge production. Reflecting on a series of questions at various stages in the research project may support continuous praxis. Photo-elicitation is not enough to balance power, especially when participants have unequal technical and environmental contexts for expressing themselves through Photovoice.

SUMMARY

Research as praxis, in the context of social justice, requires the practice and critique of research methodologies and methods. Through research as

Table 10.1 Question Guide for Designing Photovoice Use with Critical Methodologies

	Research Design

Planned Intentions	• What is the specific research intent in using the Photovoice method with a critical methodology?
	   o To produce research knowledge for social justice awareness
	   o To produce research knowledge for actions to address symptoms of injustice for social justice amelioration
	   o To produce research knowledge for transformative actions to address a specific systematic oppression
	• What is the intent with respect to the intended audience observations, assumptions, feelings, and beliefs from the photographs and photo-texts to support the social justice intent?
	• How are the aims, methodology, and methods aligned with social justice intent?

Unintentional Consequences	• How could the photographs and photo-text be interpreted to hinder the social just intent? • How could the photographs and photo-text negatively impact those being researched? • How could the photographs and photo-texts negatively impact the researcher? • How would observing, assuming, feeling, and believing the photograph and photo-text diminish the social power of the researcher or participants? o What reactions may result? • Could the research aims, methodology, and methods hinder the social justice intent?
	Research Implementation
Planned Intentions	• How will the researcher implement the critical research methodology and Photovoice method in practice? • How will the research participants implement the Photovoice method in practice? • How will the implementation of the Photovoice method be emancipatory not only for the research participants, but also for the researcher? • How could social justice awareness, amelioration, or transformative action get advanced in practice of the methodology and method? • How could social justice awareness, amelioration, or transformative action get hindered in practice of the methodology and method?

Table 10.1 (Continued)

Unintentional Consequences	• How could practice of the methodology and Photovoice method negatively impact or cause harm to the researcher?
	• How could practice of the Photovoice method negatively impact or cause harm to the research participants?
	• Which photographs did the researcher see but did not want to include as research data?
	  ◦ Why?
	• Identify the social justice implications.
	• Which photographs did the research participant take but did not want to show or discuss?
	  ◦ Why?
	  ◦ Identify the social justice implications.
	• How could the practice of the Photovoice method result in social oppression for the researcher or the research participants?

Research Dissemination	
Planned Intentions	• Where will the research photographs and photo-texts be disseminated to promote the social justice of awareness, amelioration, or transformative action? • How will the researcher present the research photographs and photo-texts to promote the social justice intents of awareness, amelioration, or transformative action?
Unintentional Consequences	• How could research dissemination of the photographs and photo-texts hinder social justice awareness, amelioration, or transformative action? • How could disseminating the photographs and photo-texts cause negative impacts or harm to the researcher? • How could disseminating the photographs and photo-texts cause negative impacts or harm to the research participant? • How could the dissemination venue, audience, or process result in the social oppression of knowledge?

praxis, nurses have an opportunity to recognize and minimize power relationships in the creation of knowledge. This chapter highlighted issues in the use of the Photovoice method with critical methodologies and provided a framework for methodology selection and critique for the future.

REFERENCES

1. Crotty M. *The Foundations of Social Research: Meaning and Perspective in the Research Process*. Thousand Oaks, CA: Sage Publications; 1998.
2. Freire P. *Pedagogy of the Oppressed*. London, UK: Penguin Hammondsworth; 1972.

3. Wang C, Burris MA. Empowerment through photo novella: portraits of participation. *Health Educ Q* Summer 1994;21(2): 171–186.
4. Wang C, Burris MA. Photovoice: concept, methodology, and use for participatory needs assessment. *Health Educ Behav* Jun 1997;24(3): 369–387.
5. Haque N, Eng B. Tackling inequity through a Photovoice project on the social determinants of health: translating Photovoice evidence to community action. *Glob Health Promot* Mar 2011;18(1): 16–19.
6. Carlson ED, Engebretson J, Chamberlain RM. Photovoice as a social process of critical consciousness. *Qualitative Health Tesearch* 2006;16(6): 836–852.
7. Boutain DM. Social justice and nursing: a review of the literature. In: Mary de Chesnay, Anderson BA, eds. *Caring for the Vulnerable.* Burlington, MA: Jones and Bartlett Learning; 2012: 43–58.
8. Wang CC, Redwood-Jones YA. Photovoice ethics: perspectives from Flint Photovoice. *Health Educ Behav* Oct 2001;28(5): 560–572.
9. Stevens CA. Lessons from the field: using Photovoice with an ethnically diverse population in a HOPE VI evaluation. *Fam Community Health* Oct–Dec 2010;33(4): 275–284.
10. Castleden H, Garvin T. Modifying Photovoice for community-based participatory Indigenous research. *Soc Sci Med* Mar 2008;66(6): 393–405.
11. Catalani C, Minkler M. Photovoice: a review of the literature in health and public health. *Health Education & Behavior* June 1, 2010;37(3): 424–451.
12. Hansen-Ketchum P, Myrick F. Photo methods for qualitative research in nursing: an ontological and epistemological perspective. *Nursing Philosophy* 2008;9(3): 205–213.
13. Racine L, Petrucka P. Enhancing decolonization and knowledge transfer in nursing research with non-western populations: examining the congruence between primary healthcare and postcolonial feminist approaches. *Nurs Inq* Mar 2011;18(1): 12–20.
14. Basch LG, Schiller NG, Szanton Blanc C. *Nations Unbound: Transnational Projects, Postcolonial Predicaments, and Deterritorialized Nation-States.* London: Gordon and Breach; 1994.
15. Thomas J. *Doing Critical Ethnography.* Newbury Park, CA: Sage Publications; 1993.
16. Murphy EJ, Mahalingam R. Transnational ties and mental health of Caribbean immigrants. *Journal of Immigrant Health* 2004;6(4): 11.
17. Wodak R, Meyer M. *Methods of Critical Discourse Analysis.* Thousand Oaks, CA: SAGE; 2009.
18. Van-Dijk TA. Critical discourse studies: a sociocognitive approach. In: Wodak R, Meyer M, eds. *Methods of Critical Discourse Analysis.* Thousand Oaks. CA: SAGE; 2009: 62–85.
19. Allen D, Hardin PK. Discourse analysis and the epidemiology of meaning. *Nursing Philosophy* 2001;2(2): 163–176.
20. Gustafson K, Al-Sumait, F. Photo conversations about climate: engaging teachers and policymakers through photography and narrative. University of Washington, Department of Communication. 2009. http://www.sightline.org/research/conversations-about-climate. Accessed October 23, 2010.
21. Thomson P. *Doing Visual Research with Children and Young People.* New York, NY: Routledge; 2008.
22. Washington-Asthma-Initiative. *Washington State Asthma Plan 2011–2015.* Olympia, WA: Washington State Department of Health. 2011. http://www.doh.wa.gov/Portals/1/Documents/Pubs/345-290_AsthmaPlan2011-15.pdf. Accessed June 22, 2011.
23. Barthes R. *Camera Lucida: Reflections on Photography.* New York, NY: Hill and Wang; 1981.

24. Prins E. Participatory photography: A tool for empowerment or surveillance? *Action Research* 2010;8(4): 426–443.
25. Potts K, Brown L. Becoming an anti-oppressive researcher. In: Brown L, Strega S, eds. *Research as Resistance: Critical, Indigenous and Anti-Oppressive Approaches*. Toronto, ON, Canada: Canadian Scholars' Press; 2005: 255–286.

Section III

Pedagogy of Praxis

Teaching for Social Justice

11 Social Justice

From Educational Mandate to Transformative Core Value

*Mary K. Canales and
Denise J. Drevdahl*

INTRODUCTION

This volume is committed to explicating social justice within nursing and examining the many ways social justice influences practice, research, and education. As a recent concept analysis of social justice indicates[1] such an explication is a challenge for the nursing profession because social justice is defined in myriad ways, or not at all, within the nursing literature. These variations and omissions in themselves suggest that although the profession claims "a long history of social justice,"[1(p949)] it continues to struggle with what social justice means for practicing nurses, educators, and students.

Despite these struggles, the nursing profession in the United States has reinforced the importance of social justice through its continued reaffirmation of it as a core value. Beginning in 2000, the United States (U.S.) American Nurses' Association (ANA) has included social justice in its key documents, including the *Code of Ethics for Nurses with Interpretive Statements, Nursing's Social Policy Statement*, and *Nursing: Scope and Standards of Practice*.[2] Yet, as analyses by Bekemeier and Butterfield,[2] and Fry,[3] White,[4] and Allen[5] before them demonstrate, these documents focus primarily on individual rights and the centrality of the nurse-patient relationship, and minimally address broader social determinants of health such as poverty, affordable housing, or access to health insurance, to name a few.

Because the ANA social policy documents often provide the framework for nursing's link to social justice, these critiques from the literature raised questions for us regarding other influential nursing documents. Within nursing education in general, and undergraduate education in the United States in particular, increased emphasis has been placed on accrediting documents with some concerns raised regarding their expanding and influential role in determining the direction of nursing education.[6-8] Although social justice is an element of these documents, to what degree is the concept integral to them?

We attempt to answer this question by examining how social justice is incorporated into nursing education in the United States. We recognize that although an international perspective is very valuable, it is beyond the scope and purpose of this chapter, which is a critique of U.S. documents and literature. We do however, in the concluding sections, return to the importance of learning from global nurse scholars who are engaged in social justice efforts.

Although practice is not easily separated from education, *how* students are socialized into the profession has a major impact on how they practice once they graduate and enter the workforce. The development of critical thinking skills essential for viewing the world and the values that guide nurses' professional practice often are established in their early nursing education. We therefore believe an examination of social justice within nursing education is warranted. We begin this chapter with the results of a review of U.S. nursing accrediting documents. Following this review, results of a critical analysis of the nursing literature, examining the intersection of social justice and nursing education, are presented. We conclude with our interpretation of the results of these examinations and what they may mean for nurse educators and accreditation organizations.

ANALYSIS OF NURSING EDUCATION DOCUMENTS

During the past 20 years, the American Association of Colleges of Nursing (AACN) and its accrediting agency, the Commission on Collegiate Nursing Education (CCNE), have emerged as the primary external organizations influencing U.S. nursing programs at all levels within the university. According to AACN's website, it "is the national voice for America's baccalaureate- and higher-degree nursing education," with membership expanding from 121 schools of nursing in 1969 to more than 690 today.[9] AACN has developed a series of Essentials documents that outline competency expectations for graduates of baccalaureate, master's, and Doctor of Nursing Practice (DNP) programs. "Using these documents, schools of nursing are able to ensure they adhere to the highest standards for their educational programs and meet accreditation guidelines."[9] How do these documents incorporate social justice into "competency expectations"?

We begin with an analysis of the primary documents that currently guide nursing education in the United States. Although one may argue that university-based nursing programs are guided by their respective missions and visions, in reality, external nursing organizations, in particular those directly involved in accreditation processes, have assumed a powerful and influential role in curricular decisions, especially at the graduate level.[6] Despite this increasingly visible role in nursing curricular matters, we were unable to locate published reports or analyses examining these relationships.

This analysis is intended to address this gap, beginning with an examination of social justice and its presence in these documents. Although we recognize that the technical college system educates 60% of U.S. educated registered nurses,[10] social justice is not a component of associate degree accrediting documents.[11] We therefore limited the analysis to nursing programs at the university level, as it has been repeatedly reported that social justice is included in these documents.[12,13] Table 11.1 provides a summary of this analysis in terms of the presence or absence of social justice concepts.

Table 11.1 Review of Accreditation Documents

Nursing Organization	Accrediting Agency	Programs Evaluated	Documents Reviewed	Presence of Social Justice in Documents
American Association of Colleges of Nursing (AACN)	Commission on Collegiate Nursing Education (CCNE)	Undergraduate: BSN Graduate: Masters Doctor of Nursing Practice (DNP)	Essentials of Baccalaureate Education for Professional Nursing Practice (2008)[14] Essentials of Master's Education in Nursing (2011)[15] Essentials of Doctoral Education for Advanced Nursing Practice (2006)[16]	Essential I-Liberal education for baccalaureate generalist nursing practice Essential V-Health care policy, finance & regulatory environments Essential VIII-Professionalism & professional values Essential VI-Health policy & advocacy Essential V: Health care policy for advocacy in health care
National League for Nursing (NLN)	National League for Nursing Accrediting Commission, Inc. (NLNAC)	Undergraduate: BSN Graduate: Masters Education Clinical Doctorate	Standards and Criteria: Baccalaureate (2008)[11] Standards and Criteria: Master's & Post-Master's Certificate (2008)[11] Standards and Criteria: Doctorate (2008)[11]	No reference No reference No reference
National Organization of Nurse Practitioner Faculty (NONPF)	National Task Force on Quality Nurse Practitioner Education (Accepted by AACN & NLN)	Graduate: Nurse Practitioner	Criteria for Evaluation of Nurse Practitioner Programs (2008)[18]	No reference

Summary of Analysis Results

Similar to the ANA's foundational documents,[2] the AACN's Essentials of Baccalaureate Education for Professional Nursing Practice[14] identified social justice as a professional value and defined it as "acting in accordance with fair treatment regardless of economic status, race, ethnicity, age, citizenship, disability, or sexual orientation."[14(p29)] The primary discussion of social justice occurs within Essential I, ensuring a liberal education. Although included within three essentials of the baccalaureate document, the role of the generalist nurse is limited to "accepting responsibility to"[14(p13)] "promoting"[14(pp13,21)] and "advocating for"[14(p26)] social justice. A discussion of *how* the nurse can accomplish these actions is not provided.

The Essentials of Master's[15] and Doctoral Education[16] both address social justice within the health policy and advocacy essential. In the Master's Essentials[15] glossary, social justice is presented as a "concept" that "relates to upholding moral, legal, and humanistic principles."[15(p39)] Although the Master's definition is exactly the same as the AACN Baccalaureate Essentials (see above),[14] it is interesting to note that the only references provided for the definition are previous AACN documents.[15] The AACN Essentials for Doctoral Education[16] does not include a definition of social justice. Neither document provides specific examples for enacting social justice or strategies for advocating for it. Although the documents recognize that social justice is influenced by health policy, as is equity, both are presented as health care delivery "issues" rather than desired outcomes or goals for populations.[15,16]

The National League for Nursing (NLN), along with its accrediting agency the National League for Nursing Accrediting Agency, Inc. (NLNAC), is considered the oldest U.S. organization focused on maintaining standards for nursing education, with its Standards for Curriculum for Schools of Nursing first published in 1917.[11] Unfortunately, this long history does not correspond to nursing's long history of valuing social justice because we were unable to locate any reference to social justice in our review of the 2008 edition of the NLNAC manual, which includes standards and criteria for nursing accreditation at all levels within the university.[11]

Considering the limited attention to social justice in the AACN/CCNE[14-16] documents and the omission of social justice in the NLN/NLNAC[11] document, we were not surprised when our review of the graduate education criteria of the National Organization of Nurse Practitioner Faculty (NONPF), which were developed by its subsidiary, the National Task Force on Quality Nurse Practitioner Education, also omitted any reference to social justice.[17] According to NONPF, CCNE has adopted the NONPF evaluation criteria into their accreditation standards whereas NLN has endorsed the evaluation criteria, recognizing the document as "the national standard for nurse practitioner educational programs."[17] Consequently, the only nursing organizations responsible for ensuring the educational standards for advanced practice nursing have adopted a document that disregards social justice.

ANALYSIS OF PUBLISHED LITERATURE

Considering the lack of attention to social justice in nursing accrediting documents, we then analyzed publications addressing social justice and nursing education. We reasoned that the published literature may more accurately reflect the efforts of nurses, particularly nurse educators, to integrate social justice into curricular and academic programming.

Each author conducted an independent literature search using the terms "nursing," "education," and "social justice." Based on Medical Subject Headings (MeSh), we also conducted searches using "academic" and "justice" in an effort to broaden the search and locate additional articles. The time frame was limited to 2006–2012 to build upon previous searches of social justice and nursing education conducted by Boutain[18,19] and to identify the most current publications. Other limits included English only; either published in a nursing journal or the first author was a nurse to ensure a nursing emphasis; and a focus on the United States to align with the document review, which centered on U.S. accrediting organizations. The four databases selected were those most commonly used in nursing: Cumulative Nursing and Allied Health (CINAHL), PubMed, Web of Science, and Google Scholar.

After each of us searched the four databases independently, we reviewed the list of citations generated from each database and deleted duplicate, non-U.S., and non-nursing sources. Of the six articles deleted as being written by someone outside the United States, we noted that the majority were from Canadian authors. This review process led to a single combined list of 23 articles to review for relevancy.

After reviewing the combined list of 23 articles, we deleted seven articles that did not meet the search criteria. For example, there were several papers that included social justice in the abstract yet either had no further discussion of it in the paper or simply mentioned social justice in the concluding comments. The review of the remaining 16 articles led us to expand the search to include articles related to anti-racist pedagogy as this was a reoccurring theme among several of the articles. We observed that anti-racist pedagogy often occurred within a social justice context and or incorporated socially just strategies to engage students. We therefore decided these articles were relevant to the review. A search of the databases for nursing education and anti-racist/racism yielded an additional two articles. We also reviewed the reference lists of the 18 identified articles to ensure that papers cited in relevant articles were not missed; this yielded an additional two articles. Finally, we conducted additional searches for social justice combined with other forms of oppression (e.g., homophobia, misogyny, and classism) without success. The final 20 articles included in this review are summarized in Table 11.2.

Following analysis of the reviewed articles, we more closely examined *how* social justice was addressed within the U.S. nursing classroom.

Table 11.2 Literature Review Summary

Publication Year	Author(s)	Journal	Type of Article-Research/Report	Level of Student	Presence of Social Justice in Article w/Key Results or Implications
2010	Abrums[20]	*Nursing Education Perspectives*	Research-qualitative narrative analysis	RN-BSN	Focus on discrimination, disparities, privilege, & oppression. Research focused on analysis of two-part assignment in required course on social & culture issues in health care. Analysis focused on students' ability to synthesize course content & personal experience; specific course components not included. Results suggest that autobiographical reflection useful strategy for addressing discrimination/privilege. Social justice not addressed specifically.
2011	Alexander[21]	*Journal of Nursing Education*	Report of development & implementation of collective seminar course	Doctoral & post-doctoral (PhD)	Describes development of doctoral seminar research course in health equity. Health equity conceptualized as integrating social justice & determinants of health. Definition of social justice provided. Lessons learned & areas for future efforts identified; reflective discourse of personal biases/practices recommended.

Year	Author	Journal	Description	Population	Summary
2008	Belknap[22]	*Nurse Educator*	Report of teaching a health equity course	Undergraduate BSN	Describes how faculty at private Jesuit university SON applied engagement pedagogy to teach health equity course. Social justice definition presented; discussions of class & race highlighted. Engagement pedagogy includes service learning (SL), writing assignments, & in-class activities. Social change model used to connect SL activities in community to increase students' awareness of injustice.
2008	Boutain[23]	*International Journal of Education Scholarship*	Report of how a community health clinical evaluation tool was revised	Undergraduate BSN	Describes major curricular revision aimed at integrating social justice content throughout undergraduate program including course content, clinical objectives, & creation of new clinical evaluation tool for public health senior experience.
2007	Fahrenwald et al.[24]	*Public Health Nursing*	Essay relating social justice to academic freedom	Faculty w/emphasis on public health	Reviews challenges to academic freedom that influence social justice education; explores academic freedom & duty to teach social justice within discipline of nursing. Proposes praxis-based approach to social justice education, using transformative pedagogy.

(Continued)

Table 11.2 (Continued)

Publication Year	Author(s)	Journal	Type of Article-Research/Report	Level of Student	Presence of Social Justice in Article w/Key Results or Implications
2011	Groh et al.[25]	*Nursing Education Perspectives*	Research study; examines impact of service learning (SL) on social justice & leadership	RN-BSN (senior)	Quantitative descriptive study comparing pre & post-test scores following service learning (SL) experience among 306 students at private, faith-based university. Catholic Social Teaching scale used to evaluate if SL increased interest in social justice. Results suggest that SL does increase interest in social justice although pre-test scores very high prior to SL experience (pre-test: 4.24/5; post-test: 4.6 /5).
2006	Hassouneh[26]	*Journal of Nursing Education*	Description of evolution of required human issues course employing anti-racist pedagogy	Faculty & graduate (master's)	Highlights personal & professional challenges faced by faculty of color engaged in anti-racist pedagogy in predominantly white schools of nursing. Integrates literature with own teaching experiences in graduate course to describe racism in schools of nursing & efforts to address it.

2009	Hess et al.[27]	*Multicultural Perspectives*	Description of model for integrating asset-based SL into nursing curricula to enhance cultural competence & effectiveness	Faculty, undergraduate, or graduate students	Proposes new model-Conceptual Model for Cultural Engagement (CMCE)-based on synthesis of review of literature regarding asset-based community building, SL, and cultural competence. Describes components of model, course objectives & content, pedagogical approaches, & applications. Model is in pilot phase & ready to be tested. Social justice not addressed specifically.
2008	Kelley et al.[28]	*International Journal of Nursing Education Scholarship*	Examination of how social responsibility enacted in a school of nursing	Not specified	Describes how private, religious SON incorporated social responsibility into core values, curricular design, admission standards, recruitment materials, clinical practice, & SL. Exemplars of social responsibility opportunities included. Views social justice as closely related construct of social responsibility.
2008	Lancellotti[29]	*Journal of Professional Nursing*	Examination of racism in nursing education; promotes Leininger's Culture Care Theory as curricular framework	Not specified	Addresses critiques raised about Culture Care Theory & offers contrasting view. Suggests theory has been misused & provides strategies for its application in addressing racism within nursing education. Promotes theory as way to raise awareness about social justice throughout curricula; reflection & discovery of meanings cited as specific pedagogical strategies.

(Continued)

Table 11.2 (Continued)

Publication Year	Author(s)	Journal	Type of Article-Research/Report	Level of Student	Presence of Social Justice in Article w/Key Results or Implications
2010	Pennington et al.[30]	*Journal of Nursing Education*	Describes university-community partnership clinical experience with persons who are homeless	Undergraduate BSN	Describes community health clinical experience for students attending a private, Catholic university in Denver. Project HOPE based on Jesuit pedagogy & included two nursing care sites: street outreach & homeless shelters. Personal journaling, real-time reflection, post-conferences, & classroom discussions used to process experience. Focus on meeting individual health needs of persons encountered.
2010	Schaffer et al.[31]	*Public Health Nursing*	Description of population-based competencies & examples of student projects	Undergraduate BSN	Henry Street Consortium-five BSN programs & 13 local health departments-developed Public Health Nursing (PHN) competencies & re-designed clinical experiences to be population-based. Competency #8 specific to social justice w/advocacy the associated nursing skill. Describes student project that addressed health disparities in Latino population through use of community assessment survey & interventions to increase access to health care & health education.

2010	Schroeder & Diangelo[32]	*Advances in Nursing Science*	Description of a project to change a climate of "whiteness" in a school of nursing	Targeted towards faculty, staff, & graduate students	Faculty at University of Washington describe how Whiteness is addressed through creation of a diversity project. Implemented faculty-staff workshops & developed & institutionalized an explicit, inclusive, & accountable diversity statement at the SON. Social justice addressed through creation of new online graduate antiracism course. Includes evaluation data supporting changes & reflection on lessons learned.
2008	Steffen[33]	*Creative Nursing*	Description of nursing student group presentations on the effect of stereotyping on delivery of health care	Undergraduate BSN	Describes creative group presentation developed by junior nursing students at private Lutheran college in MN. Through 30 minute exercise, addressed common stereotypes associated with class, age, immigration, & homelessness. Author concluded that students briefly "experienced" social injustices which will inform future nursing practice. Social justice not addressed specifically.

(*Continued*)

Table 11.2 (Continued)

Publication Year	Author(s)	Journal	Type of Article-Research/Report	Level of Student	Presence of Social Justice in Article w/Key Results or Implications
2008	Stys[12]	*Nursing Education Perspectives*	Offers definitions of social justice and social analysis; offers social analysis methodology	Targeted to faculty	Proposes that nurse educators gain theoretical & experiential knowledge relevant to health care injustices through intimate & sustained contact w/poor & marginalized society members. Includes social justice definitions, theories, critique, & "practical steps" for educators teaching social justice in the classroom. Social analysis identified as first step for connecting w/social justice issues & addressing existing inequities.
2008	Taylor et al.[34]	*Advances in Nursing Science*	Explains how to use racial auto-ethnography as pedagogical approach	Doctoral (PhD)	Describes how womanist feminist pedagogy applied to research elective course designed to address sociocultural perspectives in family & women's health w/focus on racism & privilege. Strategies included racial auto-ethnography & autobiography, personal journals, & seminar discussions. Includes student authors' perspectives of classroom experiences & expanding racial awareness.

Year	Author	Journal		Education Level	
2006	Vezeau[13]	*International Journal of Nursing Education Scholarship*	Discusses five professional values identified by AACN	Undergraduate BSN	Reviews role of values in nursing profession & education; links values to professional documents. Proposes several approaches for introducing values into nursing curricula; key is to introduce early w/ initial focus on students' own values. Social justice discussed as one of five AACN essential values; focus on discrimination & its effect on individual patient.
2009	Vickers[8]	*Southern Online Journal of Nursing Research*	Discusses integration of social justice issues in nursing curricula	Undergraduate BSN	Advocates for social justice as a thread throughout nursing curricula. Situates discussion within context of oppression & marginalization of nurses. Offers five discourses as guides for reframing education & integrating social justice into undergraduate curricula, w/critical pedagogy as key approach.
2009	Wilby[35]	*International Journal for Human Caring*	Offers perspectives on racial disparities in nursing & nursing education	Not specified	Critique of Whiteness within nursing education; utilizes photos to visually highlight racial disparities. Offers transcultural nursing within education as way to counter racism. Encourages research w/diverse students. Social justice not addressed specifically.

(*Continued*)

Table 11.2 (Continued)

Publication Year	Author(s)	Journal	Type of Article-Research/Report	Level of Student	Presence of Social Justice in Article w/Key Results or Implications
2008	Zauderer et al.[36]	*Journal of NY State Nurses Association (NYSNA)*	Advocates for political activism; describes a senior undergraduate capstone course	Undergraduate BSN	Describes how political engagement can lead to more just society; nurse educators can be part of process by creating political experiences for students. Students' participation in NYSNA Lobby Day as part of senior capstone project highlights this process. Includes students' comments on their experience. Social justice not addressed specifically.

Boutain[18] developed a framework that built upon the work of Holland and Henriot[37] to explicitly attend to the multiple ways social justice is conceptualized and actualized. This framework is organized according to three ascending levels: 1) awareness; 2) amelioration; and 3) transformation. According to Boutain[18] "social justice awareness entails exploring how one creates others as vulnerable or privileged."[(p26)] Awareness includes critical reflection and questioning of how systems of domination and oppression operate within society and one's role in these processes. Social justice amelioration addresses "the immediate results or antecedents to unjust conditions."[18(p26)] Although amelioration provides short-term remedies for urgent or semi-urgent concerns, it does not address the conditions responsible for unjust situations. Social justice transformation aims to eliminate or limit unjust conditions by "changing the structures that foster those unjust situations."[18(p27)] Individual actions are directed toward long-range systematic solutions.

Employing this framework, we examined a subset of the analyzed articles, targeting papers that described educational activities intended to engage students in learning about social justice. Table 11.3 presents our examination of the selected articles according to Boutain's[18] social justice framework.

Summary of Analysis Results

Our analysis of the 20 articles revealed that U.S. nurse authors writing about social justice are primarily from religious universities (8/20; 40%). This is striking; considering that social justice is a value promoted across the United States through professional, ethical, and accrediting nursing documents that guide nursing education, we expected a broader representation among publications. Religious-affiliated authors often connected their commitment to social justice to the mission and or theological underpinnings of their university. Although schools of nursing often include social justice in their mission and or vision statements, we have reservations about the authenticity of these statements. Given that there are many more secular nursing programs than religious ones in the United States, we assumed more, not fewer, secular nurse authors would be represented.

There was pedagogical consistency in how social justice was conveyed to students. A single course, usually related to culture, health equity, or disparities, was the most common approach reported. Several authors promoted social justice as a curricular thread although only Boutain[23] and Kelley and colleagues[28] described how this could be accomplished. Service learning, public health clinical, and self-reflection/personal autobiography were the most common strategies for engaging students in social justice content, with efforts primarily focused on increasing awareness of social justice issues and identifying personal biases.

In summary, social justice was constructed primarily as racism and discrimination with minimal discussion of other oppressions and injustices

Table 11.3 Subset Article Analysis

Author(s)	Awareness	Amelioration	Transformation	Injustice	Strategies
Abrums[20]	X			Race, class, gender	Single course on social/cultural issues; autobiographical reflection
Alexander[21]	X			Health equity	Single course on health equity; reflection
Belknap[22]	X			Diversity	Single course on diversity, followed by service-learning
Boutain[23]	X	X	X	Social justice	Community health clinical, reflection, curriculum integration
Groh et al.[25]		X		Social justice	Service-learning
Hassouneh[26]	X			Racism & oppression	Single course on human diversity & social issues
Hess et al.[27]	X			Cultural effectiveness	Service learning; reflection
Kelley et al.[28]	X	X		Social responsibility	Core value, curriculum integration, service learning & evaluation; reflection, direct care
Pennington et al.[30]		X		Social justice	Community health clinical; direct care for homeless population
Schaffer et al.[31]		X		Social justice	Community health clinical; health education for Latino population
Taylor et al.[34]	X			Racism & privilege	Single course; racial auto-ethnography; reflection
Zauderer et al.[36]			X	Political engagement	Single course; mandatory attendance at nurses' state lobby day

such as misogyny, homophobia, classism, or poverty. Also missing was a discussion of *how* to tackle existing injustices. Although authors often began the article with a discussion of social justice, some including a definition, the concept usually disappeared shortly thereafter, without any further explication for how their particular pedagogical approach, curricula, or experience actually addressed social justice.

DISCUSSION

Social justice rarely appears in U.S. accrediting documents or in the nursing education literature. It is striking that a basic definition of social justice is missing from the AACN DNP Essentials[16] whereas the definition provided in the Baccalaureate[14] and Master's Essentials[15] does not include gender as a category deserving "fair treatment." Considering that in the U.S. White women continue to earn only 0.79, African-American women only 0.69, and Latinas only 0.60 for every dollar earned by White men[38] and experience more violence, poverty, and income discrimination compared to men,[38–40] it is disconcerting that gender is absent from the AACN social justice definition. We are also uneasy about where social justice is addressed within the AACN Baccalaureate Essentials.[14] Positioning the most extensive, although still limited, discussion of social justice within AACN baccalaureate Essential I, ensuring a liberal education, appears to abdicate teaching of this professional value to academics outside of nursing.[14] This essential is one that nursing has minimal involvement in or control over, and placing the primary information about social justice here raises concerns for us regarding how, or even if, the professional value is taught.

When social justice appears in the U.S. nursing education literature, it is often focused on awareness, providing students with the "facts" of injustices or health disparities. If it rises to amelioration, students' energies are directed toward some type of health education. For example, students are directed to taking steps to help with immediate needs while little is done to address the broader factors that create the societal infrastructures and power dynamics of the injustices under examination. A typical amelioration approach is described by Shaffer et al.[31] in which students surveyed immigrants accessing a Latino resource center. Subsequent student activities included creating posters about the identified health needs, conducting community health assessments, and planning health education presentations.[31] Although these types of experiences may improve the health of a small group of individuals who attend the resource center and provide students with one-on-one contact, it does little to transform structural conditions in which the target population is immersed. Giving students an opportunity to work on projects that address neighborhood conditions (for example, mold in housing) would provide faculty the opportunity to more explicitly highlight the role of justice in addressing health inequities.

Some of the strongest examples of a social justice curriculum come from Canadian nurses. Browne and colleagues advocate for an explicit social justice curriculum as this "requires a philosophical commitment to a particular kind of active engagement in the exchange and translation of knowledge."[41(p175)] From their perspective, a social justice curriculum would include topics of resource allocation, health inequities, vulnerable populations, effects of globalization, and understanding relations of power.[41]

Canadian nurses also have recommended the use of non-health sector settings, such as English as a second language classes, and non-traditional community health settings, such as jails, to attain an understanding of social justice and be engaged in actions that may lead to changes in social and/or economic conditions. For example, Reimer Kirkham et al. examined the learning experiences of students in a variety of non-traditional settings and found that students were linking social justice to their practical experiences, noting that many students' "stories reflected the themes of equity and social justice in some way."[42(p4)] Students reported bearing witness to situations of injustice (*"critical awareness"*), encountering dissonance between the lives of the suffering and students' own lives (*"critical engagement"*), and then trying to set into motion some form of social change (*"social change"*). These accounts lend strength to the notion that "real" experiences are "necessary ingredient[s] of transformative learning."[42(p9)]

Abrams wondered if students should be "exposed to the realities of abject poverty, violence, hatred, or the wielding of brute political power."[43(p478)] We join Fahrenwald et al.[24] in a resounding "yes," as active engagement with social justice necessarily means facing the realities of health inequities. If students, as well as faculty, researchers, and practitioners, do not understand the world in which those who suffer live, how will they be inspired to change it?

LIMITATIONS

Because our search was specific to social justice and nursing education in the United States, we relied on the title, abstract, or key words to identify relevant articles. This approach is limited in that we may have omitted articles that incorporated social justice in the paper, such as within the context of health disparities, inequities, or ethics, yet did not include those terms as one of the searchable components. Recognizing this limitation led us to conduct the additional searches related to anti-racist pedagogy, social responsibility, and reference lists of relevant articles. Despite these efforts, the small number of articles retrieved suggests that educators writing about social justice need to explicitly identify the term in the title, abstract, or key words to increase its visibility within the nursing education literature.

Another limitation was the omission of the six articles written by nurses outside the United States. While this decision reduced the number of articles included in the review, it also limited our opportunity to highlight ongoing social justice educational efforts occurring outside the United States. Access to these efforts could remind U.S. nurse educators that social justice can be part of nursing curricula even within the confines of accreditation realities. While the increased pressure on U.S. faculty to focus on pass rates for licensure and certification examinations often work to ensure individual student success, this emphasis inadvertently ignores the broader conditions that affect the health of populations. This is an area that deserves further investigation.

RECOMMENDATIONS AND CONCLUSION

The results of this analysis suggest that Stys'[12] concerns for the future of the nursing profession may already be a reality: "Without a concentrated effort, the nursing profession risks imprisoning social justice within mission statements, departmental philosophies, and position papers."[(p367)] The minimal attention devoted to the espoused professional value of social justice by U.S. nurse educators is disconcerting considering that societal injustices clearly impact the health and wellbeing of the population.[38,43]

If nursing is serious about addressing health inequities, then social justice needs to be a core value in all accrediting documents. This means that leaders of graduate accrediting bodies should make concerted efforts to create documents that not only include, but emphasize the role social justice must play in educating future nurses. In addition, leaders of all accrediting organizations need to revise their documents to more explicitly describe activities that will assist students in understanding, ameliorating, and transforming social injustices.[18,24] Considering the power these documents have amassed in structuring nursing education and determining nursing curricular offerings, it is critical that changes begin with accreditation. For example, if the AACN Essentials were to recommend, or even suggest, the use of a theoretical framework to guide social justice teaching, such as Boutain's,[18] a shift in nursing education could ensue.

How then might nurse educators ensure that social justice moves from a professional value to one that is truly transformative? First, faculty teaching in baccalaureate and graduate nursing programs need to recognize the existence of the concept of social justice in their mission statements and accrediting documents. They must understand what is encompassed in social justice, including the attending concepts of power, oppression, and privilege. With this understanding in hand, they can then begin to develop methods for teaching about social justice and its accompanying concepts.

Second, teaching efforts need to move beyond the "awareness" level and towards amelioration and transformation. This means faculty themselves first must have knowledge of how to address injustices, including the use of intersectionality frameworks and approaches to understand how systems of privilege and oppression occur at socio-structural levels.[44] Students can then be assisted to see beyond the micro level of individual experience and begin to move towards transforming the macro-structural issues that maintain injustices.

Finally, those undergraduate and graduate faculty making concerted efforts to bring social justice to life in the classroom need to publish accounts of their efforts so that more examples are available to others, and in so doing, use "social justice" as a key term. Nursing faculty from across the globe can learn from one another on how to ensure social justice is an important element of curricula.

One cannot address health disparities if one does not understand social determinants of health; social determinants of health cannot be understood without understanding social justice. Yet understanding alone is insufficient to change the status quo. Meaningful change requires a commitment to and enactment of social justice principles; this is "not only a professional responsibility but an ethical one as well."[12(p369)] Social justice and ethics are intricately linked; social justice is a professional value that guides ethical nursing behavior.[14] It is therefore an ethical obligation, as members of the nursing profession, to attend to the social injustices that surround us, that each of us contribute to, and act to redress them. As Fahrenwald and colleagues noted, "nurse faculty members have the academic duty to plan and execute social justice education that transcends knowing and transforms by doing."[24(p194)] Individually and collectively we are obligated to move from awareness of social injustices to transformation into a more socially just society.

REFERENCES

1. Buettner-Schmidt K, Loeb ML. Social justice: a concept analysis. *J Adv Nurs* 2012;68(4): 948–958. doi:10.1111/j.1365-2648.2011.05856.x
2. Bekemeier B, Butterfield P. Unreconciled inconsistencies: a critical review of the concept of social justice in 3 national nursing documents. *Adv Nurs Sci* 2005; 28(2): 152–162.
3. Fry ST. Dilemma in community health ethics. *Nurs Outlook* 1983;31(3): 176–179.
4. White CM. A critique of the ANA Social Policy Statement: the case for elaboration of population and environment focused nursing. *Nurs Outlook* 1984;32(6): 328–331.
5. Allen DG. The Social Policy Statement: a reappraisal. *Adv Nurs Sci* 1987;10(1): 39–48.
6. Cronenwet L, Dracup K, Grey M, McCauley L, Meleis A, Salmon M. The doctor of nursing practice: a national workforce perspective. *Nurs Outlook* 2011;59: 9–17.
7. Spence DG. The curriculum revolution: can educational reform take place without a revolution in practice? *J Adv Nurs* 1994;19; 187–193.
8. Vickers DA. Social justice: a concept for undergraduate nursing curricula? *South Online J Nurs Res* 2008;8(1): 1–18.
9. American Association of Colleges of Nursing (AACN). About AACN. http://www.aacn.nche.edu. Accessed May 30, 2012.
10. Viterito A, Teich C. *Research Brief: The Nursing Shortage and the Role of Community Colleges in Nurse Education*. Washington, DC: American Association of Community Colleges; 2002.

11. National League for Nursing Accrediting Commission, Inc. *NLNAC Manual for Accreditation: Assuring Quality for the Future of Nursing Education.* Atlanta, GA: Author; 2008.

12. Stys JC. Social analysis formation for nurse educators. *Nurs Educ Perspect* 2008;29(6): 366–369.

13. Vezeau TM. Teaching professional values in a BSN program. *Internat J Nurs Educ Scholarship* 2006;3(1): 1–15.

14. American Association of Colleges of Nursing (AACN). *Essentials of Baccalaureate Education for Professional Nursing Practice.* Washington, DC: Author; 2008.

15. American Association of Colleges of Nursing (AACN). *Essentials of Master's Education in Nursing.* Washington, DC: Author; 2011.

16. American Association of Colleges of Nursing (AACN). *Essentials of Doctoral Education for Advanced Nursing Practice.* Washington, DC: Author; 2006.

17. National Task Force on Quality Nurse Practitioner Education. *Criteria for Evaluation of Nurse Practitioner Programs.* Washington, DC: National Organization of Nurse Practitioner Faculties; 2008.

18. Boutain DM. Social justice in nursing: a review of the literature. In: de Chesney M, ed. *Caring for the Vulnerable: Perspectives in Nursing Theory, Practice, and Research.* Sudbury, MA: Jones and Bartlett Publishers; 2005: 21–30.

19. Boutain DM. Social justice in nursing: a review of the literature. In: de Chesney M & Anderson B, eds. *Caring for the Vulnerable: Perspectives in Nursing Theory, Practice, and Research.* 2nd ed. Sudbury, MA: Jones and Bartlett Publishers; 2008: 39–52.

20. Abrums ME, Resnick J, Irving LL. Journey or destination? Evaluating student learning about race, class, and privilege in health care. *Nurs Educ Perspectives* 2010;31(3): 160–166.

21. Alexander KA, Dovydaitis T, Beacham B, et al. Learning health equity frameworks within a community of scholars. *J Nurs Educ* 2011;60(10): 569–574.

22. Belknap RA. Teaching social justice using a pedagogy of engagement. *Nurs Educ* 2008;33(1): 9–12.

23. Boutain DM. Social justice as a framework for undergraduate community health clinical experiences in the United States. *Intern J Nurs Educ Scholarship* 2008;5(1): 1–12.

24. Fahrenwald NL, Taylor JY, Kneipp SM, Canales MK. Academic freedom and academic duty to teach social justice: a perspective and pedagogy for public health nursing faculty. *Public Health Nurs* 2007;24(2): 190–197.

25. Groh CJ, Stallwood LG, Daniels JJ. Service-learning in nursing education: its impact on leadership and social justice. *Nurs Educ Perspects* 2011;12(6): 400–405.

26. Hassouneh D. Anti-racist pedagogy: challenges faced by faculty of color in predominanantly white schools of nursing. *J Nurs Educ* 2006;45(7): 255–262.

27. Hess DJ, Lanig H, Vaughan W. Educating for equity and social justice: a conceptual model for cultural engagement. *Multicult Perspects* 2007;9(1): 32–39.

28. Kelley MA, Connor A, Kun KE, Salmon ME. Social responsibility: conceptualization and embodiment in a school of nursing. *Internat J Nurs Educ Scholarship* 2008;5(1): 1–16.

29. Lancellotti K. Culture care theory: a framework for expanding awareness of diversity and racism in nursing education. *J Prof Nurs* 2008;24: 179–183.

30. Pennington K, Coast MJ, Kroh M. Health care for the homeless: a partnership between a city and a school of nursing. *J Nurs Educ* 2010;49(12): 700–703.

31. Schaffer MA, Cross S, Keller LO, Nelson P, Schoon PM, Henton P. The Henry Street consortium population-based competencies for educating public health nursing students. *Public Health Nurs* 2010;28(1): 78–90.

32. Schroeder C, DiAngelo R. Addressing whiteness in nursing education: the sociopolitical climate project at the University of Washington school of nursing. *Adv Nurs Sci* 2010;33(3): 244–255.

33. Steffen L. Stereotypes and social justice. *Creat Nurs* 2008;14(2): 73–74.

34. Taylor JY, Mackin MAL, Oldenburg AM. Engaging racial autoethnography as a teaching tool for womanist inquiry. *Adv Nurs Sci* 2008;31(4): 342–355.

35. Wilby ML. When the world is white. *Internat J Human Caring* 2009;13(4): 57–61.

36. Zauderer CR, Ballestas HC, Cardoza MP, Hood P, Neville SM. United we stand: preparing nursing students for political activism. *J NY State Nurses Assoc* 2008–2009;39(2): 4–7.

37. Holland J, Herriott SJP. *Social Analysis: Linking Faith and Justice*. Washington DC: Center for Concern; 1983.

38. DeNavis-Walt C, Proctor BD, Smith JC. Income, poverty, and health insurance coverage in the United States: 2011. Washington, DC: U.S. Government Printing Office, U.S. Census Bureau, Current Population Reports P60–243; 2012.

39. U.S. Bureau of Labor Statistics. *Highlights of Women's Earnings in 2009*. Report 1025. Washington, DC: Author; 2010.

40. Black MC, Basile KC, Breiding MJ, et al. *The National Intimate Partner and Sexual Violence Survey (NISVS): 2010 Summary Report*. Atlanta, GA: National Center for Injury Prevention and Control, Centers for Disease Control and Prevention; 2011.

41. Browne AJ, Varcoe C, Syme V, Reimer Kirkham S, Lynam MJ, Wong S. Cultural safety and the challenges of translating critically oriented knowledge in practice. *Nurs Philosophy* 2009;10: 167–179.

42. Reimer Kirkham SR, Van Hofwegen L, Harwood CH. Narratives of social justice: learning in innovative clinical settings. *Internat J Nurs Educ Scholarship* 2005:2(1). doi:10.2202/1548–923X.1166

43. Abrams SE. Education at the margins and beyond borders. *Public Health Nurs* 2009;26(6): 487–488.

44. Centers for Disease Control and Prevention. CDC health disparities and inequalities report-United States, 2011. *MMWR*. 2011;60(Suppl): 1–116.

45. Bowleg L. The problem with the phrase women and minorities: intersectionality-an important theoretical framework for public health. *Am J Public Health* 2012;102: 1267–1273.

12 Anti-Colonial Pedagogy and Praxis
Unraveling Dilemmas and Dichotomies

C. Susana Caxaj and Helene Berman

ANTI-COLONIAL PEDAGOGY AND PRAXIS: UNRAVELING DILEMMAS AND DICHOTOMIES

Critical, anti-colonial, and participatory research scholars often aim to build empowering spaces and to contribute to emancipatory movements.[1] For scholars who embrace these aims, project outcomes may be evaluated based on their relevance to communities, the development of meaningful relationships, and the ability to effect change.[2] Although methodological frameworks aligned with these aims exist, academic norms and institutionalized hegemonic knowledge systems may contradict or inadvertently interfere with these intentions. Within nursing, various emancipatory approaches, including critical and feminist research methodologies, have gained growing acceptance in recent years. However, graduate nursing education continues to be heavily grounded in post-positivist and interpretive paradigms. More generally, institutionalized knowledge is often based on Eurocentric readings of the world.[3] The net result is that novice nursing scholars committed to Indigenous forms of knowledge generation are left with little guidance.

The essence of critical and anti-colonial pedagogy requires that we contest, interrogate, and challenge knowledge claims and other normative structures and identities, a process that inevitably leads to some degree of discomfort, dissonance, and resistance. As cultural and social contexts shift, inequities and injustices may manifest in less familiar ways. Thus, our aim in this chapter is to reflect on the value of an anti-colonial research approach in promoting findings shaped by Indigenous knowledge systems and further, to consider the structural and contextual barriers that can limit these research intentions. Below, we will first discuss Indigenous knowledges in relation to hegemonic knowledge claims, and secondly, we will reflect on our experiences working with participants to incorporate local Indigenous knowledges into the research process. By sharing the lessons we have learned, we hope to promote further dialogue among critical and anti-colonial scholars focused on building research reciprocity, relevance, and genuine partnerships with Indigenous communities.

Knowledge Claims and Indigenous Knowledges

A shared assumption of critical and anti-colonial research methodologies is that knowledge claims are always tentative, political and contested.[4,5] From an anti-colonial perspective, the construction of neutral and/or "common-sense" knowledge is often a colonial mechanism for domination.[6] These knowledge claims may operate through the erasure of historical contexts that enable the portrayal of the colonizer as the natural inheritor of Indigenous peoples' land.[3] Through government policies, political rhetoric, and language, Indigenous peoples may be portrayed as wards of the state; beneficiaries of settlers' goodwill, while negating the inherent sovereignty of Indigenous nations and their rights to the land.[7,8] By developing culturally inappropriate programs and services that inadequately address the unique challenges and priorities of Indigenous peoples, policy makers and health professionals may articulate a systemic denial of the cultural, physical, and emotional genocide of generations of Indigenous peoples.[9,10] Thus, through a variety of ways, colonial claims to knowledge continue to impact the everyday realities of Indigenous peoples.

An anti-colonial lens emphasizes the ongoing resistance of Indigenous peoples to these hegemonic models of knowledge and champions epistemological pluralism as a means to counter colonial injustices.[11] Indigenous knowledges are typically defined as locally and experientially shaped forms of reason that guide and maintain Indigenous societies.[12] According to Castellano,[13] Indigenous knowledges encompass a diversity of ways of knowing including intuition, observations, and emotions. Often described as fluid and dynamic, these epistemologies may include circular, interconnected, and/or spiritual pathways of understanding.[14] Thus, they have the potential to interrupt hierarchical, fragmented, or static readings of truth and reality.[15]

Western institutions such as universities have been recognized both as sites of Eurocentric indoctrination and as spaces for alternative imaginings. In these settings, Indigenous knowledges are often marginalized, devalued, considered a threat to the existing system, or viewed as a "commodity to be exploited."[12(p134)] Alternatively, a growing cohort[12,14] of scholars has argued for the importance of Indigenous knowledges as a necessary counterpoint to a Western monopoly of knowledge. In essence, the standpoint of colonized peoples, albeit with diverse histories and identities, can be an invaluable resource to transform an unjust world. As a doctoral candidate (Caxaj) and research supervisor (Berman), we will share our reflections on learning through community partnerships at the intersection of academic expectations, colonial relations, and systemic inequities. Highlighting themes of holism, development, and research practice, we will discuss how local Indigenous knowledges have informed our research process.

HOLISM: INTERCONNECTED READINGS OF THE WORLD

In our research, we sought to study the impact of Canadian mining on Indigenous communities, focusing our attention on Maya Mam people of San Miguel Ixtahuacán in Guatemala. Using an anti-colonial narrative research approach, we employed a storytelling methodology compatible with assumptions of the ongoing existence of colonialism, Indigenous resistance, and aims to promote epistemological pluralism and Indigenous self-determination.[16] Yet, as researchers situated in a Canadian university, our ideas and assumptions were shaped by Western notions about knowledge—what it is, what it is not, and how it is generated. Throughout the four months we spent in the community, conversations with residents challenged and deconstructed Eurocentric dichotomies such as the secular-spiritual, technical-traditional, and the technological-sustainable. As a result, we felt a degree of dissonance throughout analysis, a fear of fragmenting and hierarchizing participants' stories that felt indivisible and complete. For instance, in conversation with participants, we were often asked to consider the indivisibility, or *holism*, of community experiences. In the words of one participant:

> The earth really is a mother. So there is a very profound relationship there and it's not so easy to disconnect. It is very difficult. So now with the mine I see it like this as well, like a cancer. They [the company] bought a little piece [of land] but then those who are beside [them] they lost all hope. In the end, those people there also had to sell and that is how they have moved along. They come with another neighbour, now that other person then also loses hope as a result of being neighbours with this person [person who sold the land]. In the end, those who remained had to sell. That is how they have progressed.

Indigenous ontologies often emphasize the interdependence of living beings and the importance of harmony for survival and well-being.[17] Similar to other Indigenous nations, the sacredness of the natural environment and the guiding principle of *mother earth* as a nurturer and giver of life[18,19] were central to these interpretations.

If an individual understands particular incidences as part of a larger relational whole, then this knowledge will inform how one understands well-being and health. In describing how the presence of local mining operations had contributed to increased alcoholism, binge drinking, and violence against women, study participant Raquel related particular experiences to a collective sense of reality:

> It's a huge mess then . . . the violence, the disintegration, the discrimination, in the end, it's everything because community life is a whole. And with one little thing, there, like a mesh, there the whole thing falls apart.

Many qualitative research methodologies with their emphasis on personal consciousness or *being* are often premised on the taken-for-granted assumption of the individual as the primary unit of analysis.[20,21] These approaches and the premises upon which they are based pose a challenge to researchers interested in understanding collective and relational readings of the world. To atomize an experience may be a form of institutionalized *untelling* as it reifies a Western hierarchy of reality construction: individualism. And, if a participant articulates their experience within a larger collective story, yet it is removed from this grand narrative, can the researcher still claim to work in *partnership with* community?

Thus, we were conscious of the need to develop a space that encourages the elicitation of collective storytelling and collective accounts of experiences, while also avoiding the pitfalls of cultural relativism, essentialism, or romanticization. In all villages, participants preferred to participate in group interviews. In a few cases, participants also accepted our offer of one-on-one interviews in order to share their particular experiences in-depth. The opportunity to share stories enables individuals to gain a sense of support, solidarity, and camaraderie as they recognize that they may face common threats and challenges.[22] Further, the collectivization of personal experiences provides opportunities for empowerment and can help communities mobilize towards resistance. As participants often did not restrict their storytelling to their particular neighborhood, interviews in other villages provided an opportunity to further enrich commonly known community stories and to exchange ideas and opinions expressed in other interviews. In this way, a community account, strengthened and enhanced by individual and familial particulars, emerged. In some cases, issues that had not been discussed in all villages became moments of realization for other villages. Sometimes, these issues, when raised, enriched the larger narrative by invoking stories of exception, difference, or distinctiveness. For instance, women might explain their increased economic precariousness in comparison to men in their village, or residents farther from the mine might discuss environmental contamination, or fear for "what is to come" by reflecting on the experiences of residents living downstream from the mine.

According to Brunanski,[20] ecological validity is the "degree to which the research is contextualized within a dynamic, holistic and interconnected Aboriginal worldview."[(p57)] Further, it serves as a criterion to evaluate the level to which culture and socio-historical context are considered throughout the research process. We strived for ecological validity by encouraging cultural positioning, reflections on historical and political events, and building spaces for diversity and collectivism. For instance, when we discussed the displacement of neighbors from their ancestral land by the mine, we asked participants how this experience was similar to, or dissimilar from, the 30-year genocide that targeted Indigenous populations in Guatemala.[23] Or, if participants discussed concerns about contamination or water depletion, we asked, "how does this relate to your culture/your spirituality?"

These issues often came up organically. We continued this process through-out analysis by sharing talking points from previous interviews and ask-ing whether participants saw them relating to a larger pattern or context and, if so, to explain more fully. These ongoing conversations informed our reading/listening of interviews through a community-informed inter-sectional lens—encompassing the spiritual, cultural, Indigenous, and rural contexts, as well as race, gender, poverty, global inequity, and immediate contexts. Through this dialogue, we worked to have community knowledge both inform the analysis and our very framework for analysis. This yielded a fair amount of participant engagement and much richer and more com-prehensive findings.

RETHINKING DEVELOPMENT: A QUESTION OF POSITION AND DEFINITION

Indigenous knowledges offer a necessary form of questioning to dominant knowledge systems enabling a logical uncertainty to hegemonic, normative, and/or passive readings of the world. Dussel,[24] for instance, writes that the knowledge of colonized peoples provides a profound critique and a basis for alternative strategies to the normalization and neutralization of unjust economic models. DeLisle[17] asserts that for some Indigenous communities, abundance may be more saliently measured in terms of biodiversity and environmental health as opposed to monetary wealth exclusively. Further, for some Indigenous communities the idea of all things having a measurable monetary value may conflict with a cosmovision (systematic view of the uni-verse) that understands the land, earth, and wildlife as sacred entities that can belong to no one.[19,25] For this reason, scholars have described global conditions of industrial expansion and consequent Indigenous opposition, as "paradigm wars"[11] as contemporary resource colonialism threatens material as well as cultural, intellectual, and spiritual survival.[18,19]

In our time spent in the community, many community participants eval-uated and deconstructed what was meant by *development* as commonly used in the mining company's propaganda. State and mainstream media often depicted residents opposed to mining as being "against development." In contrast, many residents would describe the social, environmental, and health problems that mining operations had brought to the region. "This is not development," many declared. Luz, one of the community residents and participants of the research, contrasted community priorities of sustain-able agriculture, cultural renewal, education, and capacity building with the alleged development that the mining company had offered:

> The company's development is solely infrastructure and their develop-ment, that is, buildings and buildings, and even higher buildings; that is the only thing, that's the only thing the company sees, but that is not

balanced. If there was a holistic form of development, education and other training programs would be stimulated. . . . Until now, other than academic schooling, there was also another type of training whether it be baking, carpentry, whatever, always based on the situation, and not with the idea of studying what the system imposes, that is, of capitalism, of moving up and up . . . but more so, developing oneself for the good of the community . . . well that is the development that we need as a peoples . . . in contrast, there is the ideology that the mine imposes.

Like Luz, others described the company's presence as an imposition on both their physical and cultural way of life and their own vision of development. Former workers for instance reported that when they raised concerns about co-workers/residents' health or environmental damages, they were instructed to "align with the mine" and to "focus on themselves." Many residents shared a vision of development that included protection of the natural environment, the common good, as well as cultural and spiritual continuity. Living in close proximity to mining operations they had witnessed threats to their economic systems, cultural and spiritual beliefs, traditions, and relationship to the land. Participants were acutely aware of the widespread poverty and limited access to education and agricultural support, yet they rejected the idea that mining could somehow resolve this issue. They saw it as a false solution based on exploitative and inaccurate depictions of their community, motivated solely by the company's expectations of financial gain.

As scholars working to build community-relevant initiatives in partnership with local residents, we must also navigate and confront the juncture of institutionalized assumptions and distinct or counter-hegemonic community priorities. We were aware that our academic positioning also threatened to impose values and/or misrepresent or exploit community challenges in much the same way the company had. In the words of one spiritual leader:

> They [the company] do not collaborate, they only give handouts but it's a problem that the people do not see it as a handout. And that offends the spirituality, its like a crime, it's very grave because they take advantage, they exploit the goodness of the people who are grateful for what ever thing they are given. And with those things they manipulate the situation to say: look, the people support the mine. That is awful.

For a community experiencing widespread poverty such that it limits their access to opportunities and services, this very condition may introduce a coercive element to a community's willingness to engage in a research project. Further, within the context of poverty and minimal state support in developing health and social services, researchers and professionals may feel entitled to carry out "their" projects without being accountable to the community in question. As an institutionalized practice, our research, similar to mining operations, can represent a Western articulation of privilege, development, and unequal benefit.

To further illustrate, in order to enter the community, residents and neighbors reported that mining company employees had provided false information and threatened, intimidated, and taken advantage of local landowners. In our own work, when presenting potential participants with *written* letters of information and consent forms, we were forced to see the symbolic similarities with our own consent process and the process that some residents had experienced when they had sold their land to the company. These encounters had been shaped by low literacy levels and limited formal education of many of the residents in the community. As Canadian citizens studying a Canadian mining company abroad, our privilege was foregrounded in these interactions. The written forms served as a reminder of this power misbalance; of our education, mobility across borders, and our presence as an institutional imposition. Further, many participants expressed their disappointment with previous projects that, in their view, had simply extracted their stories and left little of benefit for them.

We navigated this context with variable results. We sought to include different community-based organizations and community leaders in all phases of the research project. Before arrival in the community, through conversation with community leaders we shared a blueprint of a research proposal that we were able to further develop collaboratively once in the community. We solicited consent in an ongoing manner, through written and oral formats, at both the village level and the individual level, and we incorporated planning of how the research would be used in these first conversations. At both the village and municipality level, we reported our preliminary impressions of the research findings in order to both include participants in the co-construction of research findings and collaboratively engage in a research dissemination plan that would resonate with them. Throughout the four months we spent in the community, we strived to be honest and authentic about our privilege, our intentions, and the limitations of our work. In this way, we aimed to avoid making exaggerated/false claims or benefiting from social disadvantages by which exploitative projects claim to bring "development." Although systemic disadvantages could not be mediated, through ongoing consent processes and built-in spaces for collective decision making in regards to the research process and priorities, we strived to build an organic and trusting partnership. Ultimately, the hope is that researchers can build on and learn from community-initiated momentum. In the words of Elena:

> We eat because of our own efforts, because we are working here with our neighbor; among ourselves, we help ourselves, it has nothing to do with the company [Goldcorp] . . . we have joined our neighbors to defend their rights, our rights, and the rights of our children.

RESEARCH PRACTICE: TRANSPARENCY, PARTNERSHIPS, AND ACTION

Genuine community-academic research partnerships require not only a negotiation of different phases of research activities and techniques, but also a commitment to collaboratively reimagine research priorities, purpose(s), and even what counts as research. Shifting towards this mode of research practice entails working towards identifying and transparently addressing different ways of seeing and building a space for genuine diversity. The hope is that this process can transition the research project towards action that is both meaningful and relevant to the community.

In striving for authenticity, we sought to be clear about our personal interest in this project, our intentions, our background, as well as our political assumptions and viewpoints. The field investigator, Caxaj, the sole member of the research team residing in the community, described herself to participants as a doctoral candidate; Guatemalan-born daughter of refugees, *Mestiza*—of Quiche, Kachiquel Mayan, and European ancestry; English and Spanish speaker; and Canadian-educated registered nurse with Canadian citizenship. More important than listing these labels and identifiers were how these different identities were enacted in practice and how we collectively worked to build understanding of our differences and commonalities in these research spaces given our particular backgrounds and contexts. For Caxaj, this entailed an ongoing dialogue about privilege and oppression. This equally involved recognizing and acknowledging privileged differences such as ease of entry across borders in comparison to participants as well as shared (yet different) oppression, for instance, as persons threatened and displaced by the Guatemalan state and allied corporate interests. In reflecting on this dynamic and relational practice, it has been difficult to observe the continued emphasis in critical research on the ritualistic listing of social positions, which can have the tendency to read more as a penance than a starting place for action and reflexive practice. More so, as people with mixed, contradictory, or Mestiza backgrounds, this compartmentalization of one's identity can silence the subaltern perspectives imbedded within these listings of privilege. More nuanced thinking, and a sense of identity, as an action, strategy, and mode of resistance is important to continued political work in research areas such as ours.

Throughout the research process, acknowledging our different vantage points and our different vision for the project was important. In one village, an interview focused on health and the environment culminated in a final question directed at the investigator. Serafina asked:

So now that you are here with us, what support can you give us?

A version of this question was asked fairly frequently, often early in the process. Implied in this question was an expectation that the research team should have a sense of what could be done in the service of the community even before data collection. As outside researchers, we had strived to keep our proposal flexible and open so that the process could be as participatory and as fluid as possible. On the other hand, community members wanted to know what we were all about, perhaps fearing that a vague attempt at a democratic process could result in either a waste of time or resources, or worse, a hidden agenda. As a result, early in the research process we began not only to reflect with participants as to how the research project could develop and evolve but also to consistently bring new proposals to participants. This two-pronged planning process allowed residents to get a sense of our commitment level, the level of confidence we had in our skills and an assurance that their participation in this research project would not be in vain.

Following the data collection phase, approximately 100 people from the community, mostly participants, along with their friends and family, gathered to reach a consensus as to how we would develop research findings into a tangible resource for the community. By popular vote, the community decided to carry out The Peoples International Health Tribunal.[26] Guiding this decision was a consensus in the need for more (1) local participation and community-level awareness building, (2) outreach and education to the international community, and (3) justice, more particularly, the need to end Goldcorp's corporate impunity. Through community testimonies, participants had the rare opportunity to address an international audience via Internet streaming, engagement with an international group of experts participating as tribunal "judges," and live documentation. In this way, research findings were able to move beyond description and distress and become a platform for demands, a cry for justice, and a moral condemnation. In Ricardo's words:

> We just want to tell the company to leave us alone. [We want them] to go home, to go back to their country, that god may forgive them. But before that, they need to pay for the damages [i.e., to health, environment, community]. We need to continue this struggle, because the struggle is to defend life and defend our territories. They will be judged one day. At the end of time, they will be judged.

The tribunal also provided a venue for sharing and exchange among other communities in Guatemala affected by mining and other communities in Mesoamerica affected by Goldcorp operations. This provided a genuine forum for support, solidarity, and movement building. Throughout the two days of testimonies, a rejuvenating sense of energy and support could be felt among the room of 600 attendees. To end the tribunal, the international panel of judges, a combination of scientists, physicians, academics, and human rights specialists delivered the verdict, finding Goldcorp guilty of damaging, the health, quality of life, the environment, and the right to self-determination of Indigenous and campesino communities in Mesoamerica.[26]

FROM ACADEMIA TO ACTION AND BACK:
BLURRING THE BOUNDARIES

Although the tribunal represented a significant milestone in the conduct of this research, and was considered a success from the perspective of community members and allied communities and organizations, important questions arise. Most germane to this discussion is the relevance and appropriateness of this type of activism in critical and anti-colonial scholarship. Throughout the past decade, doctoral nursing programs have accorded increasing attention to various emancipatory research approaches, including methodologies that include at least some form and degree of participation and action. Typically, the emphasis is on the establishment of honest and authentic community partnerships and the challenges that are commonly encountered as a result of differences in power and privilege. To engage meaningfully in the field in a manner that can foster long-term social and political change requires time and resources, both of which are often in limited supply to doctoral students. How to engage in research-based activism within the context of a doctoral dissertation is a complex issue due to time constraints, financial constraints, inherent inequalities, and the question of data ownership, manuscript authorship, and so forth. In the case of this project, we were lucky to receive a grant from the Fund for Global Human Rights and Caxaj also had financial security, in part, by winning a three-year doctoral research award, the Canadian Vanier Graduate Scholarship. If one criterion for critical work is the capacity of the project to contribute to change however, can we really make claims to critical scholarship in the absence of social action and reciprocity?

Ultimately, we ask the question: does a project like the People's International Health Tribunal have a place as an academic requirement for a dissertation with emancipatory aims, for example? Is it demanded, in some sense, as evidence of the "critical" or "anti-colonial-ness" of one's work? Or is it made invisible, as an off-branch of research or an academic form of volunteerism? The tribunal was carried out through community consensus, planning, and collaboration, but most importantly, because it was identified as a community priority. In meeting academic expectations, particularly within the constraints of a nursing dissertation, it is important to acknowledge that there is an aspect of one's research that may not seem relevant to community members. This requires us to problematize conventional ways of thinking of collaborative research in order to develop research that fosters a true spirit of reciprocity. For instance, manuscript authorship may not be as important to participants as having a report of health findings that can be used in legal cases or other forms of community planning. It is important that we continue to articulate what we mean by "effect change" such that our research remains true to the ideological underpinnings we espouse and does not fall short of our participants' expectations. There is also a need to consider how we sustain researchers' commitment to this long-term vision when this type of work is generally not valued in academic settings nor funded by major agencies and organizations that provide funding for nursing research. Further, in revisiting how we as critical, anticolonial, or emancipatory scholars wish to define research itself we may enable the use of more diverse strategies to ensure research meaningfulness and relevance.

CONCLUSION AND IMPLICATIONS FOR NURSING SCHOLARSHIP

In partnerships with communities, academic researchers need to continue to develop new strategies to incorporate the unique vision and expertise of community participants. This must include collaborative efforts to incorporate "big picture" research issues in the process by re-evaluating research priorities, research objectives, what/how knowledge is valued, and how to co-construct findings in an authentic and participatory manner. In working with Indigenous communities affected by mega-projects or facing other environmental health challenges, issues of holism, development, and research-practice-as-action may be important sites of contestation requiring ongoing iterations to ensure a meaningful and democratic process. Through our experience with a Mayan Mam Indigenous community in Guatemala, we have attempted to illustrate the structural inequities and contextual barriers that limit and shape investigator's emancipatory intentions. Further, we have shared our reflections and lessons learned in attempting to maintain a commitment to an anti-colonial nursing mandate.

Continuing to expand the criteria by which we evaluate critical research traditions and other politicized approaches to research may help us maintain a high level of commitment to action with the communities that we work with. An anti-colonial approach in particular can provide a guiding framework for researchers working with Indigenous communities to incorporate the unique worldviews and knowledge systems of participants that can continue to strengthen and enrich nurses' relevance and responsiveness to diverse clients. It is important for us to continue these discussions with our students and colleagues not only to make visible these issues but further, to develop a preparedness and sense of support for students engaging in this emotional and political work. Ultimately, we need to reflect on how to develop our networks, institutions, research spaces, and mind-sets such that our research partnerships enable us to contribute to necessary social change, both for immediate and long-term impact.

REFERENCES

1. Castleden H, Garvin T, Huu-ay-aht First Nation. Modifying photovoice for community-based participatory Indigenous research. *Social Science & Medicine* 2008;66: 1393–1405.
2. Nicholls R. Research and Indigenous participation: critical reflexive methods. *International Journal of Social Research Methodology* 2009;12: 117–126.

3. Tuhiwai-Smith LH. *Decolonizing Methodologies: Research and Indigenous Peoples.* London, UK: Zed Books; 1999.
4. Kovach M. *Indigenous Methodologies—Characteristics, Conversations, and Contexts.* Toronto, ON, Canada: University of Toronto Press; 2009.
5. Perron A, Rudge T, Blais A, Holmes D. The politics of nursing knowledge and education: critical pedagogy in the face of the militarization of nursing in the war on terror. *Advances in Nursing Science* 2010;33(3): 184–195.
6. Lawrence B. Rewriting histories of the land: colonization and indigenous resistance in Eastern Canada. In: Razack S, ed. *Race, Space, and the Law.* Toronto, ON, Canada: Between the Lines; 2002: 21–46.
7. Endres D. The rhetoric of nuclear colonialism: rhetorical exclusion of American Indian arguments in the Yucca Mountain nuclear waste siting decision. *Communication and Critical/Cultural Studies* 2009;6(1): 39–60.
8. Sherman P. *Dishonour of the Crown: The Ontario Resource Regime in the Valley of the Kiji Sibi.* Winnipeg, Manitoba, Canada: Arbeiter Ring Publishing; 2009.
9. Chrisjohn RD, Wasacase T, Nussey L, Smith A, Legault M., Loiselle P. Genocide and Indian residential schooling: the past is present. In: Wiggers RD, Griffiths AL eds. *Canada and International Humanitarian Law: Peacekeeping and War Crimes in the Modern Era.* Halifax, Nova Scotia: Dalhousie University Press; 2002. http://www.nt.net/savard/pastispresent.pdf. Accessed April 3, 2014.
10. Haig-Brown C. Resistance and renewal: first nations and aboriginal education. In: Das Gupta T, ed. *Canada. In Race and Racialization.* Toronto, ON, Canada: Canadian Scholars Press; 2007: 165–191.
11. Mander J, Tauli-Corpuz V, eds. *Paradigm Wars: Indigenous Peoples' Resistance to Globalization.* San Francisco, CA: Sierra Club Books; 2006.
12. Steinberg SR, Kincheloe JL. Indigenous knowledges in education: complexities, dangers and profound benefits. In: Denzin, NK, Lincoln, YS, eds. *The SAGE Handbook of Qualitative Research.* Thousand Oaks, CA: Sage; 2008: 135–156.
13. Castellano MB. Updating aboriginal traditions of knowledge. In: Sefa GJ, Hall BD, Rosenberg G, eds. *Indigenous Knowledge's in Global Contexts.* Toronto, ON, Canada: University of Toronto Press; 2000: 21–36.
14. Bishop R. Freeing ourselves from neocolonial domination in research: a kaupapa Maori approach to creating knowledge. In Denzin, NK, Lincoln YS, eds. *The SAGE Handbook of Qualitative Research.* Thousand Oaks, CA: Sage; 2005: 109–138.
15. Shiva V. Foreword: cultural diversity and the politics of knowledge. In: Dei GJ, Hall BL, Roseberg DG, eds. *Indigenous Knowledges in Global Contexts: Multiple Readings of Our World.* Toronto, ON, Canada: University of Toronto Press; 2008: v–x.
16. Caxaj CS, Berman H, Varcoe C, Ray SL, Restoule JP. Tensions in anti-colonial research: lessons learned by collaborating with a mining-affected community. *Canadian Journal of Nursing Research* 2012;44(4): 76–95.
17. DeLisle S. A layered homeland: history, culture and visions of development. *Policy Matters* 2004;13: 212–223.
18. Gedicks A. Resource wars against native peoples in Columbia. *Capitalism Nature Socialism* 2010;14: 85–111.
19. LaDuke W. *Recovering the Sacred: the Power of Naming and Claiming.* Cambridge, MA: South End Press; 2005.
20. Brunanski DM. Counselling with Aboriginal street youth: an aboriginalizing narrative inquiry. Unpublished master's of arts dissertation. University of British Columbia, Vancouver, Canada; 2009.
21. Tilly C. (1998). *Durable Inequality.* Los Angeles, CA: University of California Press; 1998.

22. Webber-Pillwax C. Indigenous researchers and indigenous research methods. *Pimatisiwin: A Journal of Aboriginal and Indigenous Community Health* 2004;2(1).
23. Guatemalan Commission for Historical Clarification (CEH). Guatemala: memory of silence. Conclusions and recommendations of the report of the commission for historical clarification. American Association for the Advancement of Science, Science and Human Rights Program Web site. 1999. http://shr.aaas.org/guatemala/ceh/%20in%20English%20and%20Spanish. Accessed February 24, 2013.
24. Dussel E. *Hacia una filosofía crítica*. Bilbao, Spain: Desclée de Brouwer; 2001.
25. Munarriz GJ. Rhetoric and reality: the World Bank development policies, mining corporations, and Indigenous communities in Latin America. *International Community Law Review* 2008;10: 431–443.
26. Peoples International Health Tribunal. Verdict. 2012. http://healthtribunal.org/the-final-verdict/. Accessed April 1, 2013.

13 "And That's Going to Help Black Women How?"

Storytelling and Striving to Stay True to the Task of Liberation in the Academy

JoAnne Banks

> How we make our experience into story determines how we live our personal lives. . . . What we emphasize and retell in our collective story determines whether we quarrel or collaborate in our community. . . . What we preserve in larger human story determines what we believe is possible in the world.[1(ppx–xi)]

I never questioned if I should or could use academe as the context for working towards the survival of Black women. My question was how? I concluded long ago that I could take to the streets with a gun and attempt to kill those who insisted on my people living as the dregs of society, or I could become an academic and try to figure out some other options. Given my disdain for guns, and the prospect of not being able to hug a tree or play in the ocean waves whenever I wanted to do so, I concluded that academe was the better option. I recalled the excitement I felt as I waited to hear a speaker who was the first person I had ever met who was both a nurse scholar and an African-American woman. I also vividly recall the visceral level of rage I felt later after a private conversation with this same scholar in which she cautioned me not to pigeonhole myself by focusing my research on Black women. To me it was so clear: the only reason to be in *The Academy* or to pursue life as a nurse scholar was the possibility that I could do something towards the cause of keeping Black women alive.

This is a deeply personal essay. In it, I pause and evaluate where and how I had been true to my goal of using scholarship as a vehicle for promoting the liberation and well-being of Black women. Liberation is the linchpin in the struggle for social justice and health equity. Social justice requires exposing, clarifying, and eliminating societal differences that oppress some groups of people while privileging other groups.[2] Health equity is concerned with promoting social justice in the health arena.[3] Some of that justice begins with nurses and, in keeping with the purposes of this anthology, emancipatory nursing and the idea of praxis. To me this means the development and use of strategies that enhance understanding of the interlocking factors that promote or constrain the health within specific population groups. It also means paying particular attention to the ways in which my own experiences foster or inhibit my ability to effectively work with individuals and groups in an emancipatory fashion. Finally, it means being willing to stand in the crossroads, serving sometimes as a bridge and other times as a barricade between the Black women I love so dearly and academe. Two assumptions undergird the development of this essay. I assume that no individual, group, or living entity can be well in isolation. I also view movement towards health, liberation, and social justice as continuous processes with no end point, no arrival at a final destination. We are always moving towards higher levels of health, deeper levels of liberation, and more expansive views of social justice.

My published and unpublished papers served as data sources. I read each document and wrote notes about what I considered to be the most important ideas. I also recorded my thoughts about the linkages between the themes explored in these papers and my concept of liberation, which draws heavily on the work of Carlyle F. Stewart, III.[4] Stewart posits that African-American liberation is rooted in an understanding that spirituality is the core attribute of *humanness* and that freedom is spiritually and culturally determined, not dependent on social, political, or material reality. A major assumption of this perspective is that people exist as part of and in relation to the Creator and the whole of creation. *Liberation* is a progressive transformation from conditions that bind, subjugate, or constrain the freedom of individuals or groups. Emancipatory knowledge is also significant to liberation. Chinn and Kramer[5] have defined emancipatory knowledge as an outgrowth of critical analysis of the status quo and envisioning of changes integral to creating just and equitable conditions that support all humans in achieving their full potential.

Womanist theory[6] has served as the cornerstone for my academic career and provided a framework for advancing social justice and health equity through teaching and scholarship. In womanist theory, the lived experiences of African-American women are the starting point for addressing philosophical problems related to knowledge and truth.[7] Experience, consciousness, and action are defining features of womanist theory,[8] and their interdependence allows for new ways of thinking to be accompanied by new ways of acting and different experiences to be a catalyst for changed consciousness.

My reflections have kept bringing me back to storytelling as the taproot of my career as a teacher and scholar. Storytelling plays a pivotal role in promoting social justice and liberation. It is the meaning we give to events, not the facts, that guide our actions.[1,9] Storytelling illuminates injustices and promotes the development of creative solutions for correcting them.[5] This essay explores *the ways in which storytelling has undergirded my liberation efforts in the academic setting*. Although my career in academe has focused on the well-being of Black women, I have employed storytelling to promote the growth and development of students and colleagues more broadly. Below I discuss storytelling in the contexts of research and teaching. I also discuss challenges arising from my commitment to using storytelling as a liberation strategy in the context of an academic career. Personal stories culled from my journey illuminate the ideas presented in this essay. This essay concludes with a short discussion of future directions for my work. Demonstrating the value of storytelling as a culturally consistent and relevant data collection method and intervention strategy is arguably my most important contribution to promoting the liberation and well-being of Black women.

STORYTELLING IN THE RESEARCH CONTEXT

My scholarly path came into focus during the second or third quarter of my first year as a doctoral student. "Each of you has to develop a nursing therapeutic for your final paper," the instructor announced. As she went on to discuss the particulars of the paper, I found myself engulfed in a daydream or more accurately, a vision. I was back in Flint, Michigan, sitting in the library of my elementary school. It was story time and I was overwhelmed by a feeling of complete joy and peace.[10] This vision started me on a quest that continues to this day.

As a scholar, I have been particularly interested in storytelling as a tool for broadening researchers' and clinicians' understanding of the complex and nuanced lives of Black women, while exposing the diversity within and across populations of Black women. I have also explored the ways in which storytelling can be used to empower study participants by goal clarification, examination of the ways in which interpersonal and environmental factors intersect to influence health beliefs and practices, and development of alternative strategies for dealing with pressing issues.[10–12]

My view of storytelling as both a vehicle for understanding women's lives and a health promotion strategy is an outgrowth of stories collected during focus groups with Black women. Stories and storytelling reflect the language, mores, customs, and daily experiences of the people doing the telling. Collecting stories in a group setting facilitates the use of African/American storytelling as a tool for maintaining linkages between the historical past and present.[13] Group story gathering also nurtures a sense of community, fosters a unique cultural identity, and provides a foundation for spiritual and material freedom.[4,14]

Storytelling as a Tool for Self-Discovery

In the research context, storytelling is a powerful tool for prompting self-discovery. I have found the use of professional storytellers and the sharing of personal stories especially helpful strategies for gathering data while also providing women with information to enhance their lives.[10,12] As a result of political and structural realities in the United States, many Black women are not being exposed to folklore, myths, legends, familial, and communal stories that would provide them a more nuanced understanding of inter-personal and social determinants of health. In my work, professional story-tellers have shared stories that helped women see the connections between their personal story and the larger group story of Black people throughout the African diaspora. Study participants also developed and shared personal stories of the experience of living with or managing chronic health issues like hypertension. Women's stories revealed factors that promote or con-strain behavior change, as well as emotional responses to daily life.[6] I have found that emphasizing the creation of stories that move experiences to the foreground and limit discussion of job titles or roles serves to decrease development of social-economic hierarchies within group sessions.[15] I have developed an exercise that assisted women in developing and sharing stories in the context of a research study (Table 13.1). The process helps women to identify the key points they want to convey and to refine their story so that these points are highlighted and distracting information eliminated.

The narrative process used to analyze stories collected in this matter is rooted in African/American oral traditions.[16] It is consistent with womanist frameworks, which stress the role of experience, dialogue, and caring as foundations for assessing knowledge claims and developing meaning.[6] Anal-ysis includes evaluation of the ways in which storytelling is influenced by the historical context and environment in which stories are shared. The narra-tive process also explores how stories function within group process, with emphasis on trying to understand why a given story is shared at a particular

Table 13.1 Storytelling Exercise

1. Spend 5 minutes free-writing on a particular event, episode, or experience related to topic of the day that has left a lasting impression on you.
2. Decide what you think is the major lesson that your learned, most important outgrowth, or most significant change in your life that occurred in relation to this event or experience.
3. Write one sentence describing the purpose/point you hope to serve by sharing this story with the larger group gathered here today.
4. Pick and choose from the many things you recall about this event to develop a 3–5 minute story (can be a 1–2 minute story depending on time available) about this experience that best illustrates or illuminates the purpose you have in sharing the story. Write the story down on 3×5 cards (Each side of a 3×5 card = about 1 minute of conversation).
5. Review your story. Make minor revisions in it so that it better reflects the point you want to get across.
6. Tell your story to one person without looking at your note cards.
7. Reflect for a few minutes on your story and refine it to more closely reflect your primary purpose in sharing it.
8. Share story with the larger group without looking at your note cards.

time. Stories serve different purposes at different times. Uncovering why a story is told at a given point provides critical information about what is most important, "what matters," to participants at that moment.[17(p220)] The final step of the process entails attention to what things were not said that one would expect to be part of the discussion. These silences provide information about taken-for-granted knowledge in a given culture, the impact of the storytelling milieu, and the power dynamics of the larger society.[16,18,19] Some silences reflect the ways in which groups consciously or unconsciously collaborate to leave out or avoid discussing inconsistencies that would disrupt or cast doubt on the accepted communal story.[1] Breaking silences in our story about who we are as people, including silences about violence against women and girls,[20] or the continued sacrifice of women's rights at the altar of antiracist struggle,[21] is critical to development of a communal story that supports the well-being of all Black people. Development of analytic methods consistent with Black women's storytelling traditions is integral to fully comprehending the ways in which culture, values, historical contexts, and lived experiences influence women's decision making. Structuring experiences into stories packages critical information in a way that makes it infinitely more accessible to women and researchers than most other sources of information.

Storytelling as an Agent for Liberation

Storytelling also serves as an agent for liberation through its capacity to educate, inspire, promote creativity, challenge, depict gaps in logic, expose power dynamics, suggest alternative strategies, provide historical perspective, illuminate connections to the larger community, and facilitate the safe release of emotions. Ama Saran, a fellow student at the University of Washington, collaborated with me on the focus group study that later served as the basis for my dissertation. Her opening comments during the first of a series of four focus groups indicated that her understanding of group storytelling as an agent for change was much more developed than mine at the time.

> Much of the purpose of this is to see what happens when we come together. And as Black women, we know just being in the room together has its own benefits. You know very much like going to church; there *The Spirit* is. . . . We understand some things don't happen right away, and when we take a look at the process itself as intervention we're also looking at what are the ways we interrupt things and make them happen better cause [we] decided to gather together. . . . So part of the whole process of intervention is picking the things that can be enhanced in your life while you are being part of the gathering of Black women. And, a lot of times that happens informally. We are simply formalizing the way we capture what happens. So that too will be recorded. You know cause there are lots of things that you are working on. Things in

your secret heart that you haven't spoken of before and there may be people in here who can help you accomplish them.[22(p129)]

Each woman who participated in the aforementioned focus groups was given a copy of my dissertation. In subsequent studies, I have made an effort to provide participants copies of transcripts from focus groups and individual interviews. This not only gives participants an opportunity to review transcripts for errors but also allows them to garner wisdom from stories long after a particular study is completed.

Storytelling as an Instrument for Promoting Well-Being

Storytelling's potency as an instrument for promoting the individual and collective well-being of Black women is illustrated in the following quotes that were derived from my published studies. The significance of ancestral connections and historical stories is especially apparent. Remarks in parentheses in the third and fourth quotes reflect responses of women listening to the story. This call and response is a feature of Black storytelling traditions.[23,24]

> I attended the meeting where I met a large circle of African American women who shared stories about themselves. The energy in that room was awesome. . . . I knew within this group of women I would have support and this wiped out many of my fears about going to school and doing it alone.[11(p19)]
>
> Last week I questioned how storytelling would aid in lowering my blood pressure. This week, I found myself looking forward to and being excited to come and hear stories from our culture. . . . These sessions have opened my eyes to the beauty and richness that storytelling, especially oral storytelling, brings to our culture and everyday outlook on life. I am encouraged to study African-American storytelling more closely.[10(p29)]
>
> And see there's a tradition and I'm a firm believer. People think I'm crazy but I think that our mothers and our grandmothers can love us beyond the grave (Oh yeah. I believe that). I know my mother yet loves me. (I believe that too).[25(p31)]
>
> Oh, I appreciate this very much. I've learned quite a bit. I love to hear all of you talk. I got a whole lot out of it. I think about us being together. We can be some support to each other (yes) because we do need support. . . . But anyway this is great that we can get together and laugh at simple things, you know (it sure is). Because if we don't have a little humor in life, where would we be (that's right).[26(p29)]
>
> Ya know when this sista would do the story it would make you reflect back in your own childhood and the elders always carried the younger group along. And so, for me it's been great because it's lie across the board from 8 to 80 so to speak. And those stories helped me reflect

back. . . . And so we have learned from one another and it has been a real blessing for me.[12(p172)]

TEACHING THROUGH STORYTELLING

Storytelling is an important tool for facilitating the development of both students and faculty. Four years ago, I joined the faculty at Winston-Salem State University, a historically Black university. Prior to this, my opportunities to work directly with Black women as either students or faculty were minimal. I had no Black colleagues and fewer than 15 Black students during the 20 years I taught in predominant White college settings. This discussion about storytelling as a teaching strategy draws mainly on my experiences in these settings. The use of storytelling in overwhelmingly White settings allowed me to further my agenda of promoting the well-being of Black women by expanding the awareness of students and colleagues. Storytelling enhanced learning about people and perspectives that stood outside of students' and faculty colleagues' experiences and expanded the frameworks they could be used to think about health and the role of nursing in promoting health. As Baldwin noted,

> Those who would control the ear in the heart understand that if people truly discover each other, we will make a million circles and sit down and laugh and cry at our commonalities. And then we will not be so easily led to fight wars. We will not so unconsciously exploit other people's lives in order to make our own lives more comfortable. We will not be confused by the manipulation of half-truths and lies.[1(p33)]

Building Faculty-Student Connections

Early in my career at the University of Missouri, the importance of using story as a means of building connections between my students and me became apparent. I struggled desperately to connect with the students enrolled in my Community Health clinical. Finally, I sought out the assistance of Beth Geden, a senior faculty member in the School of Nursing. Dr. Geden suggested that I ask students to share stories about their first experiences with an elevator or escalator. I was extremely skeptical of this advice but thought, "What the hell, it cannot be worse than anything I have tried so far." During the next clinical preconference, I asked students to share their stories. I was amazed by their responses. It turned out that 8 of the 10 students in my clinical section had had their first experience on an elevator or escalator within the last three years as a result of moving to Columbia to attend the University of Missouri. As I listened, the gulf between their experiences and mine became clearer. I was a *dyed in the wool big city girl*, having been born in Flint, Michigan, and raised in a housing project in Chicago. In contrast, the majority of my students were from small, rural towns. They saw Columbia, Missouri, as the big city while I viewed it as a hick town. Bridging the gap between our perspectives was imperative to the creation of a safe learning/teaching environment. In future semesters, I reminded myself to stop and take time to elicit life stories from students as a central component of developing action plans to address course-related challenges.

I have used storytelling in the classroom, co-authoring papers with students, and attending research conferences with students to broaden students' perspectives. Students enrolled in an undergraduate/graduate Women's Studies course critically analyzed stories, poetry, and movies alongside, research studies, memoirs, and documentaries to better understand the social and interpersonal factors that shape women's health and well-being. Undergraduate Community Health students critiqued differences between the perspectives presented in *The Three Little Pigs* folktale and *The True Story of the 3 Little Pigs!*[27] This exercise helped them to better understand how unnamed assumptions and stereotypes can influence interactions with particular groups. Doctoral students enrolled in a Conceptual Structure of Nursing class selected one nursing and one non-nursing theory to serve as the foundation for developing strategies to address critical issues presented in Baida's collection of short stories.[28] This assignment deepened students' understanding and appreciation of how aesthetic knowledge can inform decision making. It also promoted critical thinking about the strengths and limitations of selected theories with respect to developing strategies to address identified problems in a particular context. In addition, I have used creative nonfiction by Jordan,[29] Farmer,[30] Fullilove,[31] and Perkins[32] to expose students to the stories of scholars outside the discipline of nursing who were particularly concerned about promoting social justice. The writings of these authors pushed students to consider the possibilities and implications of using a social justice framework to undergird one's actions as nurse.[33]

Three years ago, I began to use *The Danger of a Single Story* in my research classes at Winston-Salem State University (WSSU). In this video, storyteller and fiction writer Chimamanda Adichie[34] uses personal stories from her life to illustrate problems that arise when we make decisions about how to respond to people based on a single story. The video is followed by a free-write and discussion of implications for conducting and critiquing research. Nursing students at WSSU are the most diverse group on campus. Blacks from the United States along with those from various Caribbean and African countries comprise roughly 60% of the population. Approximately 38% of the students are White Americans, many from lower income backgrounds, and a few are immigrants from Eastern Europe. The remaining students are Asian-Americans or Latino-Americans. Most students work and many have children. This activity has been very effective in getting students to think more critically about the narratives they use to evaluate other groups of people, as well as the unspoken stories that frame their understanding of themselves. Clarity about the narratives that guide one's interactions with individuals and groups is integral to emancipatory clinical and scholarly practice.

Developing Voice and Community

Development of one's voice as a scholar and community building are two of the most important outcomes of storytelling with students in relation to developing papers for publication. Storytelling has been integral to my work in developing students' understanding of themselves as scholars. Women and students from groups who are underrepresented in academia frequently learn that remaining voiceless is a good strategy for decreasing tension and possible assault.[35] Development of papers for publication is a very scary thought for many of them. I have found that tape recording small group conversations, supplemented by one-on-one phone conversations and free writing about topics where there are strong differences of opinion, are an effective means of facilitating this process.[33] I have also found that sharing personal stories about the joys and struggles of becoming a scholar was crucial in creating a supportive environment for Black scholars affiliated with a predominant White institution.[36] Using telephone, Internet, and social media sources to create storytelling circles may become increasingly more important avenues for collaborating on publications and creating supportive communities for future generations of scholars. Vallar, a part-time graduate student noted,

> It is extremely difficult to get the academic assistance I need, let alone interact with other doctoral students because most campus services and program activities are limited to daytime hours. Furthermore, many community members interested in research have daytime jobs that prohibit them from attending programs or support sessions during this time.[36(p339)]

Opportunities to build collegial relationships with fellow students and faculty are also limited for students enrolled in nursing doctoral programs. Many work full time while attending school part time. Sharing stories in conjunction with developing a jointly authored manuscript can provide the context for students at different levels in the program to develop relationships with each other while advancing new knowledge about doctoral education.[33]

CHALLENGES TO USING STORYTELLING AS A TOOL FOR LIBERATION IN ACADEMIA

There are many challenges to devoting one's life to using storytelling as a strategy for promoting the liberation of Black women in academic settings. Self-liberation is a prerequisite for assisting others to become liberated. Other challenges include meeting tenure and promotion requirements, while simultaneously attending to personal and familial priorities. Before addressing these challenges, it is important to say something about the continued stranglehold of ideologies rooted in narratives of White, Western European, male, middle to upper class, *humancentric* supremacy, which is arguably the biggest challenge of all to working towards the liberation of Black women.

Benjamin and Hall[37] argue that the United States and other Western nations deliberately develop and implement policies designed to permanently subordinate the political, social, economic, and military positions of countries globally. They identify this praxis as *eternal colonialism*, noting that the subjugation of countries that began in the 15th century never ended but has simply morphed over time. Moreover, they conclude that continued colonization of people is taking place not only in other countries but inside the United States. Specific manifestations of internal colonialism include residential segregation of the colonized, exploitation in work environments, deficient material conditions as compared to non-colonized groups, stigmatization of culture, and co-optation of some of the leadership from a colonized group.[38] Bayette[39] contends that one of the most significant barriers to the liberation of Black Americans living in a colonized society is the fact that a large number of Black academics are actively participating in the development of scholarship that assists in maintaining the dominant narrative. Chinweizu[40] extends the argument, noting that the only African storytellers who are taken seriously in academic settings are those whose stories are written instead of spoken, embody the characteristic form and content of European storytelling, and are told in European languages.

People belonging to colonized groups are forced to think and communicate in the language of the people responsible for their colonization and taught to denigrate their native language and stories. This presents major challenges for individuals and groups trying to remain healthy and promote social justice. Jordan[41] illustrates the complex decisions faced by Blacks trying to use language as a tool for fighting against an oppressive system. She argues that Black people risk their ideas being dismissed by dominant society without consideration if they speak in *Black English*. However she noted, that to abandon one's own language for *Standard English* in order to be more acceptable to one's oppressors is a form of suicide.

Supremacy narratives and colonialism also have a negative impact on the ability of individuals and groups to be healthy. *Almanac of the Dead*[42] and *Ceremony*[43] are novels that vividly demonstrate the destructive impact of American Indians trying to use the dominant narrative as the basis for living their lives. They also crystallize the essential role of cultural stories as a foundation for healing and liberation of individuals and groups. Potential intersections between internal colonialism and negative health outcomes among Mexican-Americans have been articulated by Estrada.[44] Postcolonial theory has been identified by Mohammed[45,46] as a strategy for designing research that reexamines and contest colonist ideologies while creating opportunities for indigenous people to reconceptualize health issues in a culturally consistent manner. This approach holds great promise for working with subjugated people globally. However the name is misleading, given the continued presence of colonization within the United Stated and elsewhere around the world.[37]

Anti-supremacy and anti-colonialism work must be extended to also address the dominance of narratives that assume the primacy of humans over other animals, plants, and the earth itself. Environment is a core concept within the metalanguage of nursing frameworks.[5] Although the conceptualization of environment varies widely among theorists, the primacy of humans is a central characteristic of most nursing theories. An Earth Day 2007 YouTube video[47] that features the lyrics of "Rape of the World" by Tracy Chapman[48] clearly illuminates the interdependency of all life forms. The pictures of pigs and chickens raised on corporate farms and rivers polluted with runoff from such farms further illustrate the callous disregard for animals and water as beings that have the right to exist outside of their value to humans. Karen Nieto, the protagonist in *Me, Who Dove into the Heart of the World*,[49] is a savant with autism. She provides a profound explanation of why humans believe we have supremacy over other aspects of creation,

> Since humans live that way, thinking that first they think and then they exist, they also think that anything that doesn't think, also doesn't fully exist. Trees, the sea, the fish in the sea, the sun, the moon, a hill or a whole mountain range. None of that exists all the way; it exists on a second plane of existence, a lesser existence. Therefore, it *deserves* [italics in the original] to be merchandise or food or background for humans and nothing more.[49(pp30-31)]

Stories recorded by Chinweizu[40] and written by Silko[42] offer ways for nurses concerned with social justice to begin thinking about the relationship between people, environment, and health in ways that can more fully benefit both humans and the non-human world.

I am an academic, a nurse scholar, and a Black woman, part of a group that continues to be colonized within the United States. My survival depends on a willingness to continually push back against the dominant narrative and assist my students and colleagues to do likewise. However, I also have an obligation to help them develop the skills they need to effectively negotiate this world and to thrive in the midst of oppression. Working at WSSU has heightened my understanding of the critical need for giving focused attention to the development of ethnic/minority nursing students and faculty as a central component of promoting social justice and health equity. Black women represent the largest group among the students and faculty in the nursing program. Many are scarred as a result of trying to survive as colonized people and quite a few have huge deficits when evaluated by *traditional* academic standards. These deficits are frequently the results of inadequate educational systems, poor housing, economic deprivation, mediocre healthcare, and denigration of Black people within the public narratives. All these are manifestations of the persistence of colonialism within the United States.[38] However, Black students and faculty often internalize skill deficits as personal deficiencies. The students and faculty at WSSU are some of the brightest people I have had the opportunity to work with during my time in the academy. They have some of the most innovative ideas for addressing health inequities and are hungry to create a better life for themselves as well as their communities. Assisting the students and faculty to acquire the skills they need, while strengthening their personal and communal self-efficacy as scholars is a tremendous amount of work. Nonetheless, I feel privileged and humbled by the opportunity to be in their midst. My work here is informed by the wisdom of Audre Lorde,

> Those of us who stand outside the circle of this society's definition of acceptable women; those of us who have been forged in the crucible of difference—those of us who are poor, who are lesbians, who are Black, who are older—know that *survival is not an academic skill* [italics in the original] It is learning how to stand alone, unpopular and sometimes reviled, and how to make common cause with those others identified as outside the structures in order to define and seek a world in which we can all flourish. It is learning how to take our differences and make them strengths.[50(p112)]

Despite the often-repeated rhetoric of academic freedom, the formula for academic success in nursing has become more and more prescriptive during my time in the academy. A sustained history of funding from the National Institutes of Health, preferably RO1s, has become the benchmark for tenure and promotion at many research intensive universities. External funding for research is a requirement even at many institutions where teaching is the primary mission.[51] Moreover, there is an assumption that graduates from highly ranked nursing institutions aspire to be research superstars. Thus, there can be spoken and unspoken pressure from one's alma mater and current academic home to outshine one's peers. The scarcity of American-born ethnic minorities in research-intensive nursing doctoral programs raises the stakes even higher. As the second African-American graduate from the University of Washington's nursing PhD program and the only non-White faculty member in the School of Nursing at the University of Missouri, I felt this pressure immensely. I struggled and floundered, trying to figure out how to emulate my successful colleagues. I spent more and more time chasing grants and trying to get published in the *right* journals.

The turning point came during my third year on the tenure track. Beth Geden, in her role as Chair of the School of Nursing Appointment, Tenure, and Promotion Committee, sent me an email asking me to set up an appointment to discuss my progress. "It's nothing urgent. I just want to talk to you about a few things." However, what she had to say to me was in no way routine. "I don't know what you are doing," Dr. Geden announced without preamble. "But whatever it is, it is not working!" She went on to ask why I was in academia and what I was trying to do. Dr. Geden also noted, "You don't seem to have any passion for what you are doing. What are you passionate about?" I told her that all I cared about was storytelling and promoting the well-being of Black women. Her reply startled me: "Academia is not about promoting the health of people. So if you are passionate about storytelling, I suggest you find a way to get somebody to fund you to do storytelling." Dr. Geden concluded our meeting by noting that although she was not sure what I was going to do, she had faith in me and would assist me in any way she could.

During this same time period my son, William, struggled to adjust to life. I had uprooted him from his life in Washington to take the job in Columbia, Missouri. After three years, he still missed his friends and former life. Moreover, our time together was limited because of the time I spent working. Finally, one day as I sat at the computer, William approached me with a question that stopped me in my tracks: "Mommy, why do I have to make an appointment just to spend some time with you?" Things crystallized for me in that moment. I knew I could no longer live like this. My moment of self-liberation was on the horizon.

As I pondered how to proceed, two events came back to me. The first was a meeting with participants in Sisters in Session[11,22] that became the basis for my dissertation work. Sisters in Session was a series of focus groups conducted in Seattle, Washington, in the spring of 1992. The purpose of the focus groups was to explore how women of African descent conceptualized research and factors that influence their participation in research studies. The women who took part in this meeting told me that they would forever more be watching me. They informed me that how I modeled health rather than my words about health were what would help them move towards wellness.

The second event was a discussion with the renowned nurse scholar, Nancy Fugate Woods. Dr. Woods was chairperson of my dissertation committee and has provided me unwavering support since I met her on the first day of my doctoral program. Sometime during my second or third year at Missouri, she had come to speak at a conference and stayed at my house. Over tea, I shared my struggles and sought guidance. During our conversation, Dr. Woods shared two gems that altered the course of my thinking about academia. "Do not confuse your job with your work," she implored. These words echoed those of Dr. Geden. Later Dr. Woods added, "I do not think of funding as important in and of itself. One must decide what it is that one is trying to do and how much money one needs to do it. If you can do a project with little or no money, then there is no need to seek funding just for the sake of being funded. The important thing is what you plan to do with the money." Reflecting on these two events, along with the comments of my son and Dr. Geden, my path became clear. I would focus my career on using storytelling to promote the health and well-being of Black women. I would seek research funding as necessary to support the work I was trying to do, not however, just for the sake of funding. I would begin to walk my own talk, striving for greater liberation and wellness at home, at work, and in the larger community. I decided to trust Spirit, believing that if I was meant to be in academia that a way would open up to do the work I felt called to do. If not, then I would get a different job and continue my work. For me, Spirit is the life energy in the universe. Spirit is neither created nor destroyed but rather is the source of creation for the natural world. A piece of the Spirit dwells within all that is created. It is Spirit within the creation that allows it to connect with the larger Creator Spirit and Spirit within other creations. Spirit is embedded within not only humans but all creations, including non-human animals, plants, stones, and water. Though the physical manifestation of a creation may erode, Spirit lives on. A major work of Spirit is to ensure that the creation lives true to its purpose. Therefore, the primary question that guides my decision making is, "how/will this help Black women to stay alive and be healthy?"

CONCLUSIONS AND FUTURE DIRECTIONS

The refrain for the gospel song "How I Got Over" runs through my head as I write this concluding paragraph. "How I got over, how I got over. My soul looks back and wonders how I got over." I grew up listening to this song, which is a standard in African-American churches.[52] I respond to myself, "How I got over was through story!"

I have been called to be a *griot*. In traditional African societies, the *griot* was an oral historian and educator. *Griots* were charged with maintaining the cultural links between the past and present, sharing ancestral wisdom with current generations.[13,40] Storytelling has been more than a means for me to promote liberation for Black women. It has been the foundation for me to not only survive but thrive in the academy and the world beyond. Storytelling allows me to facilitate the well-being of Black women in research settings and through teaching. I continue to be in surprised awe, particularly when former research participants or young Black scholars approach me, wanting to discuss how a story I shared during a study session or in an article touched their lives and gave them courage to remain committed to their vision. In addition, the stories that scholars writing from a variety of critical perspectives are putting in the literature help me more thoroughly appreciate the transformational power of storytelling. Thus, pursuant to the goals of this anthology, storytelling is a form of emancipatory nursing. It liberates the teller and the listener. My work has been a praxis project. It pushes Black women (myself included) and others to challenge supremacy narratives that perpetuate the oppression of marginalized groups, other species, or the earth itself. It further promotes social justice in health care by encouraging the development of stories that embrace the importance of multiple perspectives, illuminate our global interdependence, promote peace, and call us to think more critically about what constitutes success and well-being.

Each day the siren call of storytelling grows stronger within me. I feel myself further and further away from academia and closer and closer to a place where I can devote the bulk of my time to storytelling pursuits. My journal entries from the past four years contain increasingly more entries reflecting this shift in direction. I am using these autobiographical stories to guide me as I plan the next stage of my journey. Although the exact nature of my new work is not yet clear, I feel strongly that the next phase will involve work that allows me to spend more time speaking to Black women and girls in my native tongue and less time crafting stories in my adopted language of the academy. I am also being led to more fully explore stories about the continued impact of colonialism on the well-being of Black women globally. Where I will be, I do not know. However, I do know I will be in a place where I can walk along the ocean shore and through deep forests, always alert to opportunities to catch and share story.

REFERENCES

1. Baldwin C. *Storycatcher: Making Sense of Our Lives through the Power and Practice of Story*. Novato, CA: New World Library; 2005.
2. Collins PH. *Fighting Words: Black Women and the Search for Justice*. Minneapolis, MN: University of Minnesota Press; 1998.
3. Braveman PA, Kumanyika S, Fielding J, et al. Health disparities and health equity: the issue is justice. *AJPH* (Published online ahead of print May 5, 2011). doi:10.2105/AJPH.2010.300062
4. Stewart CF III. *Soul Survivors: An African American Spirituality*. Louisville, KY: Westminster John Knox Press; 1997.
5. Chinn PL, Kramer MK. *Integrated Theory and Knowledge Development in Nursing*. 7th ed. St. Louis, MO: Mosby/Elsevier; 2008.
6. Banks-Wallace J. Womanist ways of knowing: theoretical considerations for research with African American women. *ANS Adv Nurs Sci* 2000;22(3): 33–45.
7. Taylor JY. Womanism: a methodologic framework for African American women. *ANS Adv Nurs Sci* 1998;21(1): 53–64.
8. Collins PH. *Black Feminist Thought: Knowledge, Consciousness, and the Politics of Empowerment*. New York, NY: Routledge, 1991.
9. McGregor I, Holmes JG. How storytelling shapes memory and impressions of relationships events over time. *J Pers Soc Psychol* 1999;76: 403–419.
10. Banks-Wallace J. There is a balm in Gilead: storytelling as a healing resource for African-American women. In: Cox AM, Albert DH, eds. *The Healing Heart-Families: Storytelling to Encourage Caring and Healthy Families*. Gabriola Island, BC, Canada: New Society; 2003: 26–31.
11. Banks-Wallace J. Emancipatory potential of storytelling in a group. *J Nurs Scholarsh* 1998;30(1): 17–21.
12. Banks-Wallace J, Barnes A, Swanegan D, Lewis S. Listen, just listen: professional storytelling and interactive learning as strategies for prompting

reflection on the importance of taking time for self. *Storytelling, Self, and Society* 2007;3(3): 161–182.

13. Kouyate D. The role of the griot. In: Goss L, Barnes ME, eds. *Talk that Talk: An Anthology of African-American Storytelling*. New York, NY: Simon & Schuster; 1989: 179–181.

14. Cannon KG. Surviving the blight. In: Wade-Gayles G, ed. *My Soul is a Witness: African-American Women's Spirituality*. Boston, MA: Beacon; 1995: 19–26.

15. Banks-Wallace J. Beyond survival: storytelling as an emancipatory tool among women of African descent. *Womanist Theory and Research* (formerly *The Womanist*) 1994;1(1): 5–8.

16. Banks-Wallace J. Talk that talk: storytelling and analysis rooted in the African American oral tradition. *Qual Health Res* 2002;12(3): 410–426.

17. Liehr PR, Smith MJ. Story theory. In: Smith MJ, Liehr PR, eds. *Middle Range Theory for Nursing*. 2nd ed. New York, NY: Springer; 2008: 205–224.

18. Etter-Lewis G. *My Soul is My Own: Oral Narratives of African American Women in the Professions*. New York, NY: Routledge; 1993.

19. Hilbert V. Preface: Shared thoughts. In: Hilbert V, ed. *Haboo: Native American Stories from Puget Sound*. Seattle, WA: University of Washington Press; 1985: ix–xvii.

20. Avery BY. Breathing life into ourselves: the evolution of the national Black women's health project. In: White EC, ed. *The Black Women's Health Book: Speaking for Ourselves*. Seattle, WA: Seal Press; 1990: 4–10.

21. Cole JB. *Conversations: Straight Talk with America's Sister President*. New York, NY: Doubleday; 1993.

22. Banks-Wallace J. The function of storytelling among women of African descent: secondary analysis of a focus group study. Unpublished dissertation. Seattle, WA: University of Washington; 1994.

23. Callahan JF. *In the African-American Grain: The Pursuit of Voice in Twentieth-Century Black Fiction*. Urbana, IL: University of Illinois Press; 1988.

24. Goss L, Barnes ME. Preface: about the art and the artists. In: Goss L, Barnes ME, eds. *Talk that Talk: An Anthology of African-American Storytelling*. New York, NY: Simon & Schuster; 1989: 9–14.

25. Banks-Wallace J, Parks L. It's all sacred: African American women's perspectives on spirituality. *Issues Ment Health Nurs* 2004;25(1): 25–45.

26. Banks-Wallace J. Staggering under the weight of responsibility: the impact of culture on physical activity among African American women. *J Multicult Nurs Health* 2000;6(3): 24–30.

27. Scieszka J, Smith L (illustrator). *The True Story of the 3 Little Pigs!*. New York, NY: Viking; 1989.

28. Baida PA. *A Nurse's Story and Others*. Jackson, MS: University of Mississippi Press; 2001.

29. Jordan, J, ed. *Some of Us Did Not Die: New and Selected Essays of June Jordan*. New York, NY: Basic/Civitas; 2002.

30. Farmer P. *Pathologies of Power: Health, Human Rights, and the New War on the Poor*. Berkeley, CA: University of California Press; 2003.

31. Fullilove MT. *Root Shock: How Tearing Up City Neighborhoods Hurts America, and What We Can Do About It*. New York, NY: One World; 2004.

32. Perkins J. *Confessions of an Economic Hit Man*. San Francisco, CA: Berrett-Kohler; 2004.

33. Banks-Wallace J, Adams-Leander S, Despin L, McBroom L, Tandy L. Re/Affirming and re/conceptualizing disciplinary knowledge as the foundation for doctoral education. *ANS Adv Nurs Sci* 2008;31(1): 67–78.

34. Adichie C. The danger of a single story. TEDTalks Web site. http://www.ted.com/talks/chimamanda_adichie_the_danger_of_a_single_story.html. Accessed August 27, 2012.

35. Hooks B. *Teaching to Transgress: Education as Practice of Freedom*. New York, NY: Routledge; 1994.
36. Banks-Wallace J, Enyart J, Lewis L, et al. Development of scholars interested in community-based health promotion research. *West J Nurs Res* 2002;24(4): 326–344.
37. Benjamin R, Hall GO. Introduction. In: Benjamin R, Hall GO, eds. *Eternal Colonialism*. Lanham, MD: University Press of America; 2010: xi–xv.
38. Benjamin R. The American internal colonial environment. In: Benjamin R, Hall GO, eds. *Eternal Colonialism*. Lanham, MD: University Press of America; 2010: 3–12.
39. Bayette AD. Going beyond the accepted: Black politics and enduring colonialism. In: Benjamin R, Hall GO, eds. *Eternal Colonialism*. Lanham, MD: University Press of America; 2010: 13–43.
40. Chinweizu. Introduction: redrawing the map of African literature. In: Chinweizu, ed. *Voices from Twentieth-Century Africa: Griots and Towncriers*. London, UK: Faber and Faber; 1988: xvii–xl.
41. Jordan J. Nobody mean more to me than you and the future life of Willie Jordan. In: Jordan J, ed. *Some of Us Did Not Die: New and Selected Essays of June Jordan*. New York, NY: Basic/Civitas; 2002: 157–173.
42. Silko LM. *Almanac of the Dead*. New York, NY: Penguin; 1991.
43. Silko LM. *Ceremony*. New York, NY: Penguin; 1977.
44. Estrada A. (2009). Mexican Americans and historical trauma theory: a theoretical perspective. *J Ethn Subst Abuse* 2009;8(3): 330–340.
45. Mohammed SA. Moving beyond the "exotic": applying postcolonial theory in health research. *ANS Adv Nurs Sci* 2006;29(2): 98–109.
46. Mohammed SA. The dynamic interplay between low socioeconomic status and diabetes for urban American Indians. *Family and Community Health* 2011;34(3): 211–220.
47. Wiegand L, Wigand R. Earth Day 2007. YouTube Web site. https://www.you tube.com/watch?v=oy6b9IGANjM. Accessed October 29, 2012.
48. Chapman T. *Rape of the World Lyrics*. *New Beginnings*. New York, NY: Elektra / Wea; 1995.
49. Berman S. *Me, Who Dove into the Heart of the World* (Dillman L, Trans.). New York, NY: Henry Holt; 2012.
50. Lorde A. The master's tools will never dismantle the master's house. In: Lorde A, ed. *Sister Outsider: Essays and Speeches*. Berkeley, CA: The Crossing Press; 1984: 110–113.
51. Banks J. Development of scholarly trajectories that reflect core values and priorities: a strategy for promoting faculty retention. *J Prof Nurs* 2012;28(6): 351–359.
52. Ward-Royster W. *How I got over: Clara Ward and the World-Famous Ward Singers*. Philadelphia, PA: Temple University Press; 1997.

14 Social Justice in Nursing Pedagogy

A Postcolonial Approach to American Indian Health

Selina A. Mohammed

INTRODUCTION

In response to ethical, social, and professional imperatives to address health inequities, discourses of social justice and the use of critical perspectives have become increasingly prevalent within the field of nursing. However, articles that exemplify social justice as praxis in nursing education are few and far between.[1] In congruence with models of health and health care constructed from the biomedical paradigm, the majority of undergraduate nursing education courses still relate health predominantly to genetics, lifestyle, behavior, or culture and, as such, ascribe responsibility for health to the individual. This perspective omits the contribution of broader social determinants of health and ignores respective root causes of health inequities, as well as the conceptualization of health as a collective issue. This decontextualization of social factors can lead to a lack of understanding of why some groups of people, such as Indigenous populations, bear a disproportionate burden of illness in comparison to members of the dominant society and has the propensity to sustain personal and institutional structures of racialized discrimination.

Since colonization, American Indians (AIs) in general have been more likely to experience poorer health than whites.[2] Although overviews of burgeoning physical and psychosocial health issues among AIs are frequently taught in nursing courses (especially at schools with proximity to such communities), they are often coupled with training focusing on "cultural competency" or the need to "treat everyone the same" as ways to address health disparities,[3] rather than challenging students to engage in critical reflection or conceptualize and respond to how white hegemony and institutionalized power have laid the foundation for the entrenched health inequities that exist among Indigenous Peoples today. Despite potentially good intentions, cultural essentialisms, "othering," and the social status quo continue to function.

In this chapter, I add to the literature written to detail the pragmatic undertaking of social justice as praxis in nursing pedagogy[1,4–9] by describing how I implement a framework of critical social justice[10] in an RN-to-BSN undergraduate nursing course examining issues in AI health. Although there are various and continually evolving forms of social justice within and across disciplines,[1,10–14] the foundational conception of social justice used in this course promotes "a form of justice within which there is an equitable bearing of burdens and reaping of benefits in society"[11(p23)] and shared responsibility for action. Achieving equity in society would require rectifying fundamental causes of injustice for the most vulnerable groups.[12] In order to engage students in a critical analysis of these injustices, "reposition social justice in a more radicalized, politicized light"[10(p332)] and promote collective participation in effectively redressing root causes of inequities that affect health and health care,[10] this introductory course is also built upon the theoretical perspective of postcolonialism.

Postcolonialism provides a way of analyzing colonialism and its historical effects on those who have been colonized. Fundamental points of postcolonial theory include disrupting structural inequities resulting from historically inscribed conditions of colonization and enduring manifestations of subjugation; deconstructing notions of race, racialization, and culture, as well as how these operate in the exclusionary effects of dominant ideologies; challenging inherent assumptions and relationships of power; and the centering of subaltern knowledge, voices, and perspectives.[10,15–18] In addition, the inherently consciousness-raising and transformative nature of postcolonialism invokes a commitment to engaging in praxis-oriented activities that support decolonization and social change. These emancipatory dimensions make it particularly relevant to contextualizing and rectifying health inequities for Indigenous Peoples.[19]

Using postcolonialism and critical social justice as a lens for teaching the class (rather than as a theory or concept that is explicitly taught), students in this course explore how various social determinants intersect to shape and sustain inequitable health conditions and delivery of care. They learn to question how health inequities among AI communities are created and can be addressed from a perspective that transcends genetics and personal choice and instead targets wider social conditions. Through a variety of learning techniques (e.g., instructor facilitation, large and small group discussions, multidisciplinary literature and research, Indigenous documentary films and literary works of fiction, and class exercises), we examine the impact of racializing and colonizing practices on the health of AIs and how historical, political, sociocultural, and economic contexts serve as locations for health inequities among this population. In addition to studying these deleterious effects, students analyze the complexities of health care practice and research with AIs and learn the importance of using decolonizing approaches when working with these communities. A goal of this course is not only to raise social consciousness by underscoring root causes of health inequities for AIs from a postcolonial perspective but to also learn how to apply local strengths and resiliencies of AI communities to the conceptualization and enactment of meaningful ways to mitigate these relevant health issues.

COURSE STRUCTURE

The course, "Issues in American Indian Health," is a 10-week elective that is offered as part of a one-year RN-to-BSN program and is designed to be introductory. It can be broken down into three primary areas of emphases, which are described in detail below. This elective course dovetails with a required class, "Cultural and Social Issues in Health Care,"[20] which focuses on increasing students' awareness of their own positions (both personally and within the structure of dominant society); understanding how social meanings are assigned; analyzing concepts of privilege and oppression; exploring issues of race, class, gender, and sexual orientation; and learning about Friedman's scripts of relational positionality.[21] These issues complement and are highly pertinent to concepts emphasized in the AI health class.

Prior to delving into the essence of the AI health course content, there are several fundamental course assumptions that are reviewed and discussed. In this course, "American Indian" does not reflect a monolithic racial category of genetic distinctiveness, but is a term (albeit a highly politicized, controversial misnomer) used to represent Indigenous Peoples of the United States (U.S.) from diverse tribal backgrounds and affiliations, each having their unique creation stories and histories, geographical locations, cultural practices, and languages, who share similar sociopolitical legacies of genocide, subjugation, oppression, and social inequality as a result of colonization. Second, although we use the term "American Indian" in the course (because there is difficulty in finding a neutral way to collectively represent people who still nationally self-identify in this manner), we consider how the label was created by the U.S. government to racially mark off Indigenous Peoples and, as such, is a contested signifier of Western colonial representations.[18]

In addition to these fundamental course assumptions, the students and I establish norms of engagement to create a safe classroom space and foster open dialogue. The norms are created using the nominal group technique,[22] where each student shares ideas regarding what he/she thinks contributes to effective interactions, and the class as a whole establishes agreed upon norms. Although each class develops specific norms (e.g., not talking over one another), what I have found over the years is that the norms are based on the premises of demonstrating a commitment to active engagement in the classroom and a collective responsibility to co-learning, showing respect to each other through thoughtful communication, valuing diverse viewpoints and each person's voice equally, and maintaining confidentiality within the classroom. The norms that students agree to adopt serve as a reference point for facilitating positive group processes, should tensions rise.

Root Causes for Health Inequities

The first part of the course includes an overview of AI demographics and the prominent physical and mental health illnesses among AI communities and importantly underscores the complexities of colonization and its lingering effects as a defining origin for these entrenched health inequities. Although strides have been made in improving health outcomes, AI communities face many health challenges at disproportionately high rates in comparison with the general population.[2] Understanding the danger of examining health morbidity and mortality rates without contextualizing them (e.g., the reification of racialized stereotypes and further stigmatization that inequities are a function of genes, culture, behavior, or lifestyle), we focus predominantly on socially determined root causes of health inequities in this section of the course. In essence, we move beyond the "what is" to examining "how it came to be that way."[23] The goal is to shift away from blaming AIs for their illnesses and towards acknowledging the historical and contemporary sources of health problems.

To situate the effects of colonialist practices on social, political, and economic determinants of health for AIs, students are provided with an abbreviated overview of the history of AIs with whites. This history is fraught with active oppression, neglect, and a denial of humanity.[24] In addition to covering notable atrocities that many students recognize, such as Manifest Destiny; military slaughters; forced migrations (e.g., the Cherokee Trail of Tears and The Long Walk of the Diné); the establishment of reservations and land allotments; the introduction of new diseases; and a complete destruction in way of life, we also cover practices that seem to be not as well known, such as the institutionalization of boarding schools; mass displacement of AI children through adoption into non-Native homes; and urbanization of AIs through U.S. termination/relocation policies created in the 1950s.

As we cover the above topics, we deconstruct the resulting intergenerational consequences of these injustices, as well as how their ongoing manifestations continue to constrain life opportunities for AIs. Students examine the impact that environmental desecrations, low socioeconomic status, historical trauma, and racialized discrimination have on the health and social status of AIs today by reading and discussing literature and research that underscore these links.[e.g.,25–32] Students also learn about these determinants of health by viewing Indigenous documentaries created from a decolonizing standpoint, such as *Bad Sugar*[33]—explicating the health effects resulting from the diversion of water away from the Pima and Tohono O'odham Indians; *A Century of Genocide in the Americas: The Residential School Experience*[34]—illustrating the institutionalization of sexual abuse in boarding schools; *Half of Anything*[35]—examining the notion of how Indian identity is constructed; *Transitions: Destruction of a Mother Tongue*[36]—exploring the consequences of language loss in AI communities; and *Without Reservations: Notes on Racism in Montana*[37]—addressing questions of racism against AIs. They then engage in free-writes and group dialogue to draw parallels between the films and contemporary health issues. A third pedagogical technique I employ to creatively engage students is to have them read an Indigenous literary work of fiction, selecting either *Ceremony*,[38]

The Lone Ranger and Tonto Fistfight in Heaven,[39] or *Fools Crow,*[40] and then complete a written assignment proposing what questions they think the author is trying to raise or answer and analyzing how the meanings conveyed relate to course concepts. Using a combination of aesthetic learning and various literary mediums helps bring course concepts to life by generating different ways of developing knowledge and applying course content.

Examining Ourselves and Mainstream Health Care

The second portion of the course focuses on having students develop critical consciousness about themselves as individuals and of Western health care as a profession. Emphasizing the mutually constitutive and dependent nature of relationships among dominant and marginalized groups, students are asked to reverse the traditional gaze of looking at others and examine their own social locations instead. This includes acknowledging whiteness[41–44] as a signifier of structural advantage and deconstructing how relationships of power seamlessly operate at each level in society to benefit some groups of people and disadvantage others.

We extend these analyses to the health care profession in the United States by examining the historically reinforcing relationship between Western medicine and imperialism and articulating how biomedicine (as a product and extension of whiteness, as well as a form of surveillance) continues to propagate dominant ideologies by deeming certain health parameters, beliefs, and practices as being valid and others as not. I challenge students (who inevitably have been disciplined within, or assimilated into, this system of whiteness) to question how these implicit norms and the complexities of race, class, and gender operate as subtexts and shape how they practice and then to dialogically deliberate the dangers of helping others to, in effect, be more like themselves.[45]

As our health care discussion becomes more focused on service delivery to AIs, we analyze how the system has simultaneously fostered dependency and dichotomization. We review the major acts that have influenced the history of health care services for AIs and the evolution of the system itself, from the organization of the Indian Health Service (IHS) to how services are becoming increasingly decentralized from governmental control to oversight by tribal communities through contracts and compacts.[46] Through this review, we also debate the numerous problems that accompany these issues, such as the argument that decentralization is an attempt by the federal government to end its responsibilities to Indigenous Peoples, as tribes are given an overstressed and severely underfunded health care system.[46,47] The class also discusses several barriers to care that alienate AIs from the mainstream health sector.[47,48] For instance, although AI tribes are sovereign governments within the U.S. that have retained their right to govern themselves, AIs who are enrolled members of federally recognized tribes may receive some non-insured health care benefits while on their reservations, as the result of a treaty obligation and the government's trustee duty to AIs.[49] This federal obligation "has given rise to resentment from members of dominant society with respect to 'free' health services and often is seen as an extension of welfare or undeserved charity."[47(p131)] We consider, through small and large group critique, how these types of perceptions contribute to broader practices of stigmatization and harmful stereotyping that have functioned to condone a range of improprieties, ranging from discriminatory health care encounters,[47] egregious medical misconduct,[50] and the appropriation of Indigenous healing practices.[51]

Crucial to all of these conversations is an examination of the functions and effects of cultural essentialisms and racialization in social positioning. Through these discursive constructions, colonialism becomes legitimized and binary categories (e.g., us/them, superior/inferior) re-inscribed. Thus, rather than reifying general descriptions about AI culture, we work in the classroom to problematize the notion that culture is a fixed entity that is preexisting and neutrally discovered.[52] We engage in conversations regarding the politics of difference, in terms of what it means to create cultural descriptions, the purposes that they serve and how they are sustained, the perspectival nature of these descriptions, and how these classifications intrinsically involve power.[44] We also discuss the perilous assumptions that unavoidably are produced when culture becomes conflated with "race" and "race" becomes a marker for certain beliefs and behaviors,[53] and consider the ramifications of this within a health care context. Because students are always quick to point out that there are "in fact" similar cultural practices across different AI groups (i.e., the notion of a pan-Indian culture), we examine the intricacies of this type of cultural representation and how it can be both a contested space, as well as a site of resistance and allegiance for Indigenous Peoples. In this way, students gain an appreciation of culture and identity as being fluid, complex, historically situated, and continually re-negotiated for different purposes, within different contexts.[18]

The goal of this part of the course is to have students examine the personal, professional, and social implications of cultural stereotyping and racialization in terms of how relations of hegemony have been formed and maintained, and how members of dominant society and AIs are changed in the process. In addition to readings and group discussions that focus on these topics, students engage in reflective journaling about the structural nature of whiteness, as well as personalize it by looking at the norms and dominant institutions in their lives and the everyday privileges that whiteness has individually afforded them. We watch additional Indigenous documentaries, such as *White Shamans and Plastic Medicine* Men[51]—regarding the exploitation of spiritual traditions by non-Indians—and also analyze how racialized discourses and identities are reinforced and contested through popular culture and media. For example, students are asked to bring in representations that are vehicles for reaffirmation, marginalization, or resistance (e.g., depictions of AIs from advertisements, song lyrics, American cinematic films, sports marketing, or newspaper articles) and then collectively deconstruct what they have seen or heard in terms of how it positions members of AI communities (and relatedly, members of dominant society), as well as how it reinforces or challenges some of their assumptions. Encouraging students to become mindful of the constructions that have defined their positioning is simultaneously reflexive, dialectic, and consciousness-raising.[54,55] It also is an important first step in generating a critical understanding of their social realities and the awareness that they can intervene to change them.[55]

Addressing Health Inequities

By the final third of the course, students have gained greater emancipatory knowledge[56] and a deeper understanding of the historically seeded inequities that shape health and health care for AIs, the effects of racialization, and how power functions in society. The concluding portion of the course focuses on how students can enact their new knowledge to promote social justice and address health inequities. We begin by studying why health is a collective issue and how inequitable conditions consequently diminish health for both marginalized and privileged groups.[57–59] We then examine specific courses of action that nurses can undertake to mitigate health and health care inequities among AIs and their effects. Emphasized throughout this discussion is the importance of cultivating attitudes of listening and learning, using decolonizing strategies, and building on local strengths when engaging in this type of transformative work.

An essential component in addressing health inequities for AIs is making these inequities and their effects within Native communities visible and documenting successful interventions in diminishing them through research that attends to both of these aspects. In recognition of past research injustices and the rights of Indigenous Peoples to advance their own agendas, Community-Based Participatory Research (CBPR) has increasingly been hailed as an ethical, emancipative, and socially just orientation to research with Indigenous communities.[60] The premise of CBPR is the formation of equitable, reciprocal partnerships between researchers and communities throughout all phases of the research process.[61] Along with learning about the principles of CBPR, we discuss the numerous benefits of this orientation to research (e.g., its decolonizing nature, which includes centering local knowledge and unpacking issues around race and power; its strength-based and community capacity-building foci; and its emphasis on co-learning, mutual ownership, and long-term commitment),[60–62] as well as some challenges.[60,63] Students also read examples of scholarly literature demonstrating how CBPR has been used to reduce health disparities in AI communities and engage in a variety of class exercises (see examples from *Developing and Sustaining Community-Based Participatory Research Partnerships: A Skill-Building Curriculum*[64]) to gain knowledge and practical experience regarding elements of this approach.

In addition to underscoring research as a viable avenue for alleviating health inequities, we examine other ways that students can engage in confronting the roots of these inequities on structural and political levels. Because many students unavoidably want to focus on strategies they can use with individuals and families in clinical encounters (their comfort zone), we briefly discuss how students can apply some of the partnership principles from CBPR within their practice, and the importance of engaging in processes of cultural humility[65] and providing meaningful care that is contextualized, relational, and responsive to how social determinants of health and marginalization operate for each client.[10,66,67] While acknowledging that these practices are instrumental at the individual and family levels, we also deconstruct their lack of effect in diminishing health inequities or their root causes on a structural level. This analysis enables us to further explore how nurses can critically address these systemic injustices and expand their realm of nursing to include challenging institutional practices and targeting conditions that create inequities. We reemphasize the value of taking action to reframe health inequities as reflections of race, class, and gender discrimination and to counter productions of "othering,"[18] and then read literature that underscores the significance of policy advocacy and political action in changing social determinants of health and provides tangible examples.[e.g.,3,10,13,66–68] Reflecting on these examples, student then deliberate innovative ways that they can work with AI communities to initiate changes that dismantle the multifaceted social, political, and economic conditions responsible for producing health inequities among AIs.

Capitalizing on these discussions, students synthesize their learning in a final paper that draws upon the concepts covered in each section of the course. They select a health problem that is prevalent in AI communities and, deemphasizing the role of genetics or individual choice, position it as a response to historical and present-day social inequities that have been generated through interactions with dominant society. As students write about the selected health problem, they consider how whiteness and the construction of "others" function in the determinants of health, how social determinants have operated to produce and sustain this health inequity, and polices that contribute to the health condition. Once they have detailed the genesis of the health problem, students propose how to work collectively with AIs to address the health inequity from a social determinants of health perspective.

REFLECTIONS

This course brings into focus how health inequities among AIs have been historically created and sustained through societal relations and underscores the interrelated nature of health and health care with the Nation's social, political, and economic climate. By analyzing root causes of these health inequities, as well as ourselves and the construction of AIs as "others," the ultimate and idyllic goal of the course is to begin disrupting the naturalness of these social injustices and the production of health inequities among AIs.

There is an abundance of means to articulate social justice and postcolonial theory as subjects, lenses, or curricular threads in nursing pedagogy. What I have presented here is one version of how I implemented these concepts to frame a course on AI health. There are many challenges in teaching a course of this nature. The name of the course itself is problematic and the mere act of teaching a course specific to AIs signals difference. There exists a clear tension in this course between exploring how colonizing relations have shaped circumstances for AIs and reifying binaries. Although we touch on issues of hybridity[69] and multiple positionalities to dissolve notions of authenticities and absolutes (and expand upon the scripts of relational positionality[21] that they learn in their other course[20]), capturing the shifting nature of subjectivities is difficult work and the question always becomes whether the class simply perpetuates the binary or promotes counterhegemonic change. Thus, the course is certainly not without its flaws and is a continuous work in progress, as I myself develop and receive feedback from students. My intent is not to add to the burden of difference but to illuminate the complexities of health and health care for AIs in order to effect change.

Throughout the course, we cover a breadth of material in a short amount of time. Students display a range of emotions, including white guilt, anger, wanting AIs to "pull themselves up by their bootstraps," and revelation. Although many students appear to gain critical awareness and embrace their opportunity for action, some students still cling to their romanticizing or debasing stereotypes of AIs. Although it is critical to acknowledge the gamut of emotions in a course such as this, we also frequently revisit the course objectives and norms of interaction to keep our focus on transformative learning and action. Evaluations reveal that many students have found the course to be "incredibly challenging" and, at times, "uncomfortable" for them. Reflexively critiquing their own privilege and examining how they themselves are complicit in reproducing relations of power is difficult work. Although students usually comprehend the hierarchical nature of a health care encounter itself, it is often difficult for them to recognize biomedicine as a cultural construction, because the tools of their education come from the same culture.[18] A few students still wish I had provided some generic, "cultural description" of AIs, and others have commented that I should have provided them with opportunities for service in Native communities (a situation that has its own pitfalls[43]). However, the overwhelming majority of students have consistently rated the course as being "excellent," providing comments that deem the course "highly valuable" and "critical to nursing education," and questioning why they have never previously learned such content.

Crucial elements in social justice pedagogy include acknowledging where students are in their education and supporting them as their awareness deepens.[1] The process of becoming critically responsive is slow and incremental, as students increasingly come to see themselves as political beings and move on from "what is" to envisioning through the ideals of social justice "what could be"[23] and contemplating ways to achieve this. The views that nurses hold can contribute to actions that are socially just or unjust.[54] To achieve transformative practice, nurses need to "engage in critical thinking, reflective practice, and political action if we are to end existing health disparities and create a more socially just healthcare environment and society for all."[3(p25)]

REFERENCES

1. Boutain DM. Social justice as a framework for professional nursing. *Journal of Nursing Education* 2005;44(9): 404–408.
2. Barnes PM, Adams PF, Powell-Griner E. Health characteristics of the American Indian or Alaska Native adult population: United States, 2004–2008. *U.S. Department of Health and Human Services, Centers for Disease Control and Prevention National Center for Health Statistics* 2010;20: 1–24.
3. Drevdahl DJ, Canales MK, Shannon Dorcy K. Of goldfish tanks and moonlight tricks: can cultural competency ameliorate health disparities? *Advances in Nursing Science* 2008;31(1): 13–27.
4. Boutain DM. Social justice as a framework for undergraduate community health clinical experiences in the United States. *International Journal of Nursing Education Scholarship* 2008;5(1)(35).
5. Fahrenwald NL, Bassett SD, Tschetter L, Carson PP, White L, Winterboer VJ. Teaching core nursing values. *Journal of Professional Nursing* 2005;21(1): 46–51.
6. Fahrenwald NL. Teaching social justice. *Nurse Educator* 2003;28(5): 222–226.
7. Leuning C. Advancing a global perspective: the world as classroom. *Nursing Science Quarterly* 2001;14(4): 298–303.
8. Reimer Kirkham S, Van Hofwegen L, Hoe Harwood C. Narratives of social justice: learning in innovative clinical settings. *International Journal of Nursing Education Scholarship* 2005;2(1)(28).
9. Redman R, Clark L. Service-learning as a model for integrating social justice in the nursing curriculum. *Journal of Nursing Education* 2002;41: 446–449.
10. Reimer Kirkham S, Browne AJ. Toward a critical theoretical interpretation of social justice discourses in nursing. *Advances in Nursing Science* 2006;29(4): 324–339.
11. Drevdahl D, Kneipp SM, Canales MK, Shannon Dorcy K. Reinvesting in social capital: a capital idea for public health nursing. *Advances in Nursing Science* 2001;24(2): 19–31.
12. Boutain DM. Social justice in nursing: a review of literature. In: de Chesnay M, ed. *Caring for the Vulnerable.* Sudbury, MA: Jones and Bartlett; 2004: 21–29.
13. Pauly BM, MacKinnon K, Varcoe C. Revisiting "who gets care?" Health equity as an arena for nursing action. *Advances in Nursing Science* 2009;32(2): 118–127.
14. Buettner-Schmidt K, Lobo ML. Social justice: a concept analysis. *Journal of Advanced Nursing* 2011;68(4): 948–958.

15. Anderson JM. Lessons from a postcolonial-feminist perspective: suffering and a path to healing. *Nursing Inquiry* 2004;11: 238–246.

16. Reimer Kirkham S, Anderson JM. Postcolonial nursing scholarship: from epistemology to method. *Advances in Nursing Science* 2002;25(1): 1–17.

17. Racine L. Implementing a postcolonial feminist perspective in nursing research related to non-Western populations. *Nursing Inquiry* 2003;10(2): 91–102.

18. Mohammed SA. Moving beyond the "exotic": applying postcolonial theory in health research. *Advances in Nursing Science* 2006;29(2): 98–109.

19. Browne AJ, Smye VL, Varcoe C. The relevance of postcolonial theoretical perspectives to research in Aboriginal health. *CJNR* 2005;37(4): 16–37.

20. Abrums ME, Leppa C. Beyond cultural competence: teaching about race, gender, class, and sexual orientation. *Journal of Nursing Education* 2001;40(6): 270–275.

21. Friedman S. *Mappings: Feminism and the Cultural Geographics of Encounter.* Princeton, NJ: Princeton University Press; 1998.

22. Delbecq AL, Van de Ven AH, Gustafson DH. *Group Techniques for Program Planning: A Guide to Nominal Group and Delphi Processes.* Glenview, IL: Scott, Foresman; 1975.

23. Thomas J. *Doing Critical Ethnography.* Newbury Park, CA: Sage; 1993.

24. Tuhiwai Smith L. *Decolonizing Methodologies: Research and Indigenous Peoples.* London, UK: Zed Books, Ltd; 1999.

25. Lewis DR. Native Americans and the environment: a survey of twentieth-century issues. *The American Indian Quarterly* 1995;19(3): 1–20.

26. Adler NE, Ostrove JM. Socioeconomic status and health: what we know and what we don't. *Ann NY Acad Sci* 1999;896: 3–15.

27. Williams DR, Mohammed SA, Leavell J, Collins C. Race, socioeconomic status, and health: complexities, ongoing challenges, and research opportunities. *Ann NY Acad Sci* 2010;1186: 69–101.

28. Brave Heart M, DeBruyn LM. The American Indian holocaust: healing historical unresolved grief. *American Indian and Alaska Native Mental Health Research* 1998;8(2): 56–72.

29. Walters KL, Mohammed SA, Evans-Campbell T, Beltran RE, Chae DH, Duran B. Bodies don't just tell stories, they tell histories: embodiment of historical trauma among American Indians and Alaska Natives. *DuBois Review: Social Science Research on Race* 2011;8(1): 179–189.

30. Williams DR, Mohammed SA. Discrimination and racial disparities in health: evidence and needed research. *Journal of Behavioral Medicine* 2009;32(1): 20–47.

31. Chae DH, Walters KL. Racial discrimination and racial identity attitudes in relation to self-rated health and physical pain and impairment among two-spirit American Indians/Alaska Natives. *American Journal of Public Health* 2009;99(S1): 144–151.

32. Whitbeck LB, Walls ML, Johnson KD, Morrisseau AD, McDougall CM. Depressed affect and historical loss among North American Indigenous adolescents. *American Indian Alaska Native Mental Health Research* 2009;16(3): 16–41.

33. Fortier JM. Bad sugar [DVD]. In: Adelman L, Smith L, executive producers. *Unnatural Causes: Is Inequality Making Us Sick?* San Francisco, CA: California Newsreel; 2008.

34. Gibbons R, Thomas D. *A Century of Genocide in the Americas: The Residential School Experience* [DVD]. Seattle, WA: The Native Voices Program at University of Washington; 2002.

35. Tomhave J. *Half of Anything* [DVD]. Seattle, WA: The Native Voices Program at University of Washington; 2006.

36. Kipp D, Fisher J. *Transitions: Destruction of a Mother Tongue* [DVD]. Seattle, WA: The Native Voices Program at University of Washington; 1992.
37. Native Voices. *Without Reservations: Notes on Racism in Montana* [DVD]. Seattle, WA: The Native Voices Program at University of Washington; 1995.
38. Marmon Silko L. *Ceremony*. New York, NY: Penguin Classics; 2006.
39. Alexie S. *The Lone Ranger and Tonto Fistfight in Heaven*. New York, NY: Grove Press; 2005.
40. Welch, J. *Fools Crow*. New York, NY: Viking Penguin, Inc; 1986.
41. Frankenberg, R. Introduction: local whitenesses, localizing whiteness. In: Frankenberg R, ed. *Displacing Whiteness: Essays in Social and Cultural Criticism*. Durham, NC: University Press; 1997: 1–33.
42. Schroeder C, DiAngelo R. Addressing whiteness in nursing education: the sociopolitical climate project at the University of Washington School of Nursing. *Advances in Nursing Science* 2010;33(3): 244–255.
43. Puzan E. The unbearable whiteness of being (in nursing). *Nursing Inquiry* 2003;10(3): 193–200.
44. Allen DG. Whiteness and difference in nursing. *Nursing Philosophy* 2006;7: 65–78.
45. Carter RT. Is white a race? Expressions of white racial identity. In: Fine M, Weis L, Powell LC, Mun Wong L, eds. *Off White: Readings on Power, Privilege, and Resistance*. New York: Routledge; 1997: 198–211.
46. Holkup PA. Big changes in the Indian Health Service: are nurses aware? *Journal of Trancultural Nursing* 2002;13(1): 47–53.
47. Browne AJ, Fiske J. First Nations women's encounters with mainstream health care services. *Western Journal of Nursing Research* 2001;23(2): 126–147.
48. Call KT, McAlpine DD, Johnson PJ, Beebe TJ, McRae JA, Song Y. Barriers to care among American Indians in public care programs. *Medical Care* 2006;44(6): 595–600.
49. Kunitz SJ. Public health then and now: the history and politics of U.S. health care policy for American Indians and Alaska Natives. *American Journal of Public Health* 1996;86: 1464–1473.
50. Lawrence J. The Indian Health Service and the sterilization of Native American women. *American Indian Quarterly* 2000;24: 400–419.
51. Macy T, Hart, D. *White Shamans and Plastic Medicine Men* [DVD]. Seattle, WA: The Native Voices Program at University of Washington; 1996.
52. Allen DG. Knowledge, politics, culture, and gender: a discourse perspective. *Canadian Journal of Nursing Research* 1996;28(1): 95–102.
53. Anderson J, Perry J, Blue C, et al. "Rewriting" cultural safety within the postcolonial and postnational feminist project: toward new epistemologies of healing. *Advances in Nursing Science* 2003;26(3): 196–214.
54. Anderson, JM, Rodney P, Reimer-Kirkham S, Browne AJ, Khan, KB, Lynam, MJ. Inequities in health and healthcare viewed through the ethical lens of critical social justice: contextual knowledge for the global priorities ahead. *Advances in Nursing Science* 2009;32(4): 282–294.
55. Jakubowski LM. Teaching uncomfortable topics: an action-oriented strategy for addressing racism and related forms of difference. *Teaching Sociology* 2001;29(1): 62–79.
56. Chinn P, Kramer M. *Integrated Theory and Knowledge Development in Nursing*. 7th ed. St. Louis, MO: Mosby Elsevier; 2008.
57. Bezruchka S. The hurrier I go the behinder I get: the deteriorating international ranking of the U.S. health status. *Annu Rev Public Health* 2012;33: 157–173.
58. Subramanian SV, Kawachi I. Income inequality as a public health concern: where do we stand? *Health Services Research* 2003;38(1 Part 1): 153–167.

59. Bezruchka S. Income inequality and population health: hierarchy and health are related. *BMJ* 2002;324(7343): 978.
60. Mohammed SA, Walters KL, LaMarr J, Evans-Campbell T, Fryberg, S. Finding middle ground: negotiating university and tribal community interests in community-based participatory research. *Nursing Inquiry* 2012;19(2): 116–127.
61. Israel BA, Schulz AJ, Parker EA, Becker AB, Allen III AJ, Guzman, JR. Critical issues in developing and following community based participatory research for health. In: Minkler M, Wallerstein N, eds. *Community-Based Participatory Research for Health*. San Francisco, CA: Jossey-Bass; 2003: 53–76.
62. Wallerstein N, Duran B. Using community-based participatory research to address health disparities. *Health Promotion Practice* 2006;7: 312–323.
63. Burhansstipanov L, Christopher S, Schumacher SA. Lessons learned from community-based participatory research in Indian country. *Cancer Control* 2005;12(S2): 70–76.
64. The Examining Community-Institutional Partnerships for Prevention Research Group. *Developing and Sustaining Community-Based Participatory Research Partnerships: A Skill-Building Curriculum*. 2006. http://www.cbprcurriculum. info. Accessed June 11, 2013.
65. Tervalon M, Murray-Garcia J. Cultural humility versus cultural competence: a critical distinction in defining physician training outcomes in multicultural education. *Journal of Health Care for the Poor and Underserved* 1998;9(2): 117–125.
66. Mohammed SA. The dynamic interplay between low socioeconomic status and diabetes for urban American Indians. *Fam Community Health* 2011;34(3): 211–220.
67. Reutter L, Kushner KE. 'Health equity through action of the social determinant of health': taking up the challenge in nursing. *Nursing Inquiry* 2010;17(3): 269–280.
68. Browne AJ, Tarlier DS. Examining the potential of nurse practitioners from a critical social justice perspective. *Nursing Inquiry* 2008;15(2): 83–93.
69. Bhabha HK. *The Location of Culture*. London, UK: Routledge; 1994.

15 Human Violence Interventions
Critical Discourse Analysis Praxis

Debby A. Phillips

INTRODUCTION

Theories of social reproduction maintain that "social structures and institutions that systematically impose harms on people *require* [emphasis added] vigorous mechanisms of active social reproduction in order to be sustained over time."[1(p276)] Social reproduction refers to continuously reproducing a society as it exists at any particular moment. Reproduced within a society at a given time are, for example, values, beliefs, and human behaviors, processes that are liberating for some and oppressive for others, and structures and institutions created by thoroughly social humans that benefit some and are detrimental to others. All that can be known about a society, its beliefs, its behaviors, the people in it, its processes, and its institutions can only be known through the language that is part of that very society. When written, spoken, behavioral, or visual (i.e., non-verbal) language is reproduced in any way, the social (humans, relationships, behaviors, values, society as a "whole") that language constructs is also reproduced. Effects of social reproduction include preserving existing social structures (i.e., particular gender, race, and class hierarchies and relations) and their underpinning social relations.

Critical discourse analysis from a poststructural psychoanalytic philosophical perspective examines societal language and its effects. It uncovers linguistic mechanisms that reproduce social structures, as well as power and privilege. Moreover, it exposes the bondages imposed by language by destabilizing the naturalness of beliefs, ordinary practices, behaviors, and subjectivities that are taken up consciously and unconsciously through participating in society. Poststructural psychoanalytic discourse analysis challenges accepted truths and shows how truths or facts obscure the range of human variations, constrain the field of possibilities, and limit full participation in social life. By so doing, it liberates possibilities and potentials. This analytical process is praxis. Praxis is emancipatory action, and praxis for critical awareness is political action in the service of justice.

This chapter is a synopsis of how poststructural psychoanalytic discourse analysis (PSPADA) has been used with emancipatory intentions in research to illuminate conscious and unconscious reproduction of society, social relations, norms, and practices. It identifies and connects key discourse analysis positions, psychoanalytic understandings of conscious, and unconscious learning and memories with contemporary neurobiology, showing how nerve networks throughout the mind and body develop, "hold," and activate previous beliefs, assumptions, emotions, behaviors, and physical sensations consciously and unconsciously. That is, how social discourses work themselves into us and then constitute the way we see the world and behave in it. The chapter highlights three discourse analysis exemplars from research on: 1) male violence against women; 2) society constructions of masculinity and practices of violence; and 3) sibling violence.

Poststructural Psychoanalytic Discourse Analysis: Key Positions

Discourse analysis from a poststructural psychoanalytic perspective investigates language.[2,3] It is a critical close-up lens allowing specificities of language constructions to be made visible and subject to analysis. It argues that there are no guaranteed structures or facts of something or someone, and that facts (what they "mean") are constituted through language that changes over time and is contingent on history, location, past experiences, and on available social discourses.[2-4] Descriptions, for example, are considered acts of reproduction, not acts of transparently representing an underlying structure, truth, or "fact" of something or someone.

Deconstruction is the analytical component of poststructural theoretical approaches. By breaking down the seemingly natural connection between a word, sound, and meaning, it shows that any unchanging, foundational relationship is constructed and illusory.[5,6] Uncovering the connection that is necessary for construction shows that the connection is binary. The positive or privileged end of the binary is contingent on and impossible without being constructed against the negative end, that is, what *it is not*. For example, one cannot distinguish "normal" behavior unless one also simultaneously differentiates it from "abnormal behavior." In written, visual, and verbal discourses, the process of constructing/differentiating occurs outside a person's awareness and without critical evaluation. This is an unconscious process triggered by incoming data from one or more of the senses activating a neural network that holds previous learning/exposure to societal discourses constructing the particular normal/not normal person dichotomy. Deconstruction poses questions such as how does one come to know and distinguish what is true or normal, false or abnormal, how have these changed, and who decides?

The above points to another key position of deconstruction and of psychoanalytic and neurobiological positions on the unconscious: individuals are not originators of their accounts about themselves, others, or the world. Individual accounts are understood as a data source among many sites of social reproduction. Critical knowledge investigation subverts the notion of original, individual knowledge by uncovering and exposing its multidimensional and complex history, its contingencies, and its instabilities. For example, "ideal masculinity and gender are not 'real' in the sense that they refer to innate capacities or potentials of a biological body, but are only real in the sense that their discursive representation continually generates a real."[7(p221)] There is no final point of origin. "Ideal ('normal') and marginalized masculinities are better understood as repetitive performances that work within a network of discourses and power relations, constructing gender identities."[7(p221)] Repetitive performances enacting societal discourses, known as performativity, are practices of social reproduction. For example, performativity of boys and men and performativity of cultural representations like Disney characters, movie heroes, TV stars, men in the news, professional sports stars, or health and social science discourses constructing theories about boys and men, all produce particular masculine identities and particular understandings of men and society. When norms of masculinity are reproduced, beliefs about innate gender with inherent personality traits that some men are born with more than others are also reproduced and reinforced.

Questioning how one comes to "know" something is another important aspect of PSPADA. Non-critical, non-questioning knowing unintentionally reproduces assumptions about concepts, such as identities and behaviors, reinforcing and stabilizing particular identities, societal arrangements, and social institutions. Through PSPADA, personal knowing is traced to discourses within which the person is, or has been, embedded. This analysis locates a particular discourse's evolution, explicating its reliance on other discourses to "make sense," and revealing its construction. Goals of PSPADA are exposing continuities, discontinuities, instabilities, and consequences in human lives and in societal and institutional arrangements.

These theoretical perspectives are underpinned by the primary PSPADA position that there is no boundary between the individual and society. People are understood as social through and through,[7,8] and no aspect of being "human" is untouched by language. This position opens up social discourses to examination and to accountability for damaging beliefs, behaviors, oppressions, marginalization, privileges, and injustices. When people verbally and non-verbally communicate and live cultural understandings, they enact the discourses that they have taken up both consciously and unconsciously. Describing the constraints of language, Wright[1] argues that beliefs that people hold about limits regarding themselves, others, and the world systematically affect what is conceived as possible for themselves, others, and the world. Moreover, one's knowledge and ways of understanding oneself, others, and the world are regulated by existing knowledge that is tied to histories of its construction.

Butler, Holloway, and Bourdieu[9–13] bring in a theory of the unconscious that is supported by contemporary psychoanalytic mind/body theory and neurobiology. These help explain how social discourse becomes "internalized" to the extent that individual behaviors and beliefs about oneself, others, and the world appear innate, as if coming from a fixed biological core and genetic make-up. These internalized ways of being enable people to "naturally" function in the particular society that is constructed by the very same discourses. PSPADA assumes that no person can stand outside of language to examine oneself, others, beliefs, phenomena, or society, because the language of examination is part of the same language that constructs the "it" (person) doing the examining.[3,9] For example, PSPADA positions enable conceptions of masculinity and practices of violence that move away from traditional views of boys and men as biological sources of masculine identities and "natural" violent or other behaviors (i.e., risk taking, athleticism, and heterosexuality).[3,7,8] PSPADA positions focus on embodied and linguistic practices (i.e., ways of walking, talking, and performing toughness, dominance, or heterosexuality, etc.) through which bodies appear biologically normal or not normal, while simultaneously reproducing dominant beliefs about, for example, innate male biology and normativity of the heterosexual, strong, and tough male, and of male dominance. Posing questions like, "who is and can be included in the category normal male, on what terms, and by whose authority?" underlies PSPADA analysis that exposes the complex relationship between society, possibilities for being masculine, and lived experience stored in unconscious mind/body neuro-networks. It shows how individual subjectivity and society are simultaneously reproduced. An emancipatory aspect of critical discourses analysis is its call for individual and societal critique, awareness, and accountability for harmful discourses reproduced at all levels, throughout all social institutions.

21ST CENTURY NEUROSCIENCE: THE CENTRAL ROLE OF THE UNCONSCIOUS, SENSES, AND EMOTIONS IN LEARNING

Contemporary neuroscience, stressing the importance of sensory data, emotions, the body, and the "nature" of learning, is producing a paradigm shift in psychology, education, and treatment of mental illness and brain injury.[14–17] Unlike traditional assumptions about learning and decision making centered in left brain conscious processing and "thinking," psychology, education, and positions on social language and rule acquisition are being reshaped by new understandings of how the brain and body take in environmental data unconsciously via non-verbal communication and emotions (i.e., images of facial expressions and behaviors, voice tones and rhythms) and "digest" that information neurologically and physiologically.

Resonating with psychoanalytic theory of conscious and unconscious brain/body memory and their effects in peoples' lives, neuroscience explains how neural networks, body/brain nerve and chemical connections, emotions, and non-verbal components of the brain house and run unconscious drives, motivations, reactions, and behaviors, and influence conscious choices.

Increasingly sophisticated technologies, like MRI, fMRI, and PET, are pushing the shift from belief in the dominance of disembodied conscious cognitive learning as the root of behaviors and knowledge acquisition to entire body learning that is in part unconscious and not accessible to conscious awareness or critical evaluation. For example, the central nervous system (CNS) perceives and interprets incoming data from all senses unconsciously and non-verbally. How a particular person's CNS perceives and interprets is based on human evolution, a person's familial evolutionary heredity, her/his past experiences laid down explicitly and implicitly (conscious and unconscious memories), and on her/his current psycho-emotional, physical context. Results of unconscious perception (i.e., neuroception, interoception) and interpretation automatically trigger emotions, thoughts, physiological processes, and behaviors.[14,17] This means that without conscious, intentional, critical evaluation or critique, humans intentionally (consciously) and unintentionally (unconsciously) take up and reproduce the society within which they are embedded. This calls into question traditional theories of cognitive development and learning that position society as separate from the biological body, such as social learning theory, socialization, and cognitive development theories. These assume that humans act as agents and decision makers through conscious processing, without unconscious guidance or interference.

Additional key insights of contemporary neuroscience demonstrating reproduction of society via individual embodied enactment of social discourses are: 1) emotional and non-verbal brain centers rapidly develop in utero, and are fully developed by eight months gestation (i.e., limbic system); 2) these unconscious parts of the brain can react to environmental stimuli in 1/12th of a second, are connected to the senses, and are able to induce biochemical changes in the body *before* conscious thought begins; 3) conscious, "thinking parts" of the brain (i.e., cerebral cortex) largely develop during the first three years of life and are much slower to interpret and react than unconscious aspects; 4) physical, emotional, verbal, and non-verbal experiences form brain neurological networks and nerve stimulated pathways throughout the body that are physically stored (explicit and implicit memories); 5) these nerve networks of stored experiences are building blocks of a person's inner world; 6) stored experiences determine how a person consciously and unconsciously interprets the self, others, and the world; and 7) consistent and repeated firing of experience-shaped nerve pathways form patterns that organize behaviors, thoughts, emotions, and understandings of experiences.[14,17]

Contemporary brain researchers and psychoanalytic and poststructural theorists call into question the notion of a "free" will and argue that "will" and agency are not free, but are encumbered by possibilities and limits constructed in society's language and internalized.[3,8–12] In these contexts, the terms internalized and embodied take on very new meanings. People develop, even in utero, within a discursive cultural context that subjugates, or limits, possible ways of understanding oneself, others, and the world. This occurs not only on a conscious level but also on a non-verbal, sense, emotional, and physiological level. The following hypothetical and simplified scenario illustrates how social understandings can become embodied.

A man and woman, believing in existence of innate gender differences based on biology that align with traditional gender norms, get pregnant. They undergo prenatal testing and learn that the fetus is male. This couple believes that males are naturally strong, tough, in control, athletic, and heterosexual, among other male-identified traits.[3,7,8] Having consciously and unconsciously taken up these societal beliefs, the parents assume the fetus is, and the son will be, innately strong and tough, heterosexual, and will have big muscles. The parents act in traditional gender defined ways toward the developing fetus, infant, and growing child. They communicate the social norms they have internalized to the fetus and child physically, non-verbally, verbally, visually, and emotionally via the fetal and child's sensory systems, where they are interpreted and physiologically digested/processed consciously and unconsciously. The parents' behaviors, interpreted by the child's nervous system, are stored in nerve networks to be triggered or activated by social contexts within which the child and subsequent man will be embedded.

PSPADA argues that neither the parents nor child are born with a "God given" knowledge about traditional or dominant understandings of being male or masculinity. Contemporary neuroscience shows that the parents' pre and postnatal conscious and unconscious decisions, their physicality, non-verbal emotional resonance, voice tone, volume (prosody) are transmitted to the fetus indirectly via the maternal physiology, as well as directly to the fetus or child.

Shapiro[17] provides another example of how the unconscious works, demonstrating how physically stored experiences (learning) can surface automatically as a truism outside of critical awareness or examination. She uses the simple poem phrase, "roses are red." She then asks, what comes to mind? Most people, having heard this poem in childhood, automatically respond "violets are blue." Shapiro uses this example to make several points about memories and learning. First and very important, not everything one learns is true. For instance, not all roses are red, and violets are not blue. She points out that the mind/body responded to "roses are red" with "violets are blue" automatically, without conscious processing or critical evaluation, and as if it were true. Thirdly, physically stored implicit memories surface, outside of one's control, without critical thinking, and are reproduced in response to verbal and non-verbal environmental stimuli. These mind/brain/body revelations about sensory data, implicit memory, and unconscious processing merge with current psychoanalytic theory and poststructural discourse analysis in ways that are fundamental for emancipatory research, education, and practice.

POSTSTRUCTURAL PSYCHOANALYTIC DISCOURSE ANALYSIS: EXEMPLARS FROM RESEARCH

A Discourse Analysis of Male Violence Against Women: "Patient Was Hit in the Face by a Fist"[18]

My first foray into discourse analysis was an investigation of the professional and lay literature on "male violence against women."[18] This project was inspired by my work with female victims of male violence and my evolving understanding of language as constituting and reproducing societal knowledge that can work against its presumed intent, and subsequently have adverse effects for the very people who are intended to benefit from the knowledge.

A literature analysis of 165 abstracts and 11 articles that explicitly or implicitly focused on male perpetrated violence against women published between January 1994 and June 1996 was performed.[18] The words "man," "woman," and "male violence against women" were counted, along with words and phrases substituted for "man," "woman," and "male violence against women" (i.e., male and female pronouns and code words). The analysis showed that female gender permeated this male perpetrated violence literature sample.[18] The sample was saturated with explicit female gender (words), including woman, female, she, and her ($N = 744$), and with code words, such as victim, wife, and battered woman ($N = 435$). Explicit male gender words, including man, male, he, and his, were used significantly less frequently ($N = 167$). Code words for the male perpetrator, such as abuser, attacker, batterer, husband, attacker, and abusive partner, were used similarly ($N = 160$). The explicit phrase "male violence" was only used eight times in the *male violence* literature sample. Code words *for male violence against women*, such as abuse, domestic violence, wife abuse, battering, violence, assault, interpersonal violence, family violence, and "the problem" were used 1,044 times.

A qualitative example taken from a report on the 1994 U.S. *Violence Against Women Act* is helpful in revealing the "naturalness" of not mentioning men and, thereby, not implicating males in male violence against women cultural discourses:

> These much needed legislative efforts [1994 U.S. *Violence Against Women Act*] are each important in their own right, but none have sought to address the problem of violence against women as a whole. When I introduced the Violence Against Women Act, I aimed to address a more general problem shared by women victimized by violent behaviors-whether it be a beating at home, a rape by a neighbor, or an assault on the street. I wanted to call this violence by a common name so that we could begin to understand that, although the particular acts may differ, the violence is a shared problem, shared by all women in America.[18(p119)]

In this brief excerpt, men are never mentioned whereas women are explicitly referred to four times, and code words for male violence against women were used 13 times, "violence against women" ($N = 3$), "problem," " general problem," "violent behavior," "beating at home," "rape by neighbor," "assault on the street, " "particular acts," "violence," ($N = 2$), and "shared problem."

The newest version of the *Violence Against Women Act* (VAWA) was signed by President Obama in February 2013. Although the importance of this act cannot be overstated, the language that constructs male perpetrated violence against females has changed very little and is implicated in the very problem it is designed to correct and prevent. President Obama, in his speech before signing the 2013 VAWA, for example, did not mention men or males, whereas he frequently mentioned women and girls. He described (male) violence with language such as "no woman has to choose between a *violent home*" and "victims of domestic abuse and assault" (http://www.whitehouse.gov/blog/2013/03/07/no-one-should-have-live-fear-violenceh). Similarly, in his 2013 VAWA pre-signing speech, Vice President Biden said the word men one time in relation to male culpability, mentioned women and girls frequently, and framed male violence using male invisible language, such as "domestic violence kills three women a day" and "this problem" (http://www.whitehouse.gov/blog/2013/03/07/no-one-should-have-live-fear-violence).

Historical analysis, an aspect of critical discourse analysis, sheds light on the linguistic sleight of hand that constructs male violence against women as a female problem without men. Before the 1960s, male violence against women was not a visible crime, and it was accepted as normal (i.e., "rule of thumb"). This began to change in the emancipatory climate of the 1970s, when feminists publically and explicitly named "male violence against women." However, within 10 years, explicitly named *male* violence against women was once again rendered essentially invisible by increasingly dominant language, such as wife beating, spousal abuse, marital violence, family violence, domestic violence, and interpersonal violence.[18] These discourses inadvertently highlight women and female victims and primarily confine the largely male perpetrated violence to the heterosexual family and "relationships."

Consequences of these cultural conversations are the normative stabilization of women as the problem with the simultaneous concealment of male culpability. Effects of this linguistic process are evidenced in the appallingly low arrest and conviction rates of male perpetrators and ineffectual minor consequences, if convicted, such as low prison sentences, especially when compared to other kinds of assault. Other consequences are naïve, prevalent, and socially sanctioned representations of male practices of violence against women in media, video, and computer games. Contemporary neuroscience and the positions on internalized and then reproduced social discourses help us understand how people, who do not consciously intend harm to women via their writings in professional and popular discourses, inadvertently, unconsciously, and without critical evaluation, reproduce the discourses that make invisible the men in male perpetrated violence and explicitly name and implicitly blame women for the male violence against them.

Exploring New Directions for Ending Practices of Male Violence Against Women: Masculinity, Adolescent Boys, and Culture[3,7,8,19,20]

Poststructural psychoanalytic discourse analysis was a very useful way to analyze cultural discourses of masculinity with an aim of contributing to societal male violence prevention.[3,7,8,19,20] Underlying this research is the assumption that boys and men are not born with an innate set of masculine personality traits including acting violently towards other humans. They are, however, born into a culture where there are continuous messages (verbal, non-verbal, written, visual, emotional, etc.) throughout all cultural institutions about the importance of being "normal," and where normative masculinity is repeatedly signified by practices of dominance, control, physical strength, heterosexuality, homophobia, athleticism, economic privilege, toughness, and violence. Moreover, being "normal" is highly rewarded.

This project involved multiple methods and discourse data sources, including adolescent male discussion groups, individual interviews, and numerous media sources (newspaper articles, television, commercials, movies, video and computer games, and professional and popular literature).[3,19] These are all considered sites of societal discourse reproduction, and each was analyzed for discourses of masculinity.

Poststructural psychoanalytic discourse analysis of interview, discussion group, and media data showed how incessantly reproduced discourses simultaneously constructed a normative and popular boy/man, as well as a non-normative or outcast or boy/man.[7,8,19,20] Identity as a popular (normal) boy was maintained by repeatedly enacting practices such as punking (verbally and physically humiliating another boy in public), heterosexuality (i.e., having an attractive/popular girlfriend), homophobia (i.e., harassing males wearing tight pants, pink clothes, who were nice to other males), athleticism (i.e., playing basketball, football, baseball), dangerous risk-taking (i.e., imitating in public dangerous moves from World Wrestling Entertainment), and violence (i.e., fighting, intimidating, weapons use). Outcast, shunned, and marginalized masculinity were repeatedly reproduced by the negative ends of the same discourses (i.e., publically humiliated victim of punking, not having an attractive girlfriend, wearing the wrong clothes, not participating in sports, walking away from fights, and not taking dangerous risks).

PSPADA also showed how being positioned as normal or as the masculine norm is an elusive achievement that requires repetition to be maintained, as it can be easily toppled.[7] A high school research participant provided an account of the instability and impermanence of normative identity versus the traditionally held notions of innate constant biological masculinity,

If a boy's popular, he's gonna do anything to keep that popularity . . . once you get something like that, you don't want to lose it. . . . If you're popular, it could go away just like that. All it takes is one wrong thing. . . . Then it's over and you're an outcast. . . . You could get dumped by the prettiest girls in school . . . in front of the whole school. . . . It's over, just like that.[7(p224)]

Within a social context that repeatedly signifies normative masculinity as heterosexual, this young man shows that he has taken up and internalized the dominant discourses constituting male heteronormativity and practices of its achievement or loss.

Central to critical PSPADA is locating and accounting for these acts within all kinds of cultural discourses (visual, auditory, policies, societal systems), showing how they regulate gender norms and identities. This type of explication destabilizes gender norms and other normative constructions, liberating their supposedly inherent and fixed biological status. It calls into question non-critical participation in and reproduction of societal discourses and points to individual and societal responsibility for both.

Rivalry, Competition, Wrestling, Playing, and Roughhousing Constituted as Benign: Sibling Violence Silenced[21]

Approximately 22 million U.S. children perpetrate violence against siblings yearly.[21-23] Societal language, however, constructs violent sibling practices with relatively benign language like conflict, rivalry, competition, wrestling, and aggression.[21,23] There is very little research on this topic, and what does exist struggles with definitions and determinations of what are "serious" practices of violence between siblings.[21,23,24] Discourses that *name* verbal, psychological, physical, and sexual violence between siblings explicitly as "violence" are barely visible in multidisciplinary professional discourses and in consumer and popular culture.

PSPADA was one aspect of a larger research project investigating violence between siblings in a sample of children ages 5 to 12 years hospitalized with psychiatric problems.[23] Retrospective review was conducted on medical charts of 135 children (with siblings) admitted to a psychiatric hospital in 2007. All patient records were the discourse analysis sample. These records included notations by multidisciplinary staff (nurses, physicians, social workers, mental health techs, etc.), as well as quotes from the patients, parents and non-hospitalized siblings. Violent acts perpetrated by a sibling against another sibling were described in 103 of the 135 patient records.

To explicate and analyze the language of sibling violence (SV), the records were reviewed for language constituting violent practices against a sibling.[23] After a pilot study was used to develop the data collection tool and establish reliability, practices of violence were categorized for quantitative and qualitative analysis. Instrument categories for violent practices, based on pilot data, included threats to harm, abuse, and/or kill; attempt to drown or smother; bite; hit, kick, punch, shove, and/or choke; sexual abuse (touching, oral, anal, vaginal penetration, pornography); destroys sibling's property; hurts sibling's pet; verbal, emotional, psychological abuse, and/or humiliation; pulls out hair; and other.

Findings showed that the word "violence" or phrase "sibling violence" did not appear in the 103 records that described violence perpetrated by a sibling.[23] The most common signification (descriptions) of violent behaviors were: aggression, threaten, hitting, assault, kicking. Each of these words was embedded in a linguistic context signifying what violent practice the particular writer was documenting related to the single word. For example, practices such as "hitting brother and sister in the eye," "attempting to stab brother and sister with a butcher knife," "stabbing sibling with a pen," "punching, hitting, and kicking," and "pulled knife at 16 year old, threw toys at 10 year old, and pushed 3 and 5 year olds down the stairs" were constituted as "aggression" in the records. "Threat" and "threatening" were embedded in linguistic context such as "threatening to kill mom and sister-assaulting them, hitting, biting, and stabbing with objects" and "threatened to kill his sister with a butter knife."

"Sibling rivalry," "conflict," and "acting out," however naïve and relatively innocent, were found to signify violent and harmful behavior as well.[23] For example, a clinician noted, "patient's mother reported that patient has tremendous rivalry with his 14-year-old sister, and goes after her aggressively in a repeated fashion. . . . He frequently says to his sister, 'I'm going to kill you.'" Similarly, a nurse described "homicidal threat and physical assault of family members [older sister]" as "acting out behavior."

In addition to not explicitly naming violent practices as violence or sibling violence, findings also show that the majority of sibling violence perpetrators were not diagnosed (DSM-IV-TR) with psychiatric diagnoses that included violent behavior as criteria for that diagnosis.[23] In other words, the violent practices documented in the records were not accounted for by a diagnosis that captured regularly perpetrated violent behavior.

From a critical discourse analysis perspective, exposing language like sibling rivalry, competition, and "boys will be boys," that masks the violence and harm of violent practices perpetrated by siblings is needed to deconstruct normalization of this human violence.[21,23] This project provides evidence that mental health professionals, parents, and children participate in and reproduce dominant social language and discursive practices constituting SV as normative and/or benign. Effects of non-critical participation and reproduction include lack of professional attention to these violent behaviors in diagnosing and in protecting victimized siblings. For example, out of the 103 patient charts documenting acts of sibling violence like those described above, only three of these records documented that child protective service (CPS) was contacted to protect victimized siblings.

Other effects of cultural and individual conscious and unconscious obfuscating of SV can be seen in cultural systems, like parent and professional growth and development education, social service and healthcare systems, and popular culture where sibling rivalry, competition, and aggression, are represented as normative and not harmful. Finally, two of the most serious immediate and long-term effects of not taking SV seriously are not protecting victimized children, thereby causing untoward physical and mental health problems, as well as not accurately or adequately addressing SV perpetrators. Consequences of the dominant sibling "violence" discourse are untold and unimagined by society and those embedded within it without critical awareness.

CONCLUSION

Societies, and people within them, can only be known and understood through the language and practices of society. Poststructural psychoanalytic discourse analysis makes social practices and language visible. PSPADA functions as an emancipatory, multi-dimensional, multi-sited social intervention. Emancipatory vision requires seeing the taken for granted, the common sense that links the privileged and the marginalized in reproducing a primarily smoothly running social system that is enabled through everyone's participation, and can largely resist contestations and collective actions. Explicating the ways in which society is reproduced, and how harmful ideological formations and subsequent practices are rendered invisible, were the focuses of this chapter. Violence comes in many forms and the violence of language should not be ignored.

REFERENCES

1. Wright EO. *Envisioning Real Utopias* New York, NY: Verso; 2010.
2. Phillips DA. Language as constitutive: critical thinking for multicultural education and practice in the 21st century. *Journal of Nursing Education* 2000;39(8): 365–372.
3. Phillips DA. Methodology for social accountability: multiple methods and feminist, poststructural, psychoanalytic discourse analysis. *Advances in Nursing Science* 2001;23(4): 49–66.
4. Phillips DA, Drevdahl D. "Race" and the difficulties of language. *Advances in Nursing* 2003;26(1): 19–31.
5. Powell J. *Derrida for Beginners*. New York, NY: Writers and Readers Publishing; 1997.
6. Derrida J. *Positions* (Blass A, Trans.). Chicago, IL: University of Chicago Press; 1972/1981.
7. Phillips DA. Reproducing normative and marginalized masculinities: adolescent male popularity and the outcast. *Nursing Inquiry* 2005;12(3): 219–230.
8. Phillips DA. Masculinity, male development, gender, and identity: modern and postmodern. *Issues in Mental Health Nursing, Special Issue: Men's Mental Health* 2006;27: 403–423.

9. Butler J. *Gender Trouble: Feminism and the Subversion of Identity*. New York, NY: Routledge; 1990/1999.
10. Butler J. *The Psychic Life of Power*. Stanford, CA: Stanford University Press; 1997.
11. Venn C. *Changing the Subject: Psychology, Social Regulation and Subjectivity*. London, UK: Routledge; 1984/1998.
12. Henriques J, Hollway W, Urwin C, Venn C, Walkerdine V. *Changing the Subject: Psychology, Social Regulation and Subjectivity*. London, UK: Routledge; 1984/1998.
13. Bourdieu P. *Outline of a Theory of Practice*. Cambridge, UK: University Press; 1977/2002.
14. Cozolino L. *The Neuroscience of Psychotherapy: Healing the Social Brain*. 2nd ed. New York, NY: W.W. Norton; 2012.
15. Porges S. *The Polyvagal Theory: Neurophysiological Foundations of Emotions, Attachment, Communication, Self-Regulation*. New York, NY: W.W. Norton; 2011.
16. Schore AN. *The Science of the Art of Psychotherapy*. New York, NY: W.W. Norton; 2012.
17. Shapiro F. *Getting Past Your Past: Take Control of Your Life with Self-Help Techniques from EMDR Therapy*. New York, NY: Rodale; 2012.
18. Phillips DA, Henderson D. "Patient was hit in the face by a fist": a discourse analysis of male violence against women. *American Journal of Orthopsychiatry* 1999;69(1): 116–121.
19. Phillips, DA. Exploring new directions for ending practices of male violence against women: masculinity, adolescent boys, and culture. *Dissertation Abstracts International* 2000;61: 5880.
20. Phillips DA. Punking and bullying: strategies in middle school, high school, and beyond. *Journal of Interpersonal Violence* 2007;22(2): 158–178.
21. Phillips DA, Phillips KH, Grupp K, Trigg LJ. Sibling violence silenced: rivalry, competition, wrestling, playing, roughhousing, benign. *Advances in Nursing Science* 2009;32(2): E1–E16.
22. Straus MA, Gelles RJ. How violent are American families? Estimates from the national family violence resurvey and other studies. In: Straus MA, Gelles R, eds. *Physical Violence in American Families: Risk Factors and Adaptations to Violence in 8,145 Families*. New Brunswick, NJ: Transaction Publishers; 1990: 95–112.
23. Phillips DA, Bowie B, Wan DC, Yukevich K. *Sibling Violence in Child Inpatient Psychiatric Population*. In press.
24. Eriksen S, Jensen V. A push or a punch: distinguishing the severity of sibling violence. *J Interpers Violence* 2009;24(1): 183–208.

16 Teaching, Research, and Service Synthesized as Postcolonial Feminist Praxis

Lucy Mkandawire-Valhmu, Patricia E. Stevens, and Peninnah M. Kako

In this chapter, we discuss how the tripartite academic mission of teaching, research, and service can be synthesized as postcolonial feminist praxis. Praxis is here defined as acting collectively to eliminate oppressive conditions and foster emancipation, empowerment, and health. Our engagement with women in the East African countries of Malawi and Kenya is not to satisfy intellectual curiosity but to further praxis. Our goal is to engage students in educational activities that raise their consciousness about marginalizing structures and practices, both locally and globally, so that in their nursing careers they are prepared to recognize, name, and oppose the social inequalities that drive health disparities.

In coalescing teaching, research, and service it is possible to create opportunities for social justice[1] as praxis to occur. Central to this discourse is the idea that in order to promote social justice[1] healthcare providers need to gain a deeper consciousness of the realities lived by the majority of the world's population. As Weedon[2] asserts: "Because racism is so ingrained in Western societies-often taking non-conscious and institutionalised forms-anti-racist strategies require a working through, at an individual and personal level, of often unacknowledged assumptions, prejudices and practices."[2(p1)] Without this consciousness, nurses will continue to engage in racialization by providing standard nursing interventions that are often irrelevant and impractical in addressing the complex health concerns of populations marginalized by race, class, gender, and colonization.[3,4] A postcolonial feminist worldview propels critique and agency in the face of gendered realities and the racism and other long lasting economic, social, and political effects of colonialism in postcolonial contexts. With commitment to dialogue across boundaries and guidance in developing collaborative relationships to address key issues of solidarity and citizenship,[5] nursing students can gain the insights necessary to step outside their own experiences and positively recognize difference. In building our praxis, the continual challenge for us and for our students is to avoid the Eurocentric tendency to see U.S. capitalistic society as the model for the rest of the world.

BACKGROUND AND POSITIONING

We begin by articulating our positioning as authors in relation to the women who are central to our teaching, research, and service. The first author is a native Malawian. The second author is a Euro-American. The third author is a native Kenyan. All authors are academics based in the United States with ties to colleagues at universities in Malawi and Kenya. We acknowledge that our writing is based not only on our scholarly experiences but also on our sociopolitical situatedness, and these often inform one another. Asher[6] asks how teaching, research, and service can be balanced, particularly for women academics of color advancing a leadership role. Our response[7] is that to be responsible, particularly where women of color are concerned, leadership must culminate in alliances that foster the emancipation, empowerment, and health of the communities from which we come. We claim our teamwork is enriched by third world and first world feminist wisdoms. It is important to point out here our recognition that the terms "first" and "third" world are contested while noting that feminist scholars such as Chandra Mohanty use the term *third world* to speak of those occupying spaces with limited resources not only in postcolonial nations but also in wealthier nations where they may be excluded from the benefits and opportunities of modern capitalist states.[8] We use these terms to define the places we inhabit in western academia and to convey a postcolonial resistance to oppression of indigenous peoples.

For a number of years, we have collaborated in scholarly efforts with women in East Africa. Our projects are community based and participatory, providing students with unique immersion opportunities. The teaching, research, and service span a number of issues including HIV prevention and care,[9] HIV testing, reducing violence against women,[10] women's empowerment,[11] income generation activities, orphan care, and food security. Postcolonial feminism, located within the genealogy of a critical paradigm, sharpens our sight on geopolitical and historical influences, helping us grasp how interlocking forms of race, class, and gender oppression can contribute to poor health outcomes.[12] A postcolonial feminist approach to teaching, research, and practice emphasizes the value of understanding the sociopolitical and historical context in which marginalized peoples experience health and invokes praxis that would lead to better outcomes for those who are marginalized.

TEACHING

Although the face of nursing is changing with efforts to encourage and embrace diversity within the profession, the majority of nursing students in the United States continue to be white, female, and middle class. Without concerted efforts, they may graduate unprepared to provide culturally safe, appropriate, and effective health care to an increasingly diverse U.S. popu-lace. Cultural safety implies openness and respect for what can be learned from recipients of care about their beliefs, values, strengths, and burdens. Facilitating the education of culturally safe nurses requires from educators and learners a deep and intricate understanding of the reality of those who occupy marginalized spaces and are the recipients of our nursing care.[13] For example, comprehending the lived experience of a low-income single mother and tailoring nursing care to her reality comes easily for some; many others are unable to envision the challenges that this mother might face.

Poor health outcomes for members of marginalized populations are often preceded by health care providers' lack of awareness or inaccurate under-standing of those deemed "other."[14] Indeed, it is only through direct and continued engagement with the "other" that one comes to deeply under-stand one's own privilege. It is in this context that we created the oppor-tunity for nursing students to become familiar with the everyday lives of people in Malawi and Kenya, who occupy social spaces far removed from their own. We focus our study abroad program on community health. The Institute of Medicine's[15] recommendations for the future of nursing edu-cation emphasize a shift from acute care settings to community settings. When students engage with individuals and families in the community, they are able to see where they live, who they affiliate with, how they manage their affairs, and what stands in their way of achieving health, safety and productivity.

We employ a practical pedagogical approach to facilitate transformative learning and social justice goals. Assigned readings and discussions prompt a postcolonial analysis of political and historical effects on health and health challenges in Malawi and Kenya, helping us avoid colonizing practices that may further oppress communities.[16] Socioeconomic conditions are a case in point. Whereas, in much of the western world, poverty is often hidden and some students may live without ever encountering its ramifications, in most African countries poverty is far from hidden. Malawi is one of the very poorest countries in the world. By studying in Malawi and Kenya, students come into contact with the realities faced by the majority of Malawians, where over half of the population lives below the national poverty line of less than $1 a day.[17] Similarly in Kenya where 43.4 percent of its citizenry live on less than $1.25 a day, nearly half of the Kenyans struggle to provide daily food for their families and 46 percent of those who live in rural areas lack access to clean water.[18,19] Women and children walk miles in search of daily drinking water and often go to sleep without an evening meal. An important learning outcome for students is an understanding of how such scarcity of food and clean water came to be and how it affects families.

Assignments place students in situations where they have to engage with women and children in their environments, performing individual and com-munity nursing assessments and coming up with intervention plans based on a postcolonial analysis. In their postcolonial analysis, students are able to come to an understanding of the impact of colonialism on migration of family members from urban to rural environments resulting in for instance, child-headed households when orphaned children cannot be absorbed into the extended family that has disintegrated due to migration. Students not only benefit by achieving their own learning outcomes, but they also give back to the communities who enable their education.[20] Students pair up with women and their families to identify health needs and make key assessments. On one trip, students uncovered the need for guidelines to facilitate HIV status disclosure to orphaned children infected and affected by HIV and responded to the unique needs of child-headed households left parentless by AIDS. Faculty and doctoral student research projects were spawned by these student discoveries and are currently underway, demonstrating how teaching, research, and service can be effectively synthesized in nursing academia. One example of a clinical project completed by three master's students focused on the "Implementation of On-Site Rapid HIV Testing among Orphaned Children in Southern Malawi." Another example of a dissertation in progress by a doctoral student is "The Integral Relationship between Virtue and the Self-Appraised Subjective Well-Being of Vulnerable Youth Heads of Households in Rural Southern Malawi."

RESEARCH

As feminist scholars, the research we engage in is driven by needs of the communities with whom we interact. We value our partnership with women throughout the research process, which results in narratives about women's experiences that emphasize their subaltern knowledge and their capacities and strengths. Our recommendations for health and social policy are thereby grounded in the realities of women's lives.[21] The writing of women's experiences needs to be done thoughtfully to ensure that it advances liberation and does not contribute to the further marginalization of women. Our feminist research in East Africa explicates the harsh realities and limitations that third world women face while avoiding the negation of women's agency in their own health promotion. This is indeed not an easy feat.

Compared to most mainstream women in higher income countries, East African women are disproportionately disadvantaged. The economic disparities between high-income and low-income nations are vast; and from these economic disparities health disparities follow, disproportionately affecting women. To illustrate, the Gross Domestic Product (GDP) in the United States is $48,100 per capita. The GDP in Kenya is equivalent to $1,600 per capita, and in Malawi it is equivalent to $1,000 per capita.[22] Coupled with race and gender oppressions historically and politically situated in colonial and imperialistic dynamics, these economic facts translate into very real challenges for women that have significant health implications. To provide an example, globalization can have negative implications for the health of women, particularly poor women in low-income countries.[23] Prior to western domination, cultural norms placed power in extended family members to protect women from violence and destitution. These cultural practices have eroded as individual family members attempt to survive in an increasingly capitalist society where education is key. But women's ability to achieve an education is hampered by gendered responsibilities and structural factors that do not favor women. HIV vulnerability is further increased by limited power to negotiate safe sex and limited livelihood options for meeting basic needs apart from dependence on male partners. Despite these intersecting oppressions, women innovatively leverage limited resources, including reliance on one another, to promote their own health and that of their children and their communities.

Grassroots women's movements and their impact on health have seldom been studied in low-income nations. However, our studies of women living with HIV in Malawi and Kenya continuously demonstrate that women can and do provide one another with emotional and material support in communities where infrastructure is missing. Participants in our studies often attribute their survival to other women who recognized their HIV symptomatology and provided them the necessary support to seek out HIV testing and access lifesaving medications. In research like this, third world women can be heard and engaged in a rewriting of history so that their accomplishments do not go unrecognized. Future generations of women can believe in their own abilities and have hope for their futures if such narratives are available to them and to those caring for them. As academics in the nursing profession, our role in documenting these grassroots feminist movements is to ensure that African women's history and their pivotal roles in the era of HIV/AIDS are not erased. Further, as nursing academics we have the opportunity and obligation to partner with women in these movements to help facilitate their effectiveness in health promotion. This is true not only of grassroots women's movements on the African continent, but it is true of grassroots movements for all the women we encounter who occupy spaces on the margins of society and whose history of struggle and victory in the face of daunting challenges is yet to be acknowledged and documented.

We involve undergraduate and graduate students in our research, facilitating their travel to Malawi and Kenya for data collection purposes. As students enter into spaces very unlike those they regularly occupy in the United States, they develop a deeper consciousness of the realities faced by the majority of the world's citizens. They come to see how knowledge is constructed communally, rather than by a privileged few, and learn of the collective responsibility for knowledge construction that we all have as global citizens.[24] In their research activities, students come to recognize that Malawian and Kenyan women are very cognizant of the realities of HIV infection, including how it is transmitted and the particular personal risks they face. The discussions that ensue between students and women living with HIV are often not about how HIV is spread but rather how women can negotiate safe sex given their gendered limitations and how they can use their collective power as women to facilitate the health of other women in their communities. These immersion experiences with those who had formerly been considered "other" prepare students for future interactions in which they have the skills to tailor nursing assessments, nursing interventions, and nursing research because they understand that sociopolitical factors like poverty, stigma, and social role expectations are central to the health of individuals, communities, and populations.[12]

SERVICE

We involve students in service learning through collaborations with U.S. and local non-governmental organizations (NGOs) in Kenya and Malawi that have community-based feeding programs for women living with HIV and their families and through helping to bring needed supplies to health centers. Our longest running service projects to date are in partnership with an NGO supporting orphaned children in rural Southern Malawi. These projects have resulted in hundreds of orphaned and vulnerable children being HIV tested with treatment referrals for those with positive results. Such service activities provide strategic, much needed health care and also give students chances to develop their skills at trust building, community negotiation, and responsible follow-through on delivered services.

Mohanty[25] speaks of the need to form strategic partnerships across race lines, class lines, and geographic borders. To initiate and maintain trust in these partnerships, observable actions are required. Communities must be able to see nurses' willingness to meet face-to-face, their ability to listen and speak at the appropriate times, and their generosity of time and self.[13] Students learn these lessons firsthand. Other insights come from learning about collective identity and shared decision making. Socialized in a western individualistic orientation where personal autonomy is valued above all, students traversing geographic and social borders learn from communities where collectivism and cooperation are the norm.

The collective capacity that ensues from synthesized teaching, research, and service facilitates stronger partnerships between academia and communities.[12] Our partnership with women and children across the world creates a space for their voices to be heard, helping to ensure that women's issues are addressed in policy and practice.[26] These kinds of partnerships, based on feminist solidarity, are not akin to historical colonial and hegemonic relationships between developed and developing nations. Rather, they offer critique of globalization and policies enforced by primarily western-based international conglomerates that disadvantage women in developing nations.[5] It is through service informed by postcolonial feminist consciousness that students develop as nurses who will advance social justice agenda for the betterment of humanity in the generations to come.

CONCLUSION

As nurse scholars, we are committed to a collective responsibility to work with and for women to ensure the articulation of subaltern knowledge. From a feminist perspective, it is vital to our collective liberation to leverage the power of our resources in the western world, such as knowledge production outlets, with the strengths and creativity of the women whom we serve. In an era of dwindling resources, transnational feminist organizing is key to this liberation movement. As we move forward, we need to take advantage of the porosity of borders to forge alliances and capitalize on what we have to offer each other.

We support the emancipation, empowerment, and health of all peoples. Such praxis is not accomplished by pity or rescue efforts but through authentic relationships. In today's global village where borders are porous and communities who are recipients of nursing care are no longer homogenous, nurses must engage in analysis of the positions they themselves occupy and consider how they are privileged and/or marginalized. With a postcolonial feminist praxis grounded in women's agency, nurses can rewrite a history that has nullified the experiences of developing world women or depicted them as victims in need of western intervention in order to survive. Together with women and their communities, as we also advance the education of a future generation of nurses so can we write the realities of complex and courageous characters who occupy positions on the very margins of society yet act ingeniously to raise their children, stay healthy, and contribute to their communities.

REFERENCES

1. Buettner-Schmidt K, Lobo ML. Social justice: a concept analysis. *Journal of Advanced Nursing* 2012;68(4): 948–958.
2. Weedon C. Key Issues in Postcolonial Feminism: A Western Perspective 2002. Gender Forum Web site. http://www.genderforum.org/issues/genderealisations/key-issues-in-postcolonial-feminism-a-western-perspective/. Accessed April 8, 2014.
3. Racine L. Implementing a postcolonial feminist perspective in nursing research related to non-western populations. *Nursing Inquiry* 2003;10(2): 91–102.
4. Tang SY, Browne AJ. 'Race' matters: racialization and egalitarian discourses involving Aboriginal people in the Canadian health care context. *Ethnicity & Health* 2008;13(2): 109–127.
5. Reilly N. Cosmopolitan feminism and human rights. *Hypatia* Fall 2007;22(4): 180–198.
6. Asher N. How does the postcolonial, feminist academic lead? A perspective from the US South. *International Journal of Leadership in Education. Theory and Practice* 2010;13(1): 63–76.
7. Mkandawire-Valhmu L, Kako P, Stevens PE. Mentoring women faculty of color in nursing academia: creating an inclusive environment that supports scholarly growth and retention. *Nursing Outlook* 2010;58(3): 135–141.
8. Mohanty CT, Russo A, Torres L. *Third World Women and the Politics of Feminism*. Indianapolis, IN: Indiana University Press; 1991.

9. Kako PM, Stevens PE, Karani AK. Where will this illness take me? Reactions to HIV diagnosis from women living with HIV in Kenya. *Health Care for Women International* 2011;32(4): 278–299.

10. Mkandawire-Valhmu L, Stevens PE. Applying a feminist approach to health and human rights research in Malawi: a study of violence in the lives of female domestic workers. *Advances in Nursing Science* 2007;30(4): 278–289.

11. Mkandawire-Valhmu L, Stevens PE. The critical value of focus group discussions in research with women living with HIV in Malawi. *Qualitative Health Research* 2010;20(5): 684–696.

12. Reimer-Kirkham S, Varcoe C, Browne AJ, Lynam MJ, Khan KB, McDonald H. Critical inquiry and knowledge translation: exploring compatibilities and tensions. *Nursing Philosophy* 2009;10(3): 152–166.

13. Woods M. Cultural safety and the socioethical nurse. *Nursing Ethics* 2010;17(6): 715–725.

14. Brondolo E, Gallo LC, Myers HF. Race, racism and health: disparities, mechanisms, and interventions. *Journal of Behavioral Medicine* 2009;32(1): 1–8.

15. The future of nursing. Focus on education. Institute of Medicine Web site. 2010. http://www.iom.edu/Reports/2010/The-Future-of-Nursing-Leading-Change-Advancing-Health/Report-Brief-Education.aspx. Accessed April 8, 2014.

16. Racine L, Perron A. Unmasking the predicament of cultural voyeurism: a postcolonial analysis of international nursing placements. *Nursing Inquiry* 2012;19(3): 190–201.

17. Malawi at a glance. 2010. http://devdata.worldbank.org/AAG/mwi_aag.pdf. Accessed April 17, 2013.

18. Kenya National Bureau of Statistics (KNBS) and ICF Macro. *Kenya Demographic and Health Survey 2008–09*. Calverton, MD: KNBS and ICF Macro;2010.

19. United Nations Human Development Report. Country Profile: Human Development Indicator (Kenya). 2013. http://hdr.undp.org/en/countries/profiles/KEN. Accessed April 8, 2014.

20. Mkandawire-Valhmu L, Doering J. Study abroad as a tool for promoting cultural safety in nursing education. *Journal of Transcultural Nursing* 2012;23(1): 82–89.

21. Mkandawire-Valhmu L, Wendland C, Stevens PE, Kako PM, Dressel A, Kibicho J. Marriage as a risk factor for HIV: learning from the experiences of HIV-infected women in Malawi. *Global Public Health* 2013;8(2): 187–201.

22. The World Factbook: Malawi. 2011. https://www.cia.gov/library/publications/the-world-factbook/geos/mi.htm. Accessed April 8, 2014.

23. Anderson JM. Lessons from a postcolonial feminist perspective: suffering and a path to healing. *Nursing Inquiry* 2004;11(4): 238–246.

24. Ntseane PG. Culturally sensitive transformational learning: incorporating the Afrocentric paradigm and African feminism. *Adult Education Quarterly* 2011;61(4): 307–323.

25. Mohanty CT. Under western eyes. *Feminist Review* 1988;30: 61–88.

26. Sadiqi F. Facing challenges and pioneering feminist and gender studies: women in post-colonial and today's Maghrib. *African & Asian Studies* 2008;7(4): 447–470.

Section IV

Critical Practice Approaches and Methodologies

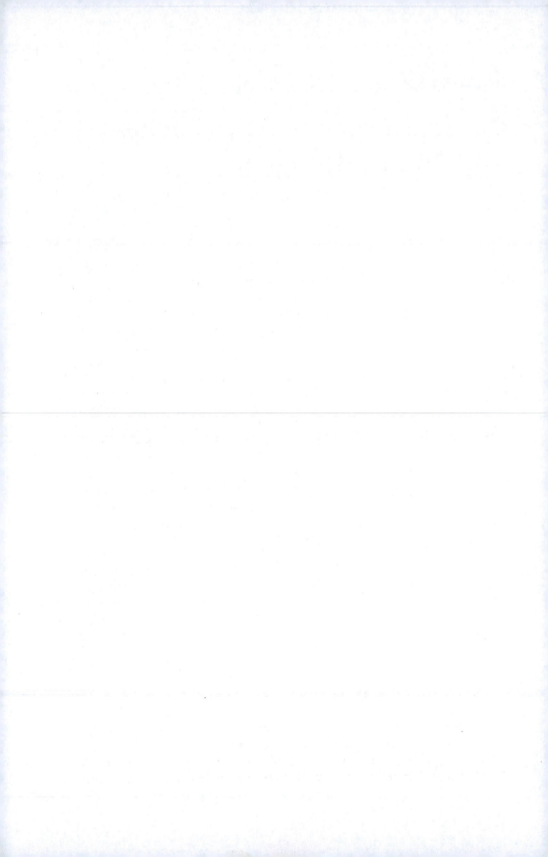

17 Cultivating Relational Consciousness in Social Justice Practice

Gweneth Hartrick Doane

When I was invited to write this chapter on social justice I felt much as I did several years ago when I was invited to join a research team focused on ethics. Confessing to the colleagues who had extended the invitation that ethics was not really my area, they replied, "all of the relational stuff you write about is ethics." Having read the ethics literature I was not convinced. However, once we began conducting focus groups with practicing nurses, hearing their stories of trying to "do good" in the midst of complex health care situations,[1] the connection between what my colleagues described as "ethics" and my own "relational" concerns and interests became apparent.

In a similar vein I confess that I do not really come from the community of scholars who devote their attention to social justice. Yet I share a kinship—something like a close relative who shares a bloodline—and I am deeply committed to compassionate, socially just action. However, as a visiting relative (the position from which I write this chapter) I am aware that my "different" background shapes my frame of reference, my interpretations, and my language. I am not fully apprised of the family intricacies within the social justice world, yet as someone who shares a kinship I am interested in furthering the relational connections. In this chapter I focus my attention on that site where social justice and my own relational concerns intermingle in an attempt to loosen the boundaries between the two conceptual domains. My intention is to explore how, in the urgencies of health care practice, social justice and the "relational" imperative that orients my work might be more intricately interwoven. I begin this exploration by recalling a conversation I had with a nurse, Allie (pseudonym), a few months ago while doing a research project on an acute medical unit.[2]

"I'M AFRAID OF WHO I AM GOING TO BECOME"

I had never actually met Allie before but she told me that she had graduated from the B.S.N. program at my university. The program has a particular emphasis on social justice and relational inquiry, which is what I believe sparked her telling me this story. She began by saying that she had graduated two years before and had been working on the medical unit since that time. She described how much she loved nursing and working on the unit but how she was struggling.

> The staff here are really caring but I have watched people change—people who graduated from the same program who really believed in everything the program teaches (compassionate, critically informed, socially just care) now treat patients in ways that I find so distressing. Yesterday I was at the nursing station and one of the senior nurses was in a room across from the station with one of the nurses who graduated a year ahead of me. The patient was a man who was homeless and had been brought in quite ill. I heard the senior nurse tell the more junior nurse to strip his clothes off and just throw them out because who knew where they had been. She said it in a tone of such disgust and the man was right there hearing everything. They didn't even acknowledge his presence. The other nurse just said ok as though there was nothing wrong with what had just happened. And the worst part is I didn't do anything about it. I just stood there feeling stunned and powerless. To them the only problem was the patient, they didn't see anything wrong with their actions. As I looked at the nurse who had just graduated a year ahead of me I felt sick—how is that possible that she doesn't see what happened as a problem, that she didn't respond to the patient in some way? And how is it that I just stood there letting it happen? There are so many experiences like that on the unit. I know my colleagues aren't bad people so is that just what happens over time? It makes me so afraid of who I am going to become!

Listening to Allie and witnessing her distress I felt my own angst surface. As an educator who had indirectly participated in educating Allie to be a critically aware, compassionately engaged, socially just nurse—schooling her to take up, integrate, and enact that identity—I was brought face-to-face with the enormous responsibility and obligation we had bestowed upon Allie and what that obligation was costing her in that moment. Of course, this was not the first time I had heard such a story about the complex realities health practitioners face in contemporary health care milieus. But as William James described, "experience has ways of boiling over, and making us correct our present formulas."[3(p107)] As I sat with Allie, the enormity of the elephant was directly in front of me, so to speak. As the rawness of her emotion and the fear she felt for her very personhood spilled over, the limitations of educational approaches and the knowledge she had been given became glaringly real. Allie had been offered theoretical and critical tools and even some behavioral technologies to assist her in dealing with issues of social justice. She was clearly able to recognize injustices and was committed to practicing in a socially just manner. However, the knowledge and practices she had developed had not sufficiently prepared her for the situation at hand. While armed with some helpful tools, she did not seem to have *a way of being in the midst of* social injustice. Perhaps an analogy would be to say that she knew she was a boat (identity as a socially just nurse) with an array of workable parts (nursing ideals, critical tools, theoretical frameworks, and epistemologies) but was not sure how to assemble the navigational system and/or connect to the power source in stormy weather.

It is this relational assemblage that has been at the heart of my own scholarly work and that was called into question as I sat listening to Allie. I began to wonder how the distress she was feeling might at least in part be a consequence of the way she was relationally orienting within the situation. Two specific elements seemed significant: (a) the subject-object relational stance that appeared to underpin her practice and (b) the mismatch between the complexity of the situation and her own relational complexity.

The Subject-Object Relational Stance

As Allie described her experience it was possible to hear the social justice orientation that shaped her interpretations of the situation. For example, she described her concern about the treatment of the man whom she saw as a "marginalized person" and her alarm that her colleagues were seemingly oblivious to their "demeaning and disrespectful" actions. Within the story it was also possible to hear one of the most powerful ideologies underlying health care practice, one that has a profound impact on relational comportment: the ideology of "change."[4] Situated in powerful discourses of problem solving, alleviation, and cure, change tends to be a primary goal of health care practice. Relationally, this goal can at times translate into an "other" orientation. That is, relational attention becomes focused on something other than "what is"—on changing "what is" into something else (unhealthy people into healthy people, unjust practices into just ones, and so forth). This focus on change sets up a very particular relational stance— namely a subject-object stance in which subjects (health care practitioners) operate on objects (patients, injustices, and so forth) to affect change. In this relationship, subjects are "identified with, tied to, fused with, or embedded in"[5(p32)] particular values and concerns. Objects include those elements "that we can . . . be responsible for . . . take control of . . . or otherwise operate on."[5(p32)] Allie's words reflect this ideology of change and the subject-object relational stance it gives rise to. As subject, Allie's relational attention was oriented toward the objects that she felt obligated to "operate on" as a socially just nurse (she clearly wished to address the injustice by acting to affect change). This subject-object stance shaped the way she related to the situation, to her colleagues, and to herself. When she did not act to change what was happening, the focus of Allie's attention became her failure to act, which sparked a fleet of emotions and questions about herself as a nurse and the person she was becoming.

Within Allie's story the insufficiency of a subject-object relational stance becomes apparent. The stance of subject operating on object was, quite simply, insufficient for the complexities at hand. For example, the nurses Allie worked with were good people, as was she, yet they did not act in accordance with the tenets of social justice. These and other complexities in the situation served to blur the distinction between subject and object and Allie had difficulty identifying a clear object she could "operate" upon. While an injustice toward the man needed to be addressed, what of her colleagues? Moreover, what of her own inaction? By not acting, she had in essence become another object that needed to be addressed. As she became both subject and object her confusion and dismay grew.

The Complexity Mismatch

Allie's story illustrates the complexity mismatch between contemporary health care situations and the subject-object relational stance. With inequities, constraints, and injustices being part and parcel of many health care situations,[6] health practitioners frequently find themselves in incredibly complex and at times conflicted relational spaces. As they are bombarded with decreased staffing ratios, the escalating pace of practice, and competing values, interests, and obligations, a subject-object relational stance cannot correspond (quite literally) with the challenges they face. From a relational perspective a crucial question needs to be asked: what might help health practitioners to effectively navigate *within* the complex relational spaces of contemporary health care practice? Drawing upon John Caputo's contention that "reason is to respond to things, to keep up a correspondence with them"[7(p228)] might a reasonable way to proceed be that of enhancing our own relational complexity to help us negotiate the realities of contemporary milieus?

Enhancing Our Relational Complexity: Developing Relational Consciousness

Kegan and Lahey contend that "When we experience the world as 'too complex' we are not just experiencing the complexity of the world. We are experiencing a mismatch between the world's complexity *and our own at this moment*. There are only two logical ways to mend this mismatch—reduce the world's complexity or increase our own."[8(p12)] The diversity of cultures, values, interests, and ideologies make health care milieus incredibly complex spaces of care. Given this reality, and the fact that the complexities are in all likelihood only going to grow, health practitioners need a relational orientation that matches that reality—that is able to correspond to/ with that level of complexity. The ideological emphasis on change and the subject-object relational stance it gives rise to is not only too linear but also too simplistic. As such, it serves to limit our capacity to relate to and within the complex realities of health care situations. Subsequently we need to enhance our own relational complexity if we are to effectively correspond and relate within the complex spaces of contemporary health care.

Increasing our relational complexity requires the development of a *relational consciousness*, a consciousness that involves paying close attention to how we are relating *within* situations, and inquiring into our own relational comportment—to the how, what, where, why, and when of the situation we find ourselves in.

A View from Beneath the Boulder

Vaclav Havel (the Czech Republic's first president), in his 1990 address to the United States Congress,[9] spoke to the form of relational consciousness I am suggesting. Having been imprisoned "beneath the pall of a totalitarian system," Havel asserted that that experience had enabled "a special capacity to look from time to time somewhat further than someone who has not undergone this bitter experience. A person who cannot move and lead a somewhat normal life because he is pinned under a boulder has more time to think about his hopes than someone who is not trapped that way."[9] In describing the instruction this experience offered, Havel claimed that it gave him "one great certainty: consciousness precedes being, and not the other way around, as the Marxists claim."[9]

Certainly the idea of consciousness is not new—it has been integral to the social justice mandate. Yet Havel's words embody an interesting *relational* twist. Having experienced years of living in a situation in which the realities were such that change and/or transformation (the central tenets of social justice practice) were curtailed, Havel was faced with his own human fallibility. Pinned under a boulder and unable to affect change and/or to relate in the world in his normal way, Havel was ultimately called to look to the one thing he could affect—namely the consciousness that was governing who/how he was *within* the situation. His emphasis on consciousness preceding being speaks of a consciousness that *is* a way of relating. Moreover, it points to a way of relating when one is unable to move or act in the desired way—a consciousness that *is* a navigational system (a way of being/relating) while *in* constraining situations.

The relational consciousness that Havel alluded to has conscious presence at its core. Similar to Berman's description of the nomad who dwells in the mid-region, *inhabiting a world presence that is oriented toward awareness of oneself in relation*,[10] it is a consciousness that takes the form of an ongoing question: how am I inhabiting and relating, how am I present within the current circumstances? This calls forth a *relational consciousness*, in which one moves out from behind the social justice text to *stand in front of it*.[11] Standing *in front* of the social justice text the focus becomes how one might inhabit social justice ideals and values within the complexities of the current moment. In contrast to orienting through a subject-object stance and attempting to enact social justice values and ideals by taking oneself up as a change agent, one *relates to* the social justice text as a question that can *inform* action. As Rorty asserts, the temporal circumstances of human life are difficult enough "without sado-masochistically adding immutable, unconditional obligations."[12(p76)] Shifting our relationship with the social justice text (by standing in front rather than behind it), the focus of our attention becomes that of relating with ever more sensitivity to ourselves, to the people we care for, and to the situations we find ourselves in.[12] This shift in attention—this relational consciousness—focuses on more whole-heartedly relating to who, where, and how we *are* in any particular moment, thus orienting us in our own and others' complexity and in the in-between spaces: in the gaps between ourselves and each other, between real and ideal health care situations and our world. In this way, this relational consciousness can provide a way of moving when it seems there is no way to go. Our attention and action shifts from what "should be" to *what is* actually happening.

When we are pinned under a boulder and feeling unable to change the circumstances of a situation, this *relational consciousness is our source of power and system of navigation for social justice practice.* That is, in "thinking of everything as relational through and through,"[12(p72)] the focus of our conscious attention moves to what is and is not happening *relationally*. One orients through a relational consciousness by asking: (a) How am I relating within what is happening? (b) What am I *not* wanting to relate to? and (c) How might I relate more fully? As a practice of attention, this orientation increases our imaginative power to responsively form our social justice practice within the complex realities of existing health care situations.

Relational Consciousness: Relating within What Is

While social justice action is most often oriented toward lessening fallibility, relational consciousness requires that we go a bit against the grain and more intentionally *be in* the emotionally laden seas of human frailty and imperfection. In essence it involves relating in a way that allows us to see the complex intermingling of people, experiences, needs, values, and so forth—to know and relate to and in the situation more fully. This does not mean we do not want to affect change and/or aspire toward social justice ideals. We are just shifting *how we relate* to the social justice text. It involves more intentionally relating to "what is"—to the present realities of the situations we need to respond to and act within. This includes relating to those aspects we may not want to relate to, for example, the shadow elements in ourselves and others. A relational consciousness asks: who/what am I primarily relating to? What is dominating my attention, including my interpretations, emotions, and responses? What am I privileging? What am I *not wanting to* relate to? And how is my relational orientation shaping my experience and my action? Central to this inquiry process is *letting things be* without adding our own by-lines that result in static still shots and bounded views of people and situations. It includes noticing and exercising the skill of holding our by-lines of good/bad, right/wrong in abeyance and focusing our attention on engaging more concertedly.[4] As we step out of the subject-object stance and relate more wholeheartedly through this inquiry process, it is possible to see beyond the dualism of letting be or change (and beyond the assumption that to "let be" means everything stays the same).[4] By extending ourselves to know and relate to "what is," we are better able to correspond within and to the situation at hand.

To be clear, I am not suggesting that a social justice framework is not a good thing or that we should not address injustices and/or work to affect change. I am proposing a particular form of *relational consciousness to be lived* while in the midst of social justice practice. It is a way of *being in* the multifaceted emotions, angst, and fallibilities of health care situations that can heighten our connectedness, address the complexity mismatch, and enhance our response-ability. As Holecek contends, "Knowing there is a light at the end of the tunnel keeps us going through it, but understanding the darkness in the tunnel helps us to negotiate it."[13(p32)] Cultivating our relational consciousness may enable more effective negotiation of the tunnels we find ourselves within.

Unclouding Our Relational View

One of the central aspects of relational consciousness is that of noticing and interrupting thing-thinking.[13] Comparable to the distinction between still shots and moving pictures, we often relate to people and situations by freezing or "thinging" them. We look through our own interpretive frames and shape the complex relational flow of living experience into still shots[14,15] as we define, judge, and assign meaning to people and circumstances. Regardless of whether our interpretations are accurate, what is significant relationally is the way in which this process of "thinging" solidifies relational matter[13] and hinders our relational responsiveness. While the practice of naming/distinguishing can create order and help us see things more clearly (for example, the naming of social inequities), the concern is that by relating in such bounded, static ways our vision can be clouded.[13] Moreover, as the relational flow is halted by bounded understandings our relational response-ability is constrained. As Holecek describes, ignorance is not only a result of being uninformed. It can also come from being too *informed*. "Ignorance is made of the fabric of cognition, of that which knows."[13(p241)] Thus any interpretive framework can serve to form what we see in ways that are limiting—can bring clarity that clouds our view. Relational consciousness brings attention to the way our thing-thinking and the still shots we create can shape and potentially limit our view. It shifts attention to the complex interplay among people, health care situations, and our own responses.

As we engage in this relationally conscious manner, we are also called to engage with the dark shadows that are part and parcel of social justice practice. Highlighting the importance of this shadow engagement, Palmer points out that if we look at leaders such as Vaclav Havel or Nelson Mandela we can very clearly see the choices that determined not only their own futures (and who they were/became) but that of their worlds.[16] "Isn't it remarkable how Nelson Mandela took 30 years in prison to prepare himself for leadership rather than for despair? He went down, and he went in, and he dealt with the violence and terror, and he emerged a leader of amazing strength able to lead people toward our complex and inexplicable caring for each other."[16(p36)] Palmer's description of Nelson Mandela exemplifies the power of relational consciousness. Mandela made the intentional choice to address the violence and terror by relating to it more whole-heartedly. As Caputo[7,15] might say, he struck up a correspondence with the darkness. By purposefully relating *with* the darkness, he was subsequently able to lead his country on a very intentional and explicit journey. The Truth and Reconciliation process was in essence a relational process that enabled the deep shadows of pain, suffering, and violence to be witnessed and the compassion and potential of the South African people to be expressed and realized. Mandela cultivated a *relational consciousness* by grounding the process in a common suffering (compassion). This relational consciousness served to forge relationships with and between people, atrocities, and possibility. Other examples of people who have made the intentional choice to address social injustices and discrimination by relating to them more fully include celebrated poet, novelist, and civil rights activist Maya Angelou and Supreme Court Justice Sonia Sotomayor. For example, in a recent interview Justice Sotomayor described how she used the disadvantages—the social injustices—as a base from which to open to her own sense of vulnerability and fear of failing (http://paw.princeton.edu/issues/2013/03/06/pages/4558/index.xml).

Central to each of these people's lives has been the willingness to relate more fully to darkness and human imperfection. While critical consciousness directs health practitioners to examine and get to know themselves, what I have long found missing in the discussions of consciousness in social justice is the question of *how* we relate to ourselves. I was reminded of this missing element as I listened to Allie. Do we offer the same compassion and inclusivity to ourselves as we attempt to offer to others? Do we relate in a wholehearted way, listening to the contradictory and/or unseemly elements within ourselves? Do we marginalize and "other" aspects of ourselves that do not fit within the bounded identity of the socially just practitioner? Are we as authentic and compassionate with ourselves as we require ourselves to be with others? Relational consciousness rests in the understanding that our unfavorable elements cannot be argued out of existence or rationalized into harmlessness.[17] Most often they are deeply ingrained patterns and habits that cannot be simply unpacked or discarded. Thus, *the crucial aspect, relationally, is to associate with those hidden elements, not dissociate from them.*[17] As Mayes asserts, when we face the hidden and imperfect aspects of ourselves—the shadows and dark recesses—we are more able to relate to them in others. Awareness of our own fallibility somehow serves to temper our "sanctimonious responses" and extend our relational responsiveness.[18(p33)] A relational consciousness includes a good inner chairperson who provides hospitality to all feelings and aspects, even (and perhaps especially) those we tend to deprecate.[19] Whether we are relating to ourselves or to others, it is this relational quality of openness and compassion that is crucial.

CONCLUSION

Caputo describes how, as we attempt to reconcile our experience with our lofty ideals and best laid theories, we are brought face to face with the limitations of any concept or theoretical construct.[7] "We are faced with the problem not only of what we know but what we are to do."[7(p236)] It is this site between what we know and what we are to do where social justice and relational practice are intimately connected. Caught between what is happening and what should be happening, between health care realities and social justice ideals, it is possible to lose our moorings and become alienated from who and what we aspire to be, from others, and from the situations in which we find ourselves.[20] Rorty contends that what is required in such moments is faith in our ability to redescribe ourselves, to reimagine and recreate ourselves.[12] I would suggest that cultivating a relational consciousness can support us in that reimagining process. In their analysis of the Nursing Manifesto, Kagan et al. quote Hagedorn, Chinn, and Cowling, "We believe that it is possible to find connection in the midst of alienation, to find inspiration in the midst of cynicism."[21(p13)] It is this finding of connection that relational consciousness provides a pathway toward.

REFERENCES

1. Varcoe C, Doane G, Pauly B., Rodney P, Storch, J, Mahoney K, et al. Ethical practice in nursing: working the in-betweens. *J Adv Nur* 2004;45(3): 316–325.
2. Stadjuhar K, & Hartrick Doane G. *Knowledge Translation in Action: Improving the Quality of Care at the End of Life*. Ottawa, Canada: Canadian Institute for Health Research; 2008.
3. James W. *Pragmatism. A New Name for Some Old Ways of Thinking*. New York, NY: Longmans, Green and Company; 1907.
4. Hartrick Doane G. Beyond behavioral skills to human-involved processes: relational nursing practice and interpretive pedagogy. *J of Nurs Edu* 2002;41(9): 400–404.
5. Kegan R. *In Over Our Heads. The Mental Demands of Modern Life*. Cambridge, MA: Harvard University Press; 1994.
6. Woods M. Exploring the relevance of social justice within a relational nursing ethic. *Nurs Phil* 2012;13(1): 56–65.
7. Caputo JD. *Radical Hermeneutics. Repetition, Deconstruction, and the Hermeneutic Project*. Bloomington, IN: Indiana University Press; 1987.
8. Kegan R, Lahey L. *Immunity to Change*. Boston, MA: Harvard Business Press; 2009.

9. Havel, V. Address to the U.S. Congress, Knihovna Vaclav Havel Library. February 21, 1990. http://www.vaclavhavel-library.org/en/vaclav-havel/works/speeches. Accessed April 20 2012.
10. Berman M. *The Wandering God.* Albany, NY: State University of New York Press; 2000.
11. Ricoeur P. *From Text to Action.* Evanston, IL: Northwestern University Press; 1991.
12. Rorty R. *Philosophy and Social Hope.* London, UK: Penguin Books; 1999.
13. Holecek A. *The Power and the Pain. Transforming Spiritual Hardship into Joy.* Ithaca, NY: Snow Lion Publications; 2009.
14. Caputo JD. *Against Ethics.* Bloomington, IN: Indiana University Press; 1993.
15. Caputo JD. *More Radical Hermeneutics. On Not Knowing Who We Are.* Bloomington, IN: Indiana University Press; 2000.
16. Palmer P. Leading from within. *Noetic Sciences Review* 1996;40: 32–42.
17. Singer J. *Boundaries of the Soul. The Practice of Jung's Psychology.* New York, NY: Random House; 1994.
18. Mayes C. Ten pillars of a Jungian approach to education. *Encounter: Education for Meaning and Social Justice* 2005;18: 30–41.
19. Daloz L, Keen C, Keen J, Parks S. *Common Fire. Leading Lives of Commitment in a Complex World.* Boston, MA: Beacon Press Books; 1996.
20. Hartrick Doane G. Am I still ethical? The socially mediated process of nurses' moral identity. *Nurs Ethics* 2002;9(6): 623–635.
21. Kagan PN, Smith MC, Cowling WR, Chinn PL. A nursing manifesto: an emancipatory call for knowledge development, conscience, and praxis. *Nurs Phil* 2009;11: 67–84.

18 Facilitating Humanization

Liberating the Profession of Nursing from Institutional Confinement on Behalf of Social Justice

Danny Willis, Donna J. Perry, Terri LaCoursiere-Zucchero, and Pamela Grace

INTRODUCTION

Social injustice, or the societal conditions that lead to dehumanization for certain populations, has a significant impact on human health. The profession of nursing has a critical potential—and mandate—to advance social justice in order to further health for vulnerable communities. But realizing this potential requires the nursing profession to liberate itself from prevailing conventional views that nursing is practiced mainly within the confines of medical institutions and is consequently largely subject to the rules and structural constraints imposed by others.

As we argue below, nursing's mandate to advance social justice emerges from the ontological, epistemological, and ethical foundations of the profession as well as its own historical development. Nursing responsibility includes recognizing and addressing social injustices; this is an historical role of nurses that seems to have lost its visibility contemporarily. Yet abandoning this duty destabilizes the profession's ability to direct its own practice in accord with its own goals related to well-being and deprives vulnerable populations of an important advocate. When this duty is abandoned, we have removed ourselves as players in the larger social realm by not focusing on those forces that impact human well-being, leaving us and the populations we serve at the mercy of social forces and rendering us powerless. The destabilizing occurs because we remove ourselves from fundamental disciplinary goals of attending to the whole person and their environments. For example, only attending to the presenting signs and symptoms associated with cirrhosis of the liver in a person suffering with alcoholism, without addressing the underlying circumstances, origins, and contributing factors, leaves us unable to promote human well-being from a nursing perspective for such individuals.

This chapter discusses the philosophical underpinnings of nursing action and argues that the profession is responsible for envisioning the full range of nursing actions (education, research, investigating root causes, sociopolitical activity) needed to fulfill its goals of furthering health and well-being. Moreover, this is a moral responsibility of the discipline for reasons given shortly. We use the terms moral and ethical interchangeably in the context of fulfilling professional aims.

In this chapter we first discuss the link between determinants of health and social justice and then discuss nursing's mandate to address these determinants as emerging from ethical, ontological, epistemological, and historical foundations. We examine reasons for nursing's failure to fulfill this mandate as partially due to institutional confinement and discuss a philosophical approach to liberation of the profession. We also discuss social injustice as a process of dehumanization and nursing social justice action in terms of facilitating humanization.

SOCIAL DETERMINANTS OF HEALTH

Social conditions have a profound bearing on human health and well-being. Several social factors have been linked with adverse human health outcomes including the corporate concentration of wealth and power,[1] environmental hazards,[2] collective violence,[3] and discrimination.[4] Moreover, research has shown that the negative health effects of social ills are not borne equally throughout society.

The landmark 2002 report *Unequal Treatment: Confronting Racial and Ethnic Disparities* brought the issue of health disparities to the forefront of the national health care agenda.[4] This report made clear that unequal health outcomes were not only due to problems within the health care system but also to social factors such as socio-economic differences and cultural bias against racial and ethnic groups.

The global impact of social factors on health inequality has been further articulated by the World Health Organization's (WHO) Commission on Social Determinants of Health.[5] The report of the Commission explicitly links health inequities with social inequalities in power distribution, earnings, shelter, access to education, health care, climate change, and other living conditions. The Commission argues that unequal social conditions can be remedied and that remediating these inequalities is an issue of social justice—and presents the global community with associated ethical imperatives.

> Social justice is a matter of life and death. It affects the way people live, their consequent chance of illness, and their risk of premature death . . . avoidable health inequalities, arise because of the circumstances in which people grow, live, work, and age, and the systems put in place to deal with illness. The conditions in which people live and die are, in turn, shaped by political, social, and economic forces. (iii, not numbered)[5]

THE FOUNDATION OF NURSING PROFESSIONAL RESPONSIBILITY FOR SOCIAL JUSTICE ACTION

The issue of social justice, what constitutes social justice, what the warrants for social justice are, and how to achieve it within and across societies remains a controversial philosophical and practical question. However, we argue that this question need not be answered fully in order for the nursing profession to understand that social obstacles to equitable human health constitute injustices of varying kinds. This chapter contributes to that ongoing dialogue by discussing social injustice/justice in terms of dehumanization/facilitating humanization processes. Purposeful consideration and action regarding social justice is a logical extension of nursing's own ethical-ontological-epistemological-historical foundation. The sections below highlight the important underpinnings of our professional mandate.

Nursing's Social Mandate: The Profession's Ethical Responsibility to Address Injustices

Ethics is the study of the good; what the good is, and how we go about choosing it. Nursing's moral foundation is based on the duty to do good for persons and society. When we cannot achieve this good, further moral deliberation leads us to reflect on what factors might be preventing this good and what actions must be taken to address those barriers. Such a deliberation leads us to consider root causes in the social structure.

In the United States, nursing's social mandate to care for vulnerable populations has been outlined in the American Nurses Association's *Social Policy Statement*.[6] This responsibility is also acknowledged by the International Council for Nursing Code of Ethics,[7] which represents nurses globally and acknowledged by numerous scholars internationally.[8–10] "The nurse shares with society the responsibility for initiating and supporting action to meet the health and social needs of the public, in particular those of vulnerable populations."[7(p3)]

The basis for asserting this as an ethical responsibility of the profession is that nursing cannot fulfill its "promises" to promote a good for society[11,12] if social conditions cause recurring problems or there are other obstacles to well-being anchored in societal arrangements.

Nursing's Social Policy Statement[6] calls for nursing to influence public policy to promote social justice. One of the key themes of the Social Policy Statement is that nursing is an *evolving* profession with an obligation that is *responsive* to changes in society. In the absence of attention to the grounds in which health issues arise, nursing cannot fulfill goals of optimizing human health.[13] The profession's social mandate means that we must include attention to this aspect of the human condition in all of our endeavors: the education of nurses, research, and practice endeavors. The evolution of nursing practice to include knowledge and action for social justice is not only a reasonable and responsible progression of these core perspectives in response to society's needs but also it is an obligation.

Ontology

Ontology is a branch of philosophy that considers the existence of objects, including but not limited to life-forms. That is, it is a field of inquiry about what it means for an entity to exist within the world. Nursing's ontology is about the reason that nursing needs to exist as a profession. Implicit in nursing's coming into existence first as an occupation and then as a profession is that human beings need a certain type of service that they cannot provide for themselves. Nursing's ontology is informed by a perspective of human beings as whole, and in relationships with self, others, and environment. Health, according to the ANA's Code of Ethics is "understood as being broader than delivery and reimbursement systems, but extending to health-related sociocultural issues such as violation of human rights, homelessness, hunger, violence, and the stigma of illness."[14(p25)] Following WHO, the National Institute of Nursing Research (NINR) has defined health as, "not merely the absence of disease, but an optimal state of physical, mental, and social well-being."[15]

Inherent in these definitions is the notion that health cannot be achieved within the confines of a health care institution. Neither can nursing actions be so confined. A growing body of research as noted above makes clear that the sources of suboptimal physical, mental, and social well-being lie in the social structure itself. In order to assist populations to maximize well-being in the fullest sense we must, as a profession, move our attention beyond the boundaries of the health care infrastructure to the broader society as a whole.

Epistemology

Epistemology is the study of knowledge, how we come to know things, and what it means to claim that we know something. Nursing's epistemological development has been shaped by its holistic ontology and includes multiple ways of knowing. Carper's seminal work on patterns of knowing included the empirical, personal, ethical, and aesthetic patterns. White proposed adding a fifth sociopolitical pattern to capture the environmental context that "lifts the gaze of the nurse from the introspective nurse-patient relationship" to the broader socio-political context.[16(p83)] However Spenceley, Ruetter, and Allen[9] proposed that rather than adding a new pattern of knowledge that those patterns could be brought to bear on policies and systems. Chinn and Kramer[17] have suggested a new pattern called "emancipatory knowing" that notices and critically examines social injustices and identifies the changes needed to effect social and structural change. Emancipatory knowing in this sense is akin to our discussion of liberation. Similarly, Butterfield[2] calls for nursing to expand its knowledge base and use strategic advocacy to advance from individual to collective public interests at an "upstream" level. Grace[12] proposes the concept of "professional advocacy" through which nurses can address both the needs of the individual patient in the immediate practice environment as well as the wider society. The work of these scholars points to the need for a broader epistemological lens through which nursing can address larger antecedents of health while still maintaining the commitment to individual care.

HUMANIZATION/DEHUMANIZATION AND SOCIAL JUSTICE

Concern about social issues affecting health brings nurses into such arenas as health disparities, environmental injustice, collective violence, and human rights—ideas that ultimately move us beyond the limitations of institutional confinement in our thinking and actions. Although these realms entail distinct bodies of scholarship, we suggest that they can be linked together through the lens of social justice. Below we build on the previous work of Willis, Grace, and Roy[18] to discuss their proposed central unifying focus for nursing as "facilitating humanization" and a broader application of this focus towards achieving social justice.

Humanitarian nurses in the late 19th century as discussed above, for example Florence Nightingale and Lillian Wald (among others), set the stage for nursing's humanistic ethic and professional advocacy. They intentionally investigated and subsequently articulated the underlying social, political, and economic conditions—such as war and poverty—negatively influencing individual, family, and community health and developed and implemented action plans to help those most in need. They focused their efforts, if not solely, on improving environments not conducive to health, alleviating suffering, and promoting optimal conditions for those injured in war, the poor, children, families, etc. Contemporarily, we find threads of their humanistic ethic toward social injustices in the leading documents of the discipline. The ANA's *Social Policy Statement* posits the goal of nursing as "the protection, promotion, and optimization of health and abilities, prevention of illness and injury, and alleviation of suffering through the diagnosis and treatment of human responses and advocacy in the care of individuals, family, community, and populations."[6(p10)] The actions of social-reforming nurses, like Nightingale and Wald, significantly influenced how people in their time lived and died. They took whatever means necessary to pursue good solutions to immediate health problems and addressed the social determinants of health, or what contemporary public health scholars term "upstream"[2] determinants of health; that is, those social, psychological, economic, and political factors impeding the health of individuals, families, communities, and populations. At this time in our evolution as a profession, we believe that nursing *must* re-invigorate its role in social reformation, building on the legacy of Nightingale, Wald, and others. In the 21st century, the nursing profession *must return to its roots*, liberating itself from the narrow confines of practice within medical institutions and medicalized healthcare systems as discussed later. To aid this process of liberation, we believe that a conceptualization of social justice in nursing that accounts for our professional goals is required, and this conceptualization must include two key aspects of social justice—outcomes and process. Thus, we identify outcomes of social justice on behalf of health and well-being and propose an action-oriented process for achieving social justice in nursing.

Definitions of Social Justice: Outcomes and Process

We have been challenged to find a conceptualization in nursing of social justice that is consistent with nursing's primary goal of optimizing human health (described above, ANA Social Policy Statement). From within a nursing perspective and specific to the outcomes of social justice for health and well-being, we recently proposed that Powers and Faden's[19] public health model of social justice is constructive for understanding universal human needs for well-being.[20] They propose six essential dimensions of well-being necessary for living a "minimally decent" human life. We refer readers to our discussion of their model where we discuss social justice outcomes, noting that their outcomes are broad in scope and congruent with nursing's goals.[20] Thus, nurses are provided with outcomes of social justice (Powers and Faden's six essential dimensions): (a) health, (b) personal security, (c) reasoning, (d) respect, (e) attachment, and (f) self-determination.

Although Powers and Faden have advanced a careful examination of social justice outcomes that are relevant for nursing, they have not provided a process for actualizing such outcomes, leaving nurses to take on that challenge from within our unique disciplinary perspective. Thus, a critical next step in nursing's professional evolution towards fully embodying social justice practice is our articulation of a process for achieving social justice outcomes. We propose a process for undergirding and actualizing social justice practice within nursing; namely, that of *facilitating humanization*, a central unifying focus of the discipline.[18] The thinking of two of the authors (Danny G. Willis, Pamela Grace) who originally proposed "facilitating humanization" as part of a group of scholars has evolved over time. In concert with the two co-authors of this chapter, we now view facilitating humanization as the overarching essence for nursing scholarship and practice, constituting a new metaparadigm concept. Facilitating humanization is different from the related concept of caring by explicitly linking nursing knowledge and professional obligations with social justice, of which caring is a critical dimension. From a nursing perspective, facilitating humanization has as its fundamental aim the provision of respect and moral worth for every individual as human. As such, it necessarily involves the nurse entering into a trusting, humanistic, caring relationship with the recipient of care, thus being related to caring, but going beyond caring by exploring the patterns and underlying origins of threats to health and of health and well-being that manifest from person-and-environment mutual interactive processes.

Facilitating humanization stems from the ontology of the nursing discipline and, by its very nature, mirrors the underlying precept of universal human rights. That is, each human being is to be considered an important individual with values and concerns that should be respected. No human being should be used as a means by which other persons realize their goals, a form of dehumanization. This means that if we accept anything as a universal precept it is that every human being should be considered of equal moral consideration, thus facilitating humanization. Many philosophical and religious foundations have been offered as a basis for this claim but perhaps the least controversial is that we all have interests in living and thriving. If those interests are not respected for any one of us then we are all at risk for dehumanization and of having our interests disrespected.[13] Facilitating humanization constitutes a nursing perspective and process that aids nurses in meeting a fundamental moral obligation of the profession, whereby social injustices are addressed.

Facilitating humanization is a nursing process for achieving social justice. It is "manifested when the nurse works with all human beings grounded in an ontology of human beings as relational, experiential, valuable, respect-worthy, meaning-oriented . . . vulnerable, complex, and capable of [experiencing] health and healing even if not capable of being cured."[18(pE34)] The major goal of facilitating humanization is ensuring an environment whereby human beings (persons) can actualize their potential for well-being, especially in those circumstances where dehumanizing conditions thwart these potentials. Unfortunately, scholars have described diverse domains of dehumanization stemming from individual and intergroup beliefs, fears, motivations, and attitudes, including, but not limited to, ethnicity/race (immigration, genocide, human rights violations), objectification of women, disability, homophobia/heterosexism, technology, social stigma (mental illness, etc.), and deterministic and instrumental approaches to persons.[21] Referring to these domains of dehumanization, it becomes clear that none of them include an in-depth complex understanding of the meanings of individual and societal well-being. That is, the domains of dehumanization, by their very nature, are described in ways that point to their lack of privileging the other's humanization, meanings, choices, quality of life, and overall needs pertaining to experiences of health and healing. Whenever human beings' sense of personal and social well-being and their qualities and experiences associated with meaning, choice, quality of life, and healing are not addressed, dehumanization occurs.

Dehumanization is a primary concern for nursing's social justice mission as dehumanization thwarts human beings' potentials for well-being. It could be argued that dehumanization constitutes the primary need for social justice practice in nursing. In accordance with nursing's social mandate, nurses *must* thoughtfully act in the face of dehumanizing conditions. Dehumanizing conditions like violence, social health disparities, discrimination, and wealth and power struggles should be some of the major concerns for contemporary public health scholars and nurse educators and clinicians. Additionally, nurses themselves may hold biases and prejudices thereby contributing to social injustice when they fail to recognize their prejudicial attitudes and subsequently engage in any of the -isms and forms of institutional violence, racism, classism, etc. Such conditions are directly and indirectly related to human health and well-being. For example, scholars have identified avenues by which social, environmental, and economic factors have an effect on health including neighborhood conditions, working conditions, education, income and wealth, race and racism, and stress.[22] Thus, a process for achieving social justice in nursing, facilitating humanization requires nurses to think and act beyond the narrow confines of the medical institutions and medicalized healthcare systems in which they find themselves. This broadens their perspectives and spheres of influence beyond the proximal health problems of care recipients, or what some scholars refer to as "downstream" social determinants of health, toward action directed at "upstream" social determinants of health.[22,23]

The process of facilitating humanization is characterized by multiple nursing actions. Facilitating humanization is the expression of great concern by nurses for human well-being, in which they assure, through whatever ethical means necessary, that human beings are accorded socially just, humanistic, caring environments in which their needs, meanings, choices, quality of life, and healing are privileged in living and dying.[18] The process of *facilitating humanization by the nurse* is characterized by:

- drawing upon the multiple patterns of knowing in nursing as described earlier and exercising critical consciousness to identify and rectify dehumanizing circumstances and oppressive power dynamics interfering with human well-being;
- collaborating with other nurses, healthcare professionals, and interested stakeholders (politicians, business owners, philanthropists, teachers, community organizers, lawyers, engineers, etc.) to develop multi-pronged strategies for addressing social injustices;
- collaborating with those directly affected by social injustices to discover the root social, environmental, educational, and economic issues associated with injustices and their influence on well-being;
- intentionally humanizing everyone encountered in the professional nursing situation entrusted to our care, especially those most affected by dehumanization and social injustices, by carefully attending to each individual as worthy of equal moral respect;
- privileging questions pertaining to life world, meanings, choices, quality of life, and healing of individuals, families, communities, or populations;
- developing (as necessary), implementing, evaluating, and revising (as necessary) strategies, action plans, and interventions—including education and social or health policy—to promote individual, family, community, and population well-being;
- identifying existing positive strengths and traits among those individuals, families, communities, and populations affected by socially unjust situations;
- building upon human strengths to leverage action and transformation in unhealthy, socially unjust situations;
- educating, articulating, and demonstrating the unique role nursing plays in substantive knowledge development and utilization of knowledge on behalf of individual and societal well-being; and
- modeling and advocating humanistic relating for others.[18]

AN UNREALIZED POTENTIAL

Despite the social mandate of nursing enshrined in normative documents such as codes of ethics and social policy statements of the associated countries of practice and even the inspiring examples of individual nurses, the full potential—and responsibility—for nursing social justice action remains unrealized. This calls for us to transcend the barriers imposed by institutional confinement.

This unrealized potential is highlighted in one nursing study that examined the influence of nursing advocacy on Massachusetts state legislators.[24] The study showed that a nursing presentation focused on asthma and the relationship between environmental hazards and health disparities significantly increased legislators' favorability towards an environmental justice bill. However, when questioned about the topics of nurse advocacy, the legislators were significantly more likely to perceive nursing testimony to be more often about issues related to the nursing profession (such as staffing ratios) as compared to general health issues. Qualitative comments supported this perception and also indicated that general health testimony from nurses would be welcomed on issues such as the link between housing and health. Thus the results suggested that nurses' testimony can effectively influence public policy yet nurses are not fully using their power to effect social policy change that could advance health.[24]

A number of reasons have been postulated regarding nursing's inadequate efforts to address larger social issues, particularly at the level of policy. Spenceley et al.[9] provide a comprehensive analysis of the research and scholarly reflection on nursing political advocacy dating back several decades. Some of the writings they reviewed identified barriers related to feelings among nurses that larger problems are outside their domain of influence,[25] perceived powerlessness and lack of peer support,[26] and the potential for risk engendered by advocacy activities.[12] Other authors' works reviewed for this paper, some of which Spenceley et al.[9] refer to, have identified barriers, such as: (a) insufficient time/intellectual space due to competing work demands[27]; (b) tension between individually focused care versus community focused care[10,12]; (c) nursing's history as a largely female and disempowered group[28]; (d) lack of understanding of health policy[27]; (e) need for greater knowledge about upstream issues that impact health[2]; (f) an overly introspective focus within the discipline of nursing[28]; (g) the "tyranny of the research industry" marginalizing "the higher goals and ideals in nursing scholarship"[29(p239)]; and (h) a detachment that has lost sight of nursing's origins as agents of social change.[1]

Emphasizing that nursing education alone will not address these barriers, Spenceley et al.[9] categorize these obstacles as existing: within the nursing profession, within the context of nursing practice, and at the discourse interface between nursing and policy. They note that many nurses lack opportunities to participate in policy processes and to gain experience in policy discourse. A study by Warner[30] suggests that successful nurse policy activists took advantage of opportunities to build networks and relationships that helped them to advance their political expertise. Warner argues that nursing leaders, practitioners, and educators must expand their political competence in order to advance the political development of the profession as a whole.

In an analysis of key American Nurses Association's documents, Bekemeier and Butterfield[24] charge that there is an inadequate framework for nurses to address broader social justice issues. They reviewed the *Code of Ethics for Nurses with Interpretive Statements, Nursing: Scope and Standards of Practice* and *Nursing's Social Responsibility Statement* and noted that despite references to the historical role of nursing in social reform the documents were largely focused on individual patient care.

A similar disconnect can be viewed in the NINR definition of health as including "social well-being" while articulating that nursing research develops knowledge to: "Build the scientific foundation for clinical practice"; "Prevent disease and disability"; "Manage and eliminate symptoms caused by illness"; and "Enhance end-of-life and palliative care."[31] The NINR foci as stated do not make explicit the context of social justice, however implicit within these foci are social injustices as root causes or obstacles to good care. In order to advance nursing knowledge development for social justice, funding is critical. Therefore it is important for nurse scholars to interpret these NINR foci in light of social injustices. It is incumbent on nurse scholars to emphasize the critical point that underlying NINR research goals are issues of social injustice.

We suggest that nursing as a profession is limited by its longstanding confinement within the medical and social institutions of health care. A medical and disease model has certainly been the predominant focus of nursing education, practice, research, and funding. This medicalized and institutionalized focus has contributed to the internal and external constraints noted above and impedes nursing from fulfilling its potential to facilitate humanization. Although nursing has long regarded health from a broad ontological perspective there has been an ontological disconnect in which "health" has been conflated with "health care."

The meaning expressed by the word "patient" in ANA documents is not only reflective of *individual* nursing care but also connotes nursing practice in a health care *institution*. Nurses are socialized from the very beginning of their careers to practice in health care institutions. For example, practical training is typically done in "clinical rotations" that are for the most part conducted within medically dominated institutions. Even community health rotations are largely focused on care of "patients" who are at home but still within an institutionalized medical context of illness. Once nurses begin practice they are plunged into a world in which they need to master the technical art of clinical nursing practice in order to become competent practitioners. Although social justice is mentioned as an essential concept in leading U.S. nursing education documents, it is unclear if courses in individual schools of nursing address the full scope of social change needed to actualize social justice, health policy, and social policy affecting health. The nursing profession has largely developed within an institutionalized medical milieu that has profoundly influenced the internal development of the profession. In fact, Bekemeir and Butterfield[23] argue that nursing roles have themselves been institutionalized by those in power and embedded within a corporatized health care structure.

Because social justice is embedded in the institutions of the social structure, in order for nurses to address social injustice they must be able to transcend these institutions. This does not mean abandoning the care of acutely ill individuals but rather integrating that care into a broader context. Nor does it mean leaving institutions behind. It means paying attention to institutions—how they work and don't work—and collaborating with other members of civil society for positive change. This includes both health care institutions and the larger social infrastructure. We do not imply that this work is easy or without challenges. In fact, fulfilling nursing's mandate to address social injustices will require resisting all sorts of pressures not to.

A PARADIGM SHIFT IN NURSING CONSCIOUSNESS THROUGH VERTICAL LIBERTY

Flaskerud and Nyamathi call for "a new paradigm that recognizes societal factors as primary pathogenic forces in the major health problems facing the U.S. today."[8(p139)] Interestingly, we can find a similar sentiment in the writings of Lavinia Dock, over a century ago.

> Of old the nursing sisters of the religious orders, closely confined in shackles of mental subjugation and social renunciation, consciously withdrew from all participation in things of the world . . . held no radical hopes of remaking the social order around them. . . . If their paths were strewn with the wrecks of social justice they patiently and untiringly bound up the wounds and nursed the victims without a protest. We have cast off their shackles because we refuse to be cut off from the world about us . . . human society can be voluntarily and consciously built into nobler and fairer forms than those of the past. [32 (p 897)]

In the above quote, Dock twice mentions the word "consciously." The relationship between nursing and the social order is predicated on recognizing the broader social forces influencing health. This relationship can be seen on a continuum from conscious withdrawal to conscious engagement with the broader social forces influencing health. Along with Dock, we call for a collective shift in nursing consciousness to address the issues leading to social injustice. However, the historical example of Lavinia Dock along with the numerous policy statements cited above illustrates, such a shift is not *away* from nursing roots but really a *return* to our roots with a fuller embracing of nursing's understanding of the human person and health.

Bernard Lonergan, a Jesuit philosopher, was interested in how reflective conscious human understanding could be used to improve the human situation. His philosophy of freedom offers a way to think about how to simultaneously return to our nursing roots while at the same time achieve a paradigm shift in nursing consciousness. Although a full explication of his philosophy is beyond the scope of this paper an overview of his work on liberty will be discussed briefly below.

For Lonergan, responsible action is linked with knowledge obtained through attentive, intelligent, and reasonable cognition. But this is not an automatic process. "Essential freedom," for Lonergan,[33] is the dynamic structure of human cognition that entails sensory input, practical insight into possible courses of action, reflection about projected risks and outcomes, and execution of decision through action. "Effective freedom" is the operational range within which the individual can choose and carry out possible courses of action. The potential for freedom exists within human consciousness but choices emerge in an individual and community context of effective freedom that can limit the range within which essential freedom is expressed. This potential can be limited both by internal as well as external barriers. For example, external barriers might include financial limitations. Internal barriers emerge from psychoneural restrictions such as fears, limitations in one's range of practical insights for action, and unwillingness to undertake certain courses of action.

Previous research[34] has suggested that internal and external constraints are intimately connected and that external barriers can be internalized, leading to pervasive internal barriers such as internalized social stigmas. Social transformation of external barriers often requires first overcoming internal limitations such as feelings of powerlessness and fear, linking back to some of the barriers identified for nursing. Internal transformation can provide individuals and communities with the knowledge and strength to transform external social barriers in turn. As external barriers are reduced, the effective freedom is expanded for those who follow.

We would suggest then that interwoven internal and external barriers cited earlier constrain "nursing effective freedom." *Nursing effective freedom* is a term coined by Perry during our discussion for this chapter stemming from her research using Lonergan's perspective. Furthermore, these barriers prevent nursing from greater involvement in social justice concerns. Internal barriers such as feelings of professional oppression, powerlessness, and time constraints are interrelated with external barriers related to the prevailing institutional roles of nursing practice and limited opportunities and preparation for political involvement. Liberation must come from within the profession itself through the essential freedom inherent in nursing consciousness. Critical reflection on the ontological, epistemological, and ethical foundations of nursing against the prevailing social situation of human needs and the barriers that prevent nursing from social justice action can bring forth inner transformation of professional understanding along with creative practical insights to be implemented in nursing education, research, and practice.

As nursing social justice action is expanded and integrated within the scope of practice there will be a gradual corresponding expansion in nursing's range of effective freedom. Thus, liberation of the profession from institutional confinement begins with the critically reflective and creative "essential freedom" of nursing consciousness that will devise the necessary changes to expand the range of "nursing effective freedom" for social justice action. Only then will we be able to become full actors in the efforts to transform society and facilitate humanization in the fullest sense.

The notion of vertical liberty can provide further insight into the process of nursing transformation. Lonergan[35] uses the work of Joseph de Finance, a Jesuit French philosopher, to distinguish horizontal liberty from vertical liberty. Horizontal liberty occurs when choices are perceived from within a determinate horizon of reference. Vertical liberty occurs when commitment to an ideal draws a person, or persons, out of their horizon to a new understanding and actions in realization of their ideals. Previous research on issues of social transformation[34-36] has indicated that genuine commitment to an ideal such as social justice can draw an individual to new actions to realize that ideal in successive situations. This results not only in progressive action but transformation in the person themselves. As noted above, nursing is committed to ideals outlined in various policy statements. Yet our realization of these ideals remains unfulfilled. *Facilitating humanization* has been proposed as a central unifying focus for the discipline and can thus be viewed as an ideal that is only partially realized, always drawing us to deeper understanding and action. Critically reflective engagement on facilitating humanization can lead nursing to act for social justice in a manner that is both transformative and at the same time grounded in the ideals of nursing's ontological, epistemological, and ethical roots. These ideas are congruent with the *Nursing Manifesto*[37] and the subsequent conceptualization of emancipatory knowing and "praxis as simultaneous reflection and action directed toward transforming the world"[(p81)] articulated by Kagan, Smith, Cowling, and Chinn.[38]

CONCLUSION

We advocate the use of *facilitating humanization* as a perspective and process for envisioning the full range of nursing's professional responsibilities to individuals and society. Most importantly, our argument supports the idea that the nursing profession must take seriously its obligation to investigate the underlying causes of poor health and social conditions. This entails the discipline and profession of nursing liberating itself from institutional confinement.

REFERENCES

1. Schroeder C. The tyranny of profit: concentration of wealth, corporate globalization, and the failed US health care system. *Adv Nurs Sci* 2003;26(3): 173–184.
2. Butterfield P. Upstream reflections on environmental health: an abbreviated history and framework for action. *Adv Nurs Sci* 2002;25(1): 32–49.
3. Krug EG, Dahlberg LL, Mercy JA, Zwi AB, Lozano R, eds. *Collective Violence. World Report on Violence and Health*. Geneva, Switzerland: World Health Organization; 2002: 213–240. http://www.who.int/violence_injury_prevention/violence/world_report/en/. Accessed October 16, 2012.
4. National Research Council. Unequal Treatment: Confronting Racial and Ethnic Disparities in Health Care (Full Printed Version). Washington, DC: The National Academies Press; 2003. http://www.nap.edu/catalog.php?record_id=10260. Accessed October 16, 2012.
5. Commission on Social Determinants of Health. *Closing the Gap in a Generation: Health Equity through Action on the Social Determinants of Health. Final Report of the Commission on Social Determinants of Health*. Geneva, Switzerland: World Health Organization; 2008. http://whqlibdoc.who.int/publications/2008/9789241563703_eng.pdf. Accessed August 24, 2012
6. American Nurses Association. *Nursing's Social Policy Statement: The Essence of the Profession*. Silver Spring, MD: Author; 2010.
7. International Council of Nursing. *Code of Ethics for Nurses*. Geneva, Switzerland: Author; 2012. http://www.icn.ch/about-icn/code-of-ethics-for-nurses/. Accessed October 16, 2012.
8. Flaskerund J, Nyamathi A. New paradigm for health disparities needed. *Nurs Res* 2002;51(3): 139–140.
9. Spenceley, SM, Ruetter L, Allen MN. The road less traveled: nursing advocacy at the policy level. *Policy Polit Nurs Pract* 2006;7(3): 180–194.
10. Tripp-Reimer T. Critical health needs of communities and vulnerable populations: clinical nursing research for vulnerable populations. In AS Hinshaw, SL Feetham & JL Shave, eds. *Handbook of Clinical Nursing Research*. Thousand Oaks, CA: SAGE; 1999: 71–73.
11. Grace PJ. A philosophical analysis of the concept 'advocacy': implications for professional-patient relationships. Unpublished dissertation. Knoxville, TN: University of Tennessee-Knoxville; 1998.
12. Grace PJ. Professional advocacy: widening the scope of accountability. *Nurs Philos* 2001;2(2): 151–162.
13. Grace PJ. *Nursing Ethics and Professional Responsibility in Advanced Practice*. Sudbury, MA: Jones and Bartlett; 2009.
14. American Nurses Association. *Code of Ethics for Nurses with Interpretive Statements*. Washington, DC: American Nurses Association; 2001.
15. National Institute of Nursing Research. *Bridging science to life: NINR strategic plan*. http://www.ninr.nih.gov/aboutninr/ninr-mission-and-strategic-plan. Accessed April 3, 2014.
16. White J. Patterns of knowing: review, critique, and update. *Adv Nurs Sci* 1995;17(4): 73–86.
17. Chinn PL, Kramer MK. *Integrated Theory and Knowledge Development in Nursing*. 4th ed. St. Louis, MO: Mosby Elsevier; 2008.
18. Willis DG, Grace PJ, Roy C. A central unifying focus for the discipline: facilitating humanization, meaning, choice, quality of life, and healing in living and dying. *Adv Nurs Sci* 2008;31(1): E28–E40.
19. Powers M, Faden R. *Social Justice: The Moral Foundation of Public Health and Health Policy*. New York, NY: Oxford University Press; 2006.

20. Grace PJ, Willis DG. Nursing responsibilities and social justice: an analysis in support of disciplinary goals. *Nurs Outlook* 2012;60: 198–207.
21. Haslam N. Dehumanization: an integrative review. *Pers Soc Psychol Rev* 2006; 10: 252–264
22. Braveman P, Egerter S, Williams DR. The social determinants of health: coming of age. *Annu Rev of Public Health* 2011;32: 381–398.
23. Bekemeier B, Butterfield P. Unreconciled inconsistencies: a critical review of the concept of social justice in 3 national nursing documents. *Adv Nurs Sci* 2005;28(2): 152–162.
24. Perry D. Transcendent pluralism and the influence of nursing testimony on environmental justice legislation. *Policy Polit Nurs Pract* 2005;6(1): 60–71.
25. Heath H. Reflection and patterns of knowing in nursing. *J Adv Nurs* 1998;27: 1054–1059.
26. DiGaudio, KM. Nurses' participation in policy making activities. Unpublished dissertation. Buffalo, NY: State University of New York; 1993.
27. Aries N. To engage or not engage: choices confronting nurses and other healthcare professionals. In DM Nickitas, DJ Middaugh, N Aries, eds. *Policy and Politics for Nurses and other Health Professionals: Advocacy and Action.* Sudbury, MA: Jones and Bartlett Publishers; 2011: 3–23.
28. Mechanic D, Reinhard SC. Contributions of nurses to health policy: challenges and opportunities. *Nurs and Health Pol Rev* 2002;1(1): 7–15.
29. Petrovskaya O, McDonald C, McIntyre M. Dialectic of the university: a critique of instrumental reason in graduate nursing education. *Nurs Philos* 2011;12(4): 239
30. Warner JR. A phenomenological approach to political competence: stories of nurse activists. *Policy Polit Nurs Pract* 2003;4(2): 135–143.
31. National Institute of Nursing Research Web site. http://www.ninr.nih.gov/. Accessed August 29, 2012.
32. Dock L. Some urgent social claims. *Am J Nurs* 1907;7: 895–901.
33. Lonergan B. *Insight: A Study of Human Understanding.* 5th ed. In: FE Crowe, RM Doran, eds. *Collected Works of Bernard Lonergan*: Vol. 3. Toronto, Canada: University of Toronto Press. 2000; 618–56.
34. Perry, D. *Catholic Supporters of Same Gender Marriage: A Case Study of Human Dignity in a Multicultural Society.* Lewiston, NY: The Edwin Mellen Press: 2008.
35. Perry D. *The Israeli-Palestinian Peace Movement: Combatants for Peace.* New York, NY: Palgrave Macmillan: 2011.
36. Lonergan BJF. *Method in Theology.* 2nd ed. Toronto, Canada: University of Toronto Press: 2003.
37. Cowling WR, Chinn PL, Hagedorn S. 2000. A nursing manifesto: a call to conscience and action. http://nursemanifest.com/a-nursing-manifesto-a-call-to-conscience-and-action/manifesto-with-markers-for-citation/. Accessed April 3, 2014.
38. Kagan, PN, Smith, MC, Cowling, R, Chinn, PL. A nursing manifesto: an emancipatory call for knowledge development, conscience, and praxis. *Nurs Philos* 2009;11(1): 67–84.

19 Promoting Social Justice and Equity by Practicing Nursing to Address Structural Inequities and Structural Violence

Colleen Varcoe, Annette J. Browne, and Laurie M. Cender

Literature and our current research show that structural inequities and structural violence have profoundly negative health effects.[1-5] In this chapter we draw on our programs of research on ethics, equity, policy, and primary health care (PHC) for marginalized groups including women who experience violence and Aboriginal people. We use the term *marginalized* to refer to the effects of inequitable health and social policies that keep people on the margins of society and have tangible negative effects on peoples' health and quality of life. Using a critical postcolonial stance and an intersectional lens, we describe how structural inequities and structural violence shape peoples' lives and health care and offer strategies for practicing nursing to foster more equitable health and health care.[6-9]

Structural inequities refer to how policies and practices in health, social services, justice, and other systems operate to produce inequitable distribution of the determinants of health.[10,11] Structural violence increasingly is seen in public and population health as a major determinant of the distribution and outcome of health inequities and is defined as "a host of offensives against human dignity, including extreme and relative poverty, social inequalities ranging from racism to gender inequality, and the more spectacular forms of violence"[10(p8)] such as war, genocide, and terrorism. Inequities are structural because they are embedded in the political and economic organizations of our social world and they are violent because they cause injury to people.[5,10] An understanding of structural inequities and structural violence moves practitioners away from an individualistic approach to care and toward understanding how the social and material contexts of peoples' lives shape their health and health care, with differential effects based on gender, age, class, ethnicity, ability, size, and other dimensions.[12] Such understanding helps practitioners counter an individualistic approach that holds people accountable for circumstances beyond their control and blames them for those circumstances and health consequences.

The chapter is organized into three sections. First, we locate the central concepts of structural inequities and structural violence within a theoretical landscape informed by an understanding of social justice grounded in critical theoretical perspectives. This approach considers the multiple intersecting influences shaping health inequities. We offer an intersectional lens as being necessary to examine how people are affected differentially by structural influences such as sexism, racism, poverty, ability, and place.[2,7,13,14] Second, we consider how widening inequities are reflected and sustained in health care. Finally, we offer a framework for practice that emanates from our theoretical stance and analysis. We argue that nurses' efforts to promote social justice and equity are not confined to advocacy at the political or policy level. Rather, such intentions also are accomplished through day to day practices and interactions with individual patients, families, communities, and leaders. Nurses can foster social justice in everyday clinical practice through our ways of being and interacting with people/patients and each other. We use diverse examples to demonstrate how understanding the dynamics of inequity can shift practice at individual, organizational, and policy levels. We illustrate how nursing practice can be more effective using the framework we offer. We conclude by offering implications for nursing practice and education.

ANTICOLONIAL AND INTERSECTIONAL PERSPECTIVES

A critical, postcolonial stance and an intersectional lens is helpful in explicating how structural inequities and structural violence shape health and the implications for nursing practice. A postcolonial perspective draws attention to history and aims to address and challenge contemporary colonial systems of oppression by acknowledging and articulating different and often invisible viewpoints on taken for granted, normalized, and dominant perspectives and knowledges[15] and can help surface and challenge how such dynamics play out in health care. For example, privileging of western biomedical approaches has been intertwined with European colonialism so that such approaches are taken for granted as superior to non-western ones (think of acupuncture or meditation versus pharmacological treatment). A postcolonial lens acknowledges how societal and organizational structures produce and reproduce inequalities based on race, class, sexual, and gender location and necessitates questioning institutional power and privilege and the associated rationale for dominance in social relations.[16] For example, think about the race, class, and gender characteristics of medical hierarchies. In western countries, nursing tends to be dominated by women, physicians tend to be primarily from economically advantaged families, and service staff (janitorial, food) tend to be from non-white groups. Thus, such a lens draws our attention to how health care institutions and policies and professional privilege foster inequity. Moreover, a postcolonial perspective emphasizes individual agency and resistance to systems of oppression and recognizes that power and discourse not only are held by those in authority but that dominant and opposing discourses can operate simultaneously.[16,17] This draws our attention to how nurses can both be very committed to fairness yet practice in ways that discriminate unfairly. However, it also stresses how people, regardless of their disadvantage (including their relative positions within health care hierarchies), are active agents, not merely passive victims.

An intersectional perspective complements an anti-colonial lens and offers an effective tool in examining how structural inequities and structural violence shape and influence health and health care delivery. Hill Collins[18] explains that intersectionality expands the conceptualization of oppression to include a network of power relations and domination in economic, political, and ideological domains that cannot be reduced to a set of discrete sets of binary oppositions (e.g., male/female, poor/wealthy). Hankivsky and colleagues[19] underscore that intersectional analysis captures several levels of difference, recognizes the multidimensional and relational nature of social locations, and situates lived experiences, social forces, and interactive systems of discrimination and subordination at the center of analysis. So an intersectional analysis guides us to consider how "patients" experience nursing practice and health care as the key to recognizing the dynamics of inequity. Further, by paying attention to time, place, and social, economic, and political specifics, an intersectional approach resists essentializing any social groups (such as "women," the "poor," etc.)[19,20]. Rather than privileging one category of social identity (such as gender or socioeconomic status) over others, an intersectional lens allows for consideration of intersecting axes of discrimination[19] and facilitates a complex analysis of the intricate power relations inherent in dominant discourses and ideologies, social determinants of health, and among categories of difference, and how these interact to shape health and health care delivery and contribute to health inequities. For example, when considering the health of "new immigrants," an intersectional analysis directs attention to how racialization, age, class, language skills, gender, and so on interact to shape the migration experience differently for different groups and individuals. To continue the example, failure to provide interpreters, or racial or religious discrimination in health care, disproportionately disadvantage certain immigrants more than others.[21] Because an intersectional approach considers how multiple forms of oppression and resistance are enacted within given social contexts, it facilitates examination of how power relations are maintained and reproduced within health care.

An intersectional approach seeks to uncover what happens when multiple forms of discrimination and oppression converge rather than attempting to simply add social categories to understand individuals' health experiences.[19] From this perspective gender is experienced by an individual simultaneously with their experiences of class, race, sexual orientation, and other forms of social difference, without gender (or any other social category) being viewed as the primary determinant.[2] An intersectional approach embraces the complexities essential to understanding social inequities that shape health inequities, and thereby has the potential to more accurately describe the multiplicity of social locations and lived experiences of diverse people and inform responsive and socially just health systems and policies.[20]

STRUCTURAL INEQUITIES AND STRUCTURAL VIOLENCE

Inequity refers to differences that are unjust, not simply differences that are unequal. Whitehead and Dahlgren[22] identify three distinguishing features of social inequities in health: systematic patterns of differences in health across social groups (e.g., there are consistent differences in health across socioeconomic groups); social (as compared to biological) variations that create health differences; and those health differences that most people would consider unfair due to "unjust social arrangements." Health inequities are directly or indirectly created by social, economic, and environmental forces and structurally shaped lifestyles.[22] Consequently, health inequities are *structural* by definition. The World Health Organization[23,24] emphasizes that to promote equity in health care access, attention must be directed toward structural injustices that serve as barriers to health care services. This involves addressing the stigma and discrimination often experienced by people disadvantaged because of differences in social positioning related to such factors as class, gender, and ethnicity.[25] Stigma and discrimination act as barriers to health care and thus must be addressed by both organizations and individual practitioners. For example, our research[26] shows that people who are poor, especially who are poor and racialized, learn that to attempt to mitigate the disadvantages incurred by health care providers' judgmental attitudes they need to "dress for success" when going to Emergency. To promote health equity and decrease the gaps in health outcomes between groups in society, it is also necessary to focus on the broader determinants of health inequities such as poverty, inadequate housing, unemployment and food security, racializing structures, and social exclusion and how these converge with social differences such as gender and ethnicity.[25,27–29] It also is necessary to scrutinize social processes and structural injustices that contribute to and perpetuate health inequities including dominant discourses and ideologies such as biomedical and individualism discourses that foreground individual autonomy, personal rights, and self-determination over the broader contextual determinants of health.[27,30,31]

When structural conditions cause significant harm to people—for example, race-based policies that keep certain groups of people living under constant threat of imprisonment and/or in conditions of material deprivation, they can be considered violent. A long history of racist colonial policy has sustained large scale and ongoing removal of children from their families into state care,[32] policy enforced poverty,[33] confinement to reserves, and disproportionate imprisonment.[34] Hence Aboriginal people live under structurally violent conditions and routinely experience discrimination in health care.[3,35] For example, Aboriginal women have poorer access to prenatal care in part because they try to avoid harm to themselves and apprehension of their children.[36-38] Rather than understanding the root causes of access barriers, including ongoing racism, providers often draw on individualistic discourses to blame women for making "poor choices" and paradoxically contribute to negative judgments about Aboriginal women as inadequate mothers, entrenching their risk for child apprehension. Nurses must understand how structural conditions shape health and integrate such understanding in how they view, relate to, and work with patients. Importantly, how nurses practice can influence how people experience the impact of structural violence and inequities in their everyday lives. Consider the example of an Aboriginal woman who returned to Emergency repeatedly with anxiety, asthma, and chronic pain and was chastised by a nurse for presenting "thirty-three times."[3] The woman experienced this response as continuous with a lifetime of discriminatory treatment.

INEQUITIES ARE WIDENING GLOBALLY

Inequities are widening globally[39-41] with a few exceptions in Latin America.[42] A recent study of 16 countries indicated rich people tend to be healthier than poor people even after controlling for socio-demographic attributes and household income.[39] A country's overall resources and the distribution of those resources are both important; although economic resources can increase the average health of the population, they do not weaken the tie between wealth and health. On the other hand, whereas greater equity within a country does not raise the health of the population, it does weaken the tie between wealth and health.

Given the contemporary global situation, most nurses are working within contexts in which inequities are widening, poorer people are at greater health disadvantage, and certain groups are disadvantaged more than others based on gender, ethnicity, and other forms of disadvantage. As Braveman[43] notes,

> We are failing on health equity because we are failing on equity. Globally, economic inequality is rising dramatically. Safety nets in nations that historically have had relatively egalitarian policies—and in nations with less-egalitarian policies—are being eroded or threatened by responses to a global financial crisis brought on by unbridled greed. Inequalities in health by social class and by racial or ethnic group cannot be erased simply by reducing inequalities in medical care.[(p515)]

Despite the fact that nurses cannot rectify global structural inequities, we *can* practice in ways that take inequities into account, mitigate the impact of inequities on peoples' quality of life, and avoid participating in further entrenching inequities. Specifically, health care inequities are often perpetuated by placing responsibility for poor health, "lifestyle choices," or "risk factors" on individuals, rather than viewing individuals as influenced by their social contexts, life histories, personal circumstances, the lack of affordable housing, and other social policies. Inequities in health care are entrenched by practices that put responsibility on individuals for circumstances beyond their control, overlook their unique personal circumstances, and, worse, blame them for their circumstances. When nurses overlook these dynamics, their practices and ways of speaking can convey that they simply accept inequities as inevitable or part and parcel of "the way things are"—in the process, they participate in such entrenchment. Indeed, not actively addressing inequities in our everyday interactions with patients, families, and communities contributes to structural inequities and is a form of structural violence. The assumptions nurses make about patients, social judgments, and the discourses that shape those judgments function to sustain and deepen inequities. Our research shows that actively conveying respect and acceptance to individuals, and attending to power differentials has significant impact, particularly for people who experience social exclusion on an everyday basis.[5] In a recent study in PHC clinics serving populations marginalized by racism, poverty, and multiple forms of stigma, many patients claimed that the providers "saved my life" and explained what was profoundly important about care: "they know who I am," "I'm not just a number," "they helped me get housing," "they helped me get disability [income]." Treating people with positive regard and attending to the social determinants of health made significant differences, sometimes a life and death difference.

Importantly, inequities enacted in practice can lead to moral distress for nurses themselves. Thus, we offer ideas for equity-transformative potential—transformation that can promote the well-being of patients, nurses, and the systems within which care is provided.

AN EQUITY-TRANSFORMATIVE FRAMEWORK FOR ADDRESSING STRUCTURAL INEQUITIES AND STRUCTURAL VIOLENCE IN NURSING PRACTICE

Nursing has long espoused a commitment to social justice and equity.[44–48] However, what constitutes equity-oriented or emancipatory practice has received limited attention, leaving nurses in direct care with little direction about how to integrate the goals of equity and social justice in day to day clinical practice. Understanding the dynamics that give rise to inequities, and actively working to redress inequities through our actions and ways of being, provides direction for such integration. An equity lens draws attention to 1) conditions that shape health; 2) determinants of inequities; and 3) distribution of power and calls for counteracting the constant tide of inequities that shape peoples' experiences.

In order to propose an "equity-transformative" framework for nursing practice, we draw on the work of Doane,[49–51] Poole,[52] and our research. Poole explains that

> gender transformation is a relative concept that seeks to shift gender roles and relations closer to gender equity in a given context. Gender transformative approaches actively strive to examine, question, and change rigid gender structures and imbalance of power as a means of reaching health and gender equity objectives.[52]

Poole argues that because

> gender equity is likely never fully attained, gender transformation is an ongoing process toward it. What is transformative in one context, however, may not be transformative in another. Gender transformation involves identifying the ways that gender discrimination, inequality or oppression operates in a particular situation and taking feasible steps toward improving these conditions. . . . Gender transformation is therefore possible in every context, from the most repressive to the most progressive.[52]

Similarly we argue that equity is a goal that is never fully attained and varies with contexts and situations but is possible to promote in every moment, situation, and context. Through research in PHC Browne et al.[5] developed an evidence and theoretically informed framework identifying strategies for individual providers and health care organizations to enhance their capacity to provide equity-oriented services. Individual providers can: recognize and affirm the humanity and worth of each person, recognize and acknowledge the constraints to choice that individuals face (e.g., poverty, violence, racism), and seek to lessen those constraints for individuals. Contrary to dominant rhetoric about efficiencies and lack of time, data from our research[5] show that these strategies can be implemented incrementally and in "small" ways that do not require additional time or costs.[(p12)] Drawing on a postcolonial and intersectional lens, our research and analysis of the root causes of structural inequities and violence, we propose nine principles to guide nurses' practice toward equity and social justice—that is, to practice in an equity-transformative manner.

PRINCIPLES

#1: Commit to equity—offering all persons unconditional positive regard.[53]
A commitment to equity implies that all people should have the same rights, in this case, to health and health care access. Consequently, all persons are deserving of health. Equity does not imply that everyone must be treated

equally or that we provide the "same" care to all; rather, it means tailoring care to individuals and groups such that those who have greatest need are provided with more (resources, support, etc.). Nor does it mean approving of people's behaviors unconditionally; rather, it means actively recognizing when you may be relating to people on the basis of assumptions, pre-empting judgments based on gender, race, abilities, or circumstances, and disrupting discriminatory practices and policies that support them. Hence, the idea of unconditional positive regard means affirming the humanity of each person.

#2: Situate nursing practice within the context of equity and inequity. Seek to understand yourself, relationships with patients and others, and the contexts of peoples' lives (including nursing practice) as located within matrices of power and inequities. This requires continually taking stock of how you are being positioned and taking stock of your disadvantages (easiest to see) and advantages (harder to see) relative to others. "Reflexivity" is not just about reflecting on yourself[54]; it involves thinking critically about how you are positioned (by race, class, gender, ability, language, body type, education, professional positions) and how such positioning creates advantages in some context and disadvantages in others. For example, a nurse who has personally experienced racism on a daily basis may be highly attuned to others' similar experiences; if the same nurse has always had financial security she may be less likely to understand how experiences of poverty affect people's lives. Our positioning shapes our interpretative lenses— meaning, the way we view people and the taken-for-granted assumptions and biases we hold. As nurses, we must attune to our assumptions and biases, so we can be mindful of when they influence our thinking, behaviors, reactions, and practices, often in unexpected ways. Next, consider how your interpersonal relationships with patients, coworkers, and others within the health care hierarchy are shaped by power and relative advantage and disadvantage. For example, who do you most need approval from in order to act—patients? Physicians? Managers? Co-workers? This automatically draws attention to how structures and processes within wider contexts are operating and allows you to consider how health care practices, including your own, may sustain and deepen inequities.

#3: Locate vulnerability, risk, and precarity intra-personally, interpersonally, and contextually. Rather than locating vulnerability within individuals (e.g., "at risk youth"), analyze the dynamics of vulnerability. For example, consider what within your own biases and assumptions might contribute to the vulnerability of youth, what interactions with youth contribute to vulnerability (think of how youth might be treated in stores, by police, and so on), and what contextual elements foster the vulnerability of youth (e.g., employment opportunities, laws, and policies).

#4: Analyze how vulnerability, risk, and precarity are manifest in particular situations. Cautiously and thoughtfully moving between the general and the particular (for example keeping in mind population statistics while attending to specific community, family, or individuals), will help you to use knowledge effectively, test your assumptions, and avoid stereotyping. Think of a vulnerable or "at risk" group in your clinical area. Where does the vulnerability "come from"? Where is risk "located"? For example youth who are "at risk" are often put at risk by poverty and neighborhood contexts, abusive caregivers, mental health problems, or other factors beyond their control. Now consider a particular person within such a population and consider whether those assumptions apply to that individual (e.g., not all homeless youth have mental health problems despite a higher proportion of such problems among the population).

#5: Balance analysis of vulnerabilities with analysis of capacity, resistance, and resilience. Taking a capacity-oriented approach while being mindful of how structural inequities and structural violence create vulnerabilities provides a basis for a strengths-based approach to nursing practice and assists you to avoid paternalizing, pitying, or patronizing people. You can acknowledge the strengths of people while seeking to understand the disadvantages they face. Understanding and acknowledging what it takes to live with specific challenges—a disabling chronic condition, grief, homelessness—can affirm people and enhance capacities.

#6: Ensure practices are appropriate for those people who are in the most marginalized, vulnerable, precarious positions. If practice is designed to be appropriate for people in the most difficult positions, then they will be optimally helpful for all. For example, if brochures or posted signs are clear enough to be understood by people with no or very low literacy, everyone will understand them. If physical touching is approached with safety for those who have experienced violence (e.g., women, elderly or children with histories of abuse, prisoners, or refugees), that approach should work for all.

#7: Orient practice simultaneously toward individual health outcomes and broader transformation of the structures that sustain inequities. Although most nursing practice is conducted with particular individuals or families, we practice in similar patterns. Thus every instance of practice is an example of practice generally and can be transformed to enhance practice broadly. Strategies for improving practice on all levels simultaneously include:

- Disrupting discourses of egalitarianism and assumptions that there is ever a "level playing field." That is, everyone does not have the same life chances; society is not equal, so when you hear someone imply that everyone has the same opportunities, disrupt with your knowledge of inequalities. With patients, learn and acknowledge the constraints to well-being they face—"it must be very difficult." With colleagues, use questions ("do you know how far people from the campesino travel to get here?") and facts ("do you know that minimum wage is only $x per hour, and that farm laborers earn about half that amount?").

- Disrupting discourses of choice. Whenever the discourse of individual "choice" or "lifestyles" is being used, pay attention to how the speaker understands choice. The discourse of choice is a flag for blaming individuals for their life circumstances. Again, use questions ("have you thought about how domestic violence might play a role in women's access to prenatal care?") and facts ("a high percentage of unplanned pregnancies are related to forced sex").
- Disrupting discourses of "risk" and marginalization that fail to specify the root causes and dynamics of risk or fail to locate marginalization intrapersonally, interpersonally, and contextually. Again, use questions and facts ("do you know that most youth at risk of homelessness have experienced significant violence in their homes?").

#8: Treat problems as practice problems first. That is, rather than locating problems in patients (e.g., "the difficult patient"), yourself ("I am just too emotional"), or the context ("there isn't enough time), analyze each problem at all three levels (intrapersonal, interpersonal, and contextual) from the perspective of "better" practice. Ask what could happen at each level to improve nursing practice? For example, for women who do not access prenatal care, analyzing the barriers without locating the problem in the women will lead you to consider how to improve your understanding, your interpersonal approach, and the structures and processes in the health care context (e.g., racism, judgment, service hours, and locations) and the wider context (e.g., transportation, childcare).

#9: Change yourself and your organizations first. You have more potential for changing your own practice than anything else. Given that you are aiming to promote people's health, aiming to make your organization as accessible and health promoting as possible should be a higher priority than trying to change patients to suit your workload, preferences, and your organization. Practicing to promote social justice and equity requires that we each recognize that our own privileges (e.g., fluency in an official language, professional status, education) act as buffers to seeing inequity and lead us to sustain inequities unless we purposefully act to counter these dynamics. Practicing to promote social justice and equity also requires you to accept that some things have to be done differently. For example, promoting the participation of certain patients in discussions of their care often means learning to listen more, say less, and be less "expert" in your approach.

PROCESSES

There are a number of processes that can help put these principles into practice. Figure 19.1 suggests that the principles we identified above and the processes below can be combined to support strategies for equity-transformative nursing practice.

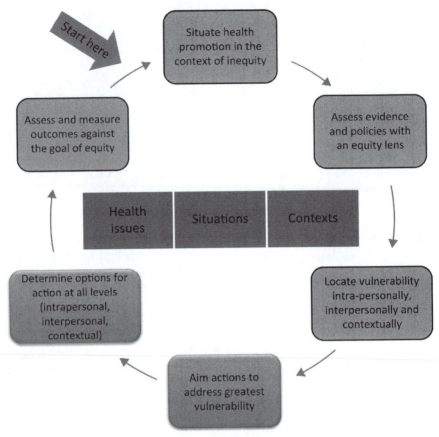

Figure 19.1   Inequity Transformative Health Promoting Nursing Practices

Learn about Your Context

First learn about the forms of inequity and structural violence that pervade the context within which you practice. Start with your health care organization, community, or country, asking:

- Who are the people most advantaged and disadvantaged in your practice setting, community, country?
- What stereotypes, assumptions, and forms of discrimination sustain inequities?
- How are those stereotypes, assumptions, and forms of discrimination sustained and reproduced? Think about some of the common stereotypes (e.g., "trailer trash," "skid kids"), where they place responsibility, what they obscure, and what new forms they take over time.
- What mechanisms (e.g., discourses of individual choice or lifestyles, policies, organizational practices) sustain inequities?

Throughout, scrutinize theory, evidence, and policies using an "equity" lens (attending to conditions that shape health, determinants of inequities, and distribution of power). For example, if you learn that certain ethnic groups are less likely than the general population to use prenatal care, an equity lens would help you consider how structural inequities such as social welfare, taxation, employment, and immigration policies might contribute. In Canada, we have immigration policies that permit employers to admit temporary workers (such as foreign-educated nurses, farm laborers, and domestic workers), but these workers do not have the same rights, including employment standards, minimum wages, or access to health care as citizens or other immigrants.

Learn about Yourself within Your Context

While learning more about the social context of your practice, analyze how you are positioned within that context. How does your social positioning advantage or disadvantage you relative to those to whom you provide care. For example, we (authors) are fluent in English, are viewed as "white," have years of university education, and above-average incomes for Canadian women. Thus, we have considerable advantages accessing health care and have to be conscious of how most others to whom we provide care do not share these advantages. Next, consider how you are positioned within health care. Again, as nurses, we often are treated as "experts," even when we do not have relevant knowledge. We have to resist the temptation to assume the stance of expert, particularly because we routinely want to "make space" for the knowledge and expertise of those to whom we are providing care.

Learn about Your Patients within Their Contexts

Practicing to promote social justice and equity requires that nurses strive to understand patients (particular patients and families and their communities) and health issues within the context of inequity. Whether you begin with a particular patient or family, a specific health issue (diabetes, HIV, cardiac disease), or a particular situation, ask questions to "contextualize"—that is, to understand how structural features, including power and inequities, are exerting influence. Again, scrutinize theories, evidence, and policy through an equity lens. For example, does funding policy better support some people with a certain health condition than others (e.g., those in rural settings, those with income to support transportation)? What are the power dynamics that sustain such inequities? Questions might include:

- What structural features (e.g., how things are organized, funding, policies) shape the lives of these patients/families, the characteristics of this health issue, or this situation?

- How is the situation being shaped by the individual involved and by influences beyond the individual (e.g., other family members, health care providers, housing policies, resources)?
- What power dynamics are involved?

Set Goals Related to Equity-Oriented Practices

Goals related to equity are required at the intrapersonal, interpersonal, and contextual levels. For example, intrapersonally, identify situations in which you are most likely to be judgmental or treat people unfairly. Everyone reacts differently to various behaviors (e.g., overeating, smoking, violence toward others) or situations (e.g., ignoring one's children while on cell phones), challenging our commitment to treat people fairly and with unconditional positive regard. Identifying areas that you find challenging can provide a basis for setting intrapersonal goals. Interpersonally, identify what practices among people that (between yourself and your colleagues, between providers and patients) contribute to and sustain inequities. For example, you might set a goal of disrupting "eye rolling" or other nonverbal signs that convey exasperation and negative judgments about specific patients (in Emergency units this might be people labelled in a derogatory manner as "return customers," "regulars," or "frequent flyers"). Finally, attending to patterns of inequity can help identify harmful practice and policies. For example, one clinic in an inner city set "women-only" hours because women felt threatened when coming to the clinic.[12]

Continuously scrutinizing practice to consider who is being advantaged and disadvantaged, how practice might sustain or mitigate inequities, and how those in the most marginalized situations might be served optimally will help you to align your practices with the goals of equity. For each individual instance in which you identify inequity there is likely an implication for how practice can be improved. For example, when you see a woman being judged negatively because she has not left her abusive partner, rather than only disrupting such judgment related to that specific person, how might you shift your colleagues' attitudes more generally?

Assess Outcomes against the Goal of Equity

Being able to evaluate practice against the goal of equity often requires different approaches to evaluation and measuring outcomes. For example, in PHC settings with which we work, "good" outcomes for people with HIV often are measured only using CD4 viral load counts. However, knowing incremental steps are required for people marginalized by stigma, poverty, and sometimes racism, staff also use "willingness to attend appointments" or "willingness to take the ARV [antiretroviral] meds" as initial indicators of good outcomes and work to engage people who have experienced the highest levels of trauma (and are therefore least likely engage). They also purposefully use patient surveys and interviews to assess how well they are achieving their goals of improving access.

PRACTICING TO TRANSFORM INEQUITY: AN EXAMPLE

I (Colleen) was working in the Emergency Department (ED) doing field work for a study of Emergency Nursing practice. The ED was packed and we were on "diversion" (ambulances diverted to other hospitals). Patients on stretchers lined both halls. Some had ambulance attendants with them because policy required them to "report off" to a nurse prior to leaving. Others had family members in attendance. Leah, the nurse with whom I was working, was assigned to the hall, which was an "unofficial" patient area. Care was provided with no privacy and only portable equipment. Some required treatment for acute problems and thus would be moved into stretcher bays with monitors as soon as available; some awaited assessment, others were stable. Decades of hospital closures, bed closures, "contracting out" of services, decreasing staff to patient ratios, and so on resulted in this pattern becoming widespread practice,[55] a pattern that persists today. Leah was relatively senior, with about five years of experience in that unit where the most senior had less than 10 years of experience. The unit had a new manager with no ER experience, and overall, staff were negative about his leadership. Leah had told me she loved the ER and prided herself on being competent in the midst of chaos. She liked it best when it was busy.

Leah had six patients. A 79-year-old woman with terminal bowel cancer had arrived by ambulance and lay on a stretcher surrounded by 5–7 family members. She was pale, her breathing was labored and very slow, occasionally apneic. The family recently emigrated from Fiji, none spoke English, and although Leah had called for an interpreter, no one had shown up. A 24-year-old man had suffered a crush injury to his leg at his construction site. He was clearly in severe pain, but trying to keep control. He was alone as the ambulance attendant had reported off. He had been seen by the physician who ordered morphine, but Leah had not had time to give it. An 82-year-old man was in a wheelchair, holding a basin, retching. He had vomited frank blood twice already. He was accompanied by an equally elderly looking woman, who was trying to comfort him, but looked like she needed a wheelchair herself. The triage nurse had said he was stable, but the ER physician had not yet seen him. A 46-year-old woman, also in a wheelchair and alone, had a severe and blinding headache. Leah had given her Demerol about 30 minutes earlier but had not yet reassessed her. This woman spoke little English, and had been conveying her pain with gestures. Another elderly man with chronic obstructive pulmonary disease was awaiting transfer to a medical unit; he spoke only Hindi, and his daughter, who had been interpreting, had left to go to work. Leah was moving her sixth patient, a 64-year-old man with abdominal pain not yet diagnosed from the hall into a stretcher bay when the ambulance attendants rolled a stretcher in to the vacated spot. I helped the nurse assigned to the stretcher bay settle him while Leah rushed off to assess the new patient who had just taken his place.

I set up an IV for the other nurse, emptied the vomiting man's basin, and took a chair from the charting station for the woman with him. Leah blasted past me, on her way to the charting station (where all physicians, nurses and other staff charted, phoned, consulted, and so on). "That's it," she said in a loud and angry tone. "No 58 year old will die in the hall on my shift." She told the unit clerk to call the supervisor and told the charge nurse she was bringing her patient into a monitor bed (there were none available) immediately. Her new patient had classic myocardial infarction symptoms, and she was not waiting for a physician to "get around" to assessing him. The charge nurse said, "you can't do that." "I'm doing it," she replied.

How do you read this situation? What draws your attention? What relationship does this scenario have to the idea of structural inequities and structural violence? We know little about the particular patients, but the patterns were commonplace. Because the hospital was situated in a community in western Canada populated by recent immigrants, it was usual for many patients to speak languages other than English. Given the aging population, the demographics of Leah's six patients were usual. The care-givers accompanying patients were usually women. The health issues with which the patients presented were representative. For example, the community served was undergoing considerable new construction and young men with workplace injuries were admitted every shift. How then might various forms of inequity be shaping this situation? How might inequities related to age, gender, ethnicity, and so on be playing out? How is immigration policy within the context of global economics playing out? How are health care funding decisions shaping this moment? How are management decisions influencing the situation? And what is a nurse to do? How do you judge Leah's actions in that moment? What do her actions suggest about her thinking? Is it satisfactory for a 79-year-old woman to die in the hallway (she was clearly dying), but not a 58-year-old man? What could Leah have done differently? Could she have done anything differently? What would allow more equitable practice, and how might that effect the wellbeing of the patient, Leah, and the unit?

CONCLUSION

Structural inequities are growing and have harmful health consequences. Without awareness, nurses can participate in sustaining inequities and their harmful effects. Conversely, with intent to foster equity and social justice, nurses can mitigate harm through their daily practices and interactions with patients, their relationships with colleagues, and their participation in developing organizational policies and practices. In the case above, the nurses were engaged in a participatory research process and through that, took multiple actions to improve their own team dynamics, work more effectively with the department management, and enhance the ethics of their care. The wider community had long been aware that the community need had outstripped the hospital resources, and a new ED has opened. Better conditions for providing care should support more equitable care. However, regardless of conditions, in every moment of care each nurse can work toward equity-transformative practice with positive consequences for everyone including nurses. Just as inequities harm entire populations (not just those most affected), equity is good for us all.

ACKNOWLEDGMENTS

The studies informing this chapter were funded by the Canadian Institutes of Health Research. We also thank Dr. Gweneth Doane for her ongoing contributions to our thinking that fundamentally shaped this chapter.

REFERENCES

1. Anderson JM, Rodney P, Reimer-Kirkham S, Browne AJ, Khan KB, JL. Inequities in health and healthcare viewed through the ethical lens of critical social justice: contextual knowledge for the global priorities ahead. *Advances in Nursing Science* 2009;32(4): 282–294.
2. Varcoe C, Hankivsky O, Morrow M. Introduction: beyond gender matters. In: Hankivsky O, Morrow M, Varcoe C, eds. *Women's Health in Canada: Critical Perspectives on Theory and Policy*. Toronto, ON, Canada: University of Toronto; 2007: 3–30.
3. Browne AJ, Smye VL, Rodney P, Tang SY, Mussell W, O'Neil J. Access to primary care from the perspective of aboriginal patients at an urban emergency department. *Qualitative Health Research* 2011;21(3): 333–348.
4. Whitehead M, Popay J. Swimming upstream? Taking action on the social determinants of health inequalities. *Social Science and Medicine* 2010;71(7): 1234–1236.
5. Browne AJ, Varcoe C, Wong S, et al. Closing the health equity gap: evidence-based strategies for primary healthcare organizations. *International Journal for Equity in Health* 2012;11(15).
6. Young IM. *Justice and the Politics of Difference*. Princeton, NJ: Princeton University Press; 1990.
7. Varcoe C, Pauly B, Laliberte S, MacPherson G. Intersectionality, social justice and policy. In: Hankivsky O, ed. *Intersectionality-type Health Research in Canada*. Vancouver, BC, Canada: UBC Press; 2011: 331–348.
8. Reimer Kirkham S, Browne AJ. Toward a critical theoretical interpretation of social justice discourses in nursing. *Advances in Nursing Science* 2006;29(4): 324–339.
9. Browne AJ, Smye VL, Varcoe C. Postcolonial feminist theoretical perspectives and women's health. In: Hankivsky O, Morrow M, Varcoe C, eds. *Women's Health in Canada: Critical Perspectives on Theory and Policy*. Toronto, ON, Canada: University of Toronto; 2007: 124–142.

10. Farmer P. *Pathologies of Power: Health, Human Rights, and the New War on the Poor.* Berkeley, CA: University of California Press; 2003.

11. Farmer PE, Nizeye B, Stulac S, Keshavjee S. Structural violence and clinical medicine. *PLoS Medicine* 2006;10(3): 1686–1691.

12. Browne AJ, Varcoe C, Fridkin A. Addressing trauma, violence and pain: research on health services for women at the intersections of history and economics. In: Hankivsky O, ed. *Health Inequities in Canada: Intersectional Frameworks and Practices.* Vancouver, BC, Canada: UBC Press; 2011: 295–311.

13. Weber L, Parra-Medina D. Intersectionality and women's health: charting a path to eliminating disparities. *Advances in Gender Research* 2003;7: 181–230.

14. Hankivsky O, Reid C, Cormier R, et al. Exploring the promises of intersectionality-type methodologies for advancing women's health research. *International Journal for Equity in Health* 2010;9(5): 1–15.

15. Hollenberg D, Muzzin L. Epistemological challenges to integrative medicine: an anti-colonial perspective on the combination of complementary/alternative medicine with biomedicine. *Health Sociological Review* 2010;19(1): 34–56.

16. Dei GJS. Rethinking the role of Indigenous knowledges in the academy. *International Journal of Inclusive Education* 2000;4(2): 111–132.

17. Shahjahan RA. Mapping the field of anti-colonial discourse to understand the issues of indigenous knowledges: decolonizing praxis. *McGill Journal of Education* 2005;40(2): 213–240.

18. Collins PH. *Black Feminist Thought: Knowledge, Consciousness, and the Politics of Empowerment.* 2nd ed. New York, NY: Routledge; 1990.

19. Hankivsky O, Reid C, Cormier R, et al. Exploring the promises of intersectionality for advancing women's health research. *International Journal for Equity in Health* 2010;9: 1–15.

20. Hankivsky O, Christoffersen A. Intersectionality and the determinants of health: a Canadian perspective. *Critical Public Health* 2008;18(3): 271–283.

21. Abraham D, Rahman S. The community interpreter: a critical link between clients and service providers. In: Guruge S, Collins E, eds. *Working with Immigrant Women: Issues and Strategies for Mental Health Professionals.* Toronto, BC, Canada: Canadian Center for Addictions and Mental Health; 2008: 103–118.

22. Whitehead M, Dahlgren G. *Concepts and principles for tackling social inequities in health: Levelling up Part 1.* Copenhagen, Denmark: World Health Organization; 2006.

23. Lee J, Sadana R, eds. *Improving equity in health by addressing social determinants.* Geneva, Switzerland: World Health Organization; 2011.

24. World Health Organization. *Closing the Gap in a Generation: Health Equity through Action on the Social Determinants of Health.* Geneva, Switzerland: World Health Organization; 2008.

25. Pauly B, MacKinnon K, Varcoe C. Revisiting "Who gets care?" Health equity as an arena for nursing action. *Advances in Nursing Science* 2009;32(2): 118–127.

26. Varcoe C, Browne AJ, Wong S, Smye VL. Harms and benefits: collecting ethnicity data in a clinical context. *Soc Sci Med* 2009;68(9): 1659–1666.

27. Raphael D, Curry-Stevens A, Bryant T. Barriers to addressing the social determinants of health: insight from the Canadian experience. *Health Policy* 2008;88: 222–235.

28. Mukherjee JS, Barry DJ, Satti H, Raymonville M, Marsh S, Smith-Fawzi MK. Structural violence: a barrier to achieving the millennium development goals for women. *Journal of Women's Health* 2011;20(4): 593–597.

29. Krieger N. Methods for scientific study of discrimination and health: an ecosocial approach. *American Journal of Public Health* 2012;102(5): 936–945.

30. Browne AJ. Clinical encounters between nurses and First Nations women in a western Canadian hospital. *Social Science & Medicine* 2007;64(10): 2165–2176.

31. Tang SY, Browne AJ. 'Race' matters: racialization and egalitarian discourses involving aboriginal people. *Ethnicity & Health* 2008;13(2): 1–19.

32. Blackstock C, Trocmé N, Bennett M. Child maltreatment investigations among Aboriginal and non-Aboriginal families in Canada. *Violence Against Women* 2004;10(8): 901–916.

33. Bennett M, Blackstock C. The insidious poverty epidemic: considerations for Aboriginal children, families, communities and other Indigenous nations. *First Peoples Child & Family Review* 2007;3(3): 5–7.

34. Welsh A, Ogloff JRP. Progressive reforms or maintaining the status quo? An empirical evaluation of the judicial consideration of Aboriginal status in sentencing decisions. *Canadian Journal of Criminology & Criminal Justice* 2008;50(4): 491–517.

35. Bourassa C, McKay-McNabb K, Hampton MR. Racism, sexism, and colonialism: the impact on the health of Aboriginal women in Canada. *Canadian Woman Studies* Fall 2004;24(1): 23–29.

36. Brown H, Varcoe C, Calam B. The birthing experiences of rural Aboriginal women in context: Implications for Nursing/Les expériences d'accouchement des femmes autochtones en région rurale, mises en contexte : les implications en matière de soins infirmiers. *Canadian Journal of Nursing Research* 2011;43(4): 100–117.

37. Varcoe C, Brown H, Calam B, Harvey T, Tallio M. Help bring back the celebration of life: a community-based participatory study of rural Aboriginal women's maternity experiences and outcomes *BMC Pregnancy and Childbirth* 2013;13(26).

38. Denison J, Varcoe C, Browne AJ. Aboriginal women's experiences of accessing healthcare when state apprehension of children is being threatened. *Journal of Advanced Nursing* in press.

39. Semyonov M, Lewin-Epstein N, Maskileyson D. Where wealth matters more for health: the wealth–health gradient in 16 countries. *Social Science & Medicine* 2013;81: 10–17.

40. Mackenbach JP. The persistence of health in equalities in modern welfare states: the explanation of a paradox. *Social Science & Medicine* 2012;75(4): 761–769.

41. Milanovic B. Global income inequality in numbers: in history and now. *Global Policy.* 2013;4(2): 198–208.

42. Lustig N, Lopez-Calva L, Ortiz-Juarez E. Declining inequality in Latin America in the 2000s: the cases of Argentina, Brazil, and Mexico. *World Development.* 2013;44:129–141.

43. Braveman P. We are failing on health equity because we are failing on equity. *Australian and New Zealand Journal of Public Health* 2012;36(6): 515.

44. Drevdahl D, Kneipp SM, Canales MK, Dorcy KS. Reinvesting in social justice: a capital idea for public health nursing. *Advances in Nursing Science* 2001;24(2): 19–31.

45. Lipscomb M. Challenging the coherence of social justice as a shared nursing value. *Nursing Philosophy* 2011;12(1): 4–11.

46. Falk-Rafael A, Betker C. Witnessing social injustice downstream and advocating for health equity upstream: "The trombone slide" of nursing. *Advances in Nursing Science* 2012;35(2): 98–112.

47. Boutain DM. Social justice in nursing: a review of the literature. In: de Chesnay M, Andersen ML, eds. *Caring for the Vulnerable: Perspectives in Nursing*

Theory, Practice and Research. 3rd ed. Burlington, MA: Jones and Bartlett Learning; 2012: 43–56.

48. Kagan PN, Smith MC, Cowling WR, Chinn PL. A nursing manifesto: an emancipatory call for knowledge development, conscience, and praxis. *Nursing Philosophy* 2009;11(1): 67–84.

49. Hartrick GH. Reflexivity as presence: a journey of self-inquiry. In: Finlay L, Gough B, eds. *Reflexivity. A Practical Guide for Researchers in Health and Social Sciences.* Oxford, UK: Blackwell Publishing; 2003.

50. Hartrick Doane GA, Varcoe C. Relational practice and nursing obligations. *Advances in Nursing Science* 2007;30(3): 192–205.

51. Hartrick Doane G. Cultivating relational consciousness in social justice practice. In this volume.

52. Poole N. *Understanding Health Promotion Approaches in the Context of Gender and Women's Health: Backgrounder.* Vancouver, BC, Canada: Phi Women; 2012.

53. Rogers C. *Client-Centered Therapy: Its Current Practice, Implications and Theory.* London, UK: Constable; 1951.

54. Nelson S. The lost path to emancipatory practice: towards a history of reflective practice in nursing. *Nursing Philosophy* 2012;13: 202–213.

55. Freeman J. The emerging subspecialty of hallway medicine. *Canadian Journal of Emergency Medicine* July 2003;5(4): 283–285.

20 Military Sexual Trauma and Nursing Practice in the Veterans Administration

Ursula A. Kelly

Women are the fastest growing group of military recruits and veterans. Among female veterans, reports of military sexual trauma (MST) and of posttraumatic stress disorder (PTSD) are each consistently 20% or higher.[1] During the past decade, the United States Veterans Administration (VA) has identified female veterans, veterans with PTSD, and veterans who have experienced MST as priority populations. Significant resources have been dedicated to clinical and research initiatives to improve care to these historically overlooked groups. In spite of these initiatives, gender and racial health disparities exist among VA patients marginalized by their gender (female), ethnicity (African-Americans), and experiences of sexual trauma.[2-4] These barriers, health disparities, and inequities reflect social injustices within the VA system. As health care professionals, nurses are called upon to address social injustice and disadvantages in their clinical practice by integrating "contextual knowledge" about inequities and social disadvantages in their patients' lives with their purely clinical knowledge.[5(p285)] To address this goal, in this chapter I will discuss contextual knowledge and social action in nursing to address health disparities in the VA system.

This chapter begins with an intersectional analysis of areas of social injustice within the VA as a single system. Next, this analysis will be applied to a specific veteran patient population, African-American female veterans who experienced MST and have PTSD. In the final section I will delineate ways in which nurses in all areas of the VA can work toward goals of social justice with individual patients and within the VA system, consistent with nurses' professional responsibilities.

INTERSECTIONALITY

Intersectionality provides a framework for considering issues of social justice within the VA system. Black feminist scholars defined intersectionality as a complex process by which people's positions of race, class, gender, and sexuality lead to inferior social status.[6,7] This scholarship has been extended to additional social groupings, for example, age and disability status.[8,9] Within the intersectionality framework, oppression and its effects are understood as multiplicative, not additive. Power is wielded by individuals to dominate and control members of disadvantaged social groups and those living and working within hierarchical institutions, such as the military and the VA. Power relationships exist at the macro level of social systems and institutions and at the micro level of interpersonal relationships. MST is an example of oppression at both the macro and micro levels in the military—it is enabled by the social structure of the military as an institution, perpetrated by individuals at the interpersonal level, and tolerated at multiple strata within the military hierarchy.

The multiplicative effects of oppression and discrimination directly affect a person's regard for one's health, access to external material resources, and participation in one's health care.[10] In order for these health disparities to be reduced and eliminated, the interlocking nature of multiple forms of oppression that contribute to poor health has to be recognized and attended to in health care and health care research.[11,12]

THE VA SYSTEM

The VA was established by Congress in 1865 to provide health care to veterans (male) of military service and benefits for their families (women and children). The VA developed as an entity within the federal government with an organizational and social structure that mirrors that of the military—viewed by many as oppressive to various social groups, for example, women, racial and ethnic minorities, and gay men and women, among others.[13–16] The disadvantaging nature of the VA and the military perpetuate injustices, such as health disparities, despite the best intentions of leaders and personnel working within these systems. Health disparities and social injustices that are derived from oppressive institutions and social structures cannot be dismantled by either individuals' good intentions or punitive action against individual perpetrators of injustice.

DISADVANTAGED POPULATIONS WITHIN THE MILITARY AND THE VA

The populations most overtly subordinated, disadvantaged, and experiencing disparities within both the military and the VA are women, racial, and ethnic minorities and those with a homosexual orientation. The status of women and racial and ethnic minorities within the military and the VA will be discussed below. While it is the antithesis of an intersectional approach, information is presented primarily using singular social categories, i.e., gender and race and ethnicity (artificially reduced to Black/White). Data that incorporate more than one social category or demographic variable are for the most part unavailable—a reflection of the uni-dimensional approach typical of the biomedical sciences and government agencies.[17] However, whenever possible within each category, the compounded effects of social disadvantage will be highlighted.

The structure of the military is intentionally hierarchical with clearly delineated strata of power and control. The rationale for this is that it is essential to the conduct of war to have a clear chain of command and power structure. Ironically, the military is viewed by some as an equalizer of power differentials in the U.S. social structure. Theoretically, once enlisted, each service member has an equal opportunity for education, training, compensation, and career development. However, the reality is that groups that are subordinate in civilian society are also subordinate and oppressed in the military, for example, Black women.

The demographic profile of the military is disproportionately 1) White men and Black women, and 2) White officers and Black active duty personnel.[18,19] This profile is particularly salient to an intersectional analysis of African-American female veterans who experienced MST and have PTSD. They experience the multiplicative effects of subordination based on race, gender, sexual violence perpetrated by men, and a stigmatized mental illness.

WOMEN AND THE VA

Gender-Based Health Care

More than a decade ago, Congress mandated the expansion of health care services to women veterans and MST-screening and provision of MST-related health care services within the VA. Women's health services included primary care and specialty services afforded to all veterans, as well as gender-specific services, including prenatal and obstetric services and infertility evaluation and treatment.[20] However, the lack of a formal structure or universal system for the creation of expanded clinical services for women resulted in inconsistent, disparate, and fragmented women's health programs within the VA. For example, only approximately 60% of VA medical centers have designated women's health clinics, although this represents an eight-fold growth over the previous decade.[21,22] Very few VA medical centers provide prenatal and obstetric services on site; these are generally subcontracted to the private sector. For some women, in order to receive VA women's health care, they literally must go elsewhere.

Similar to women's health services, the mandate to provide MST-related services resulted in the rapid expansion of specialized health care services without a universal or evidence-based approach. While every VA medical center has a designated MST coordinator who is responsible for overseeing and facilitating access to MST-related health care, there are very few specialized MST treatment teams within PTSD Clinics or residential MST-related PTSD treatment programs within the VA system. Further, many health care providers within the VA do not feel prepared or have the expertise to provide primary or specialty care to female veterans. Regardless of size, VA medical centers remain male-dominated environments in which women veterans are often invisible or, as noted above, not present, having been sent elsewhere.

VA Health Care Services Utilization

Women veterans utilize VA health care less than men, after adjusting for age and medical co-morbidity.[23] Documented barriers to health care for female veterans include being uninsured, knowledge gaps about VA care, the perception that VA providers are not gender-sensitive, and MST predicted delaying or foregoing health care,[24] despite the expressed commitment of national VA leadership to eliminate them.

Gender-Based Health Disparities

Gender-based disparities in health care quality exist among female veterans who do seek health care at the VA. For example, research conducted in 2004–2008 demonstrated that management of cardiovascular risk factors (hypertension, high cholesterol, and diabetes) was poorer for women than for men. Fewer female veterans received colorectal cancer and depression screening than did male veterans.[25] Elderly female veterans are more likely to receive inappropriate medications than male veterans, potentially due to sex bias in which providers attribute somatic symptoms to mental disorders.[26]

Physical and Mental Health

Women veterans who receive health care within the VA system have more co-morbid physical and mental health problems than do male veterans. Women veterans who experience MST have a six-fold risk for having three or more mental health conditions than those who did not experience MST.[1] The burden of mental and physical illness falls disproportionately on female veterans. Female veterans experience socioeconomic burdens as well. They are at higher risk for homelessness than male veterans and more than twice as likely to be homeless than their female civilian counterparts.

Health disparities among female veterans, particularly among those who experienced MST, are highly problematic from an intersectional perspective. Women's complex physical and mental health problems, including PTSD, have been problematized at the level of individual veterans rather than, at least in part, a reflection of male sexual violence and social subordination perpetrated system-wide in and outside of the military. Individuals are pathologized rather than the social structures that enable and tolerate their victimization. Systemic and structural causes of these health problems are noted in public discourse but have not been effectively addressed by the military or the VA.

In the next section of this chapter, I will provide an intersectional analysis of the experiences and health care needs of African-American female veterans who experienced MST and have PTSD. This population will be used as an example to illustrate the contextual knowledge that nurses need in order to work effectively with patients and to pursue social justice as part of nursing practice.

EXEMPLAR: AFRICAN-AMERICAN FEMALE VETERANS WHO EXPERIENCED MST AND HAVE PTSD INTERPERSONAL TRAUMA

In addition to MST, female veterans experience high rates of non-military service related trauma: 81%–93% report at least one lifetime trauma. These traumas include 38%–64% lifetime sexual assault, 27%–49% childhood sexual abuse, 24%–49% adult sexual abuse, 46%–51% physical assault, 35% childhood physical abuse, and 18%–19% domestic violence.[4] These estimates are higher than reported estimates among nationally representative samples of women. Research findings suggest that many women join the military in an effort to leave violent home environments.[27]

MILITARY LIFE AND MST

The military is often described as valuing dominance, assertiveness, aggression, self-sufficiency, and competitiveness in service members. These characteristics are generally considered masculine, contributing to the male-dominated image of military culture. All soldiers are trained to be physically and mentally strong and unemotional. While there is some social debate about this, many believe that these cultural norms enable and foster sexual assault and harassment of female soldiers. Ironically the military is referred to sometimes as a brotherhood, in which soldiers defend and protect each other and remain loyal, much like a family.

For those who experience MST, being victimized by fellow military service members intensifies their sense of betrayal and limits their options in responding to the trauma. Female victims of MST may believe that they should not have or show any emotional reaction to the assault or report MST, as this would reveal their vulnerability and undermine their standing in the military. Other factors associated with MST in the context of military culture are that victims may believe that escape is not possible and they may fear negative consequences and heightened harassment or violence if they disclosed the sexual trauma.[28] Unlike their civilian counterparts, military victims of sexual assault often are forced to continue to work with or report to their rapist. Similar to civilian survivors of sexual assault, women who report MST also may be re-traumatized by the responses of the institutions and individuals who should be providing them resources and prosecuting the perpetrator.

STEREOTYPES AND SUPERWOMAN

African-American women are subject to specific social narratives or stereotypes that are derived from historical and contemporary social group oppression. Thomas et al. described three stereotypes of African-American women derived from slavery—Mammy, Sapphire, and Jezebel. The Mammy and Jezebel stereotypes are particularly relevant to African-American females who experience MST and/or have PTSD.[29] The stereotype of Mammy, a congenial and non-threatening housekeeper, has led to the perception of African-American women as nurturing, strong, supportive, and selfless. This may impact African-American women's perceived need to project a façade of strength.[30] The Jezebel stereotype is derived from the historical sexual exploitation and victimization of African-American women during slavery. According to this stereotype, African-American women are seductive, promiscuous, manipulative, and have uncontrollable sexual desires.[29] This stereotype is an illustration of sexualized racism.[6] The potential impact of this stereotype on African-American women who are sexually assaulted may be to inhibit their reporting of the assault for fear of being blamed or not being taken seriously or believed.

A contemporary construct that provides the basis for African-American women's responses to their life experiences is the Superwoman schema,[31] also referred to as the Strong Black Woman[32] and the Sojourner Syndrome.[33] In this role, African-American women are obligated to demonstrate strength and resiliency, to suppress emotions, and to help others, even at great cost to themselves; they must be resistant to being vulnerable or dependent and overcome adversity despite limited resources.[31] This schema evolved in the context of the legacy of slavery, historical racism, and oppression, and experiences of trauma, abuse, and disappointment, as well as spiritual values and family patterns of self-sufficiency.[31] Being a Superwoman or Strong Black Woman is a survival strategy, with short- and long-term benefits, but also with significant costs. The chronic stress of fulfilling this role in the context of the interacting and intersecting effects of racial and sexual inequality and social, economic, and political oppression has negative physiological effects, psychological vulnerability, and stress-related illnesses and health behaviors. As Leigh Mullings noted, "While race may not be biological, racism has biological consequences."[33(p87)]

REPORTING/DISCLOSING MST AND SEEKING MENTAL HEALTH TREATMENT

These stereotypes and the Superwoman/Strong Black Woman schema create barriers for African-American women to disclosing or reporting MST as a veteran. Either action might be perceived as an admission of weakness, vulnerability, or failure or as a request for help. African-American women may also be skeptical, based on life experiences of discrimination and social group oppression, that there would be any benefits to making the MST known; the likelihood is greater that there would be negative ramifications.

Very few studies have been conducted with female veterans about barriers to disclosing MST and seeking trauma-related mental health care.[34] Researchers studying civilian populations have reported that African-American women are less likely to report sexual assault than White women.[35,36] They also may be less likely to seek and complete mental health treatment.[37,38] The image of the Superwoman/Strong Black Woman may prevent female veterans both from recognizing their symptoms of PTSD and from seeking mental health care.[39]

In studies using primarily male samples of military service members and veterans, stigma, lack of knowledge of PTSD, negative views of mental illness and mental health treatment, lack of social support, and logistic barriers are the most frequently cited factors in lack of utilization of mental health services.[40-43] Studies that included women either had a negligible number of women in the sample or women were not considered separately in the analysis. It is likely that these are all important factors for female veterans, in addition to the social and structural barriers described above. Further, for women who have been sexually traumatized, particularly while serving in the military, the male-dominated environment of the VA can be so uncomfortable as to preclude PTSD treatment seeking.[44]

The stigma against seeking mental health care in the military and among veterans is so strong that the VA has launched a campaign to appeal to veterans to seek care. The motto of the campaign is "It takes the strength and courage of a warrior to ask for help." The term warrior is strongly, if not universally, associated with men. There is no gender-neutral or parallel gender-specific campaign to reach female veterans. Campaigns such as this, while possibly effective for engaging male veterans in mental health care, serve to further marginalize female veterans and perpetuate lack of access to VA mental health services for women.

NURSING PRACTICE AND SOCIAL JUSTICE

This intersectional analysis of the VA system has significant implications for nursing practice, particularly related to social justice. Nurses in all levels of the institution have the responsibility to pursue social justice as an integral part of their nursing practice, be it clinical care, education, leadership, or research. The concept of social justice has been part of feminist nursing discourse for some time. However, there continues to be a gap in knowledge translation about the well-established social determinants of health to nursing practice, that is, operationalizing social justice into "practice ready" knowledge.[5(p284)] This link between knowledge and practice is the essence of praxis, which requires action and reflection.

Reflection in the context of socially just nursing refers to the act of critically considering, within ourselves and in encounters with others (patients and colleagues), the patient's social reality and how it was constructed. This reflection sets the stage for transformative action in nursing practice. In the final section of this chapter, I provide strategies that nurses can use in each area of practice to work toward social justice, continuing to use African-American female veterans with PTSD who experienced MST as an exemplar.

CLINICAL CARE

Integrating contextual knowledge in every step of the nursing process from assessment through evaluation can directly impact the health and well-being of patients—fostering health equity and social justice. For example, clinicians often view female veterans as being somatic and needy in their presentation. While this population is known to have complex medical and mental health problems, this disparaging view may also be a function of the long-held view that women's physical symptoms are likely to be "somatic"—attributable to depression, anxiety, or another mental disorder and thus are not taken seriously or at face value. In some cases, that may in fact be true, given the correlation between physical and mental health symptoms. However, beginning an assessment of a patient with that assumption precludes accurate assessment, presumably yielding ineffective, disrespectful care. Nurses working with all female veterans, including those who experienced MST and have PTSD, must be self-reflective to discern to what extent they may hold that bias, consciously or not. With such self-reflection, nurses would assume the validity of the veteran's report, improving their assessment of that patient. At the same time, it is important for nurses to recognize the inherent strength and resilience of female veterans and to capitalize on these in planning and implementing nursing interventions. Further, overall improvements are needed in the assessment of African-American women for depression and PTSD, a gap in clinical care that nurses can address directly.

In implementing a treatment plan, ideally co-created with the patient and her self-identified needs, nurses need to be aware of the circumstances within which the patient is living—does she have access to resources to enable her to adhere to the plan? For example, is this patient able to come to weekly mental health appointments, given her employment and childcare responsibilities and transportation needs? The nurse's role in this case is to assist the patient in addressing her resource needs as part of clinical intervention by linking the patient with local resources. Finally, clinical nurses can disseminate their contextual knowledge via professional conferences and publications, bringing attention to the disparate circumstances experienced by those in subordinate social positions and advocating for policy changes to address these inequities.

LEADERSHIP

Nurses in leadership positions have numerous opportunities to guide organizational priorities, clinical services, and policies that affect the lives of patients. Key factors in the establishment of gender-sensitive health services include local organizational culture and the quality of local leadership's support for women's health.[25] Thus, even within a large bureaucratic system, leaders at the local level can ensure changes to address disparities within the VA. Nurse leaders must be able to assess the current state of patient care services and identify and address gaps in quality care. Currently, VA health services for female veterans and those who experienced MST are inadequate to meet their needs. Nurse leaders and nurses providing clinical care must serve as advocates within the VA system to direct financial and human resources to these needs.

EDUCATION

Educational forums in academic and health care settings can be used to engage in dialogue about health and health care disparities and their root causes. This education should include self-reflection, dialogue across clinical settings and disciplines, and development of the knowledge and skill set necessary to advocate for social justice within their medical centers and national governing or administrative bodies. Traditional nursing education about diversity focuses on ethnicity-based cultural competence. Education that incorporates an intersectionality perspective would include discussion of the marginalizing experiences of at least some members of diverse ethnic minority groups and the multiplicative impact of these on their health, health care, and health behaviors, for example, African-American women. In order to incorporate social justice as praxis in education, nursing faculty and educators must first be educated about this perspective and engaged in the process of its implementation—ideally through the same dialogic approach recommended by Anderson and colleagues in translating contextual knowledge to practice.[5]

Social justice-driven education can also be incorporated in health care settings. For example, one barrier to establishing high quality women's health services within the VA has been health care providers' lack of experience and knowledge in caring for female veterans. Health care providers equipped with contextual knowledge of the multiplicative effects of multiple social group identities, for example, African-American women who experienced MST, will be able to provide more effective health care, improving health outcomes for this population.

RESEARCH

Research on women's health, MST, PTSD, and ethnically based health disparities would be strengthened by the inclusion of stakeholders in the research process using a community-based research (CBPR) approach. CBPR is a research approach that attends to broad considerations of the ethical principle of justice and is consistent with the intersectional approach to health disparities research.[11,17] Researchers who use a CBPR approach form collaborative and equitable relationships with stakeholders. In CBPR, research questions are generated by community members and stakeholders and address their self-identified needs, for example, barriers to care. CBPR with African-American female veterans with PTSD who experienced MST could result in advocacy for necessary VA health services and relevant resources.

CONCLUSION

Despite significant attention and resources devoted to women's health, MST, PTSD, and ethnically based health disparities within the VA, gaps in services, barriers to care, and health disparities continue to exist for many veterans. The intersectional analysis of the VA system provided above is useful for identifying the underlying causes of these disparities—inequitable power dynamics that result in disparate access to health resources among those who are members of subordinate and marginalized social groups based on race, gender, class, sexual trauma, etc. Within the VA, interventions that target oppressive and discriminatory policies and practices are necessary to address the health and health care disparities experienced by African-American female veterans, particularly those with PTSD and who have experienced sexual trauma while serving in the military. Nurses working within every area of the VA system, the largest health care system in the United States, have the responsibility and multiple opportunities to address these social injustices as an integral component of their nursing practice.

REFERENCES

1. Suris A, Lind L. Military sexual trauma: a review of prevalence and associated health consequences in veterans. *Trauma, Violence & Abuse* 2008;9(4): 250–269.
2. Saha S, Freeman M, Toure J, Tippens KM, Weeks C, Ibrahim S. Racial and ethnic disparities in the VA health care system: a systematic review. *Journal of General Internal Medicine* 2008;23(5): 654–671.

3. Bean-Mayberry B, Batuman F, Huang C, et al. *Systematic Review of Women Veterans Health Research 2004–2008*. Department of Veterans Affairs, Evidence-Based Synthesis Program Center for the Health Services Research and Development Service. Washington, DC.; 2010. Retrieved from http://www.hsrd.research.va.gov/publications/esp/womens-health.pdf. Accessed April 8, 2014.

4. Zinzow HM, Grubaugh AL, Monnier J, Suffoletta-Maierle S, Frueh BC. Trauma among female veterans: a critical review. *Trauma, Violence, & Abuse* 2007;8(4): 384–400.

5. Anderson JM, Rodney P, Reimer-Kirkham S, Browne A, Khan KB, Lynam MJ. Inequities in health and healthcare viewed through the ethical lens of critical social justice: contextual knowledge for the global priorities ahead. *SO—Advances in Nursing Science* October/December 2009;32(4): 282–294.

6. Collins PH. *Black Feminist Thought: Knowledge, Consciousness, and the Politics of Empowerment*. New York, NY: Routledge; 2000.

7. Crenshaw KW. Mapping the margins: intersectionality, identity politics, and violence against women of color. In: Crenshaw K, Gotanda N, Peller G, Thomas K, eds. *Critical Race Theory: The Key Writings that Formed the Movement*. New York, NY: The New Press; 1995: 357–383.

8. Chavis AZ, Hill MS. Integrating multiple intersecting identities: a multicultural conceptualization of the power and control wheel. *Women & Therapy* 2009;32(1): 121–149.

9. Cramer EP, Plummer S-B. People of color with disabilities: intersectionality as a framework for analyzing intimate partner violence in social, historical, and political contexts. *Journal of Aggression, Maltreatment & Trauma* 2009;18(2): 162–181.

10. Kelly UA. "I'm a mother first": the influence of mothering in the decision-making processes of battered immigrant Latino women. *Research in Nursing & Health* June 2009;32(3): 286–297.

11. Weber L. Reconstructing the landscape of health disparities research: promoting dialogue and collaboration between feminist intersectional and biomedical paradigms. In: Schulz AJ, Mullings L, eds. *Gender, Race, Class, and Health: Intersectional Approaches*. San Francisco, CA: Jossey-Bass; 2006: 21–59.

12. Rogers J, Kelly UA. Feminist intersectionality: bringing social justice to health disparities research. *Nursing Ethics* 2011;18(3): 397.

13. Shilts R. *Conduct Unbecoming: Gays and Lesbians in the US Military*. New York, NY: St. Martin's Griffin; 2005.

14. Death of Chinese-American Soldier Draws Attention to Racism in Military [radio broadcast]. Public Radio International: The Takeaway with John Hockenberry radio program. December 22, 2011. http://www.thetakeaway.org/story/177126-death-chinese-american-soldier-draws-attention-racism-military/. Accessed April 8, 2014.

15. Benedict H. *The Lonely Soldier: The Private War of Women Serving in Iraq*. Boston, MA: Beacon Press; 2010.

16. Herbert M. *Camouflage Isn't Only for Combat: Gender, Sexuality, and Women in the Military*. New York, NY: NYU Press; 2000.

17. Kelly UA. Integrating intersectionality and biomedicine in health disparities research. *Advances in Nursing Science* Apr–Jun 2009;32(2): E42–E56.

18. Office of the Deputy Under Secretary of Defense. *Demographics 2009: Profile of the Military Community*. Washington, DC: US Department of Defense; 2009.

19. Maxfield BD. *Blacks in the US Army: Then and Now*. Office of Army Demographics; 2004. www.armyg1.army.mil/hr/docs/demographics/BlacksThenNow 83–03.ppt. Accessed April 8, 2014.

20. Yano EM, Washington DL, Goldzweig C, Caffrey C, Turner C. The organization and delivery of women's health care in Department of Veterans Affairs Medical Center. *Women's Health Issues* 2003;13(2): 55–61.

21. Bean-Mayberry BA, Yano EM, Caffrey CD, Altman L, Washington DL. Organizational characteristics associated with the availability of women's health clinics for primary care in the veterans health administration. *Military Medicine* 2007;172(8): 824–828.
22. Yano EM, Goldzweig C, Canelo I, Washington DL. Diffusion of innovation in women's health care delivery: the Department of Veterans Affairs' adoption of women's health clinics. *Women's Health Issues* 2006;16(5): 226–235.
23. Frayne SM, Yu W, Yano EM, et al. Gender and use of care: planning for tomorrow's Veterans Health Administration. *Journal of Women's Health* 2007;16(8): 1188–1199.
24. Washington DL, Bean-Mayberry B, Riopelle D, Yano EM. Access to care for women veterans: delayed healthcare and unmet need. *Journal of General Internal Medicine* 2011;26: 655–661.
25. Bean-Mayberry B, Yano EM, Washington DL, et al. Systematic review of women veterans' health: update on successes and gaps. *Women's Health Issues* 2011;21(4): S84–S97.
26. Bierman AS, Pugh MJV, Dhalla I, et al. Sex differences in inappropriate prescribing among elderly veterans. *The American Journal of Geriatric Pharmacotherapy* 2007;5(2): 147–161.
27. Sadler AG, Booth BM, Mengeling MA, Doebbeling BN. Life span and repeated violence against women during military service: effects on health status and outpatient utilization. *Journal of Women's Health* 2004;13(7): 799–811.
28. Street AE, Vogt D, Dutra L. A new generation of women veterans: stressors faced by women deployed to Iraq and Afghanistan. *Clinical Psychology Review* 2009;29(8): 685–694.
29. Thomas AJ, Witherspoon KM, Speight SL. Toward the development of the stereotypic roles for Black women scale. *The Journal of Black Psychology* 2004;30(3): 426–442.
30. West CM. Mammy, Sapphire, and Jezebel: Historical images of Black women and their implications for psychotherapy. *Psychotherapy: Theory, Research, Practice, Training* 1995;32(3): 458.
31. Woods-Giscombé C. Superwoman schema: African American women's views on stress, strength, and health. *Qualitative Health Research* 2010;20(5): 668.
32. Beauboeuf-Lafontant T. *Behind the Mask of the Strong Black Woman: Voice and the Embodiment of a Costly Performance.* Philadelphia, PA: Temple University Press; 2009.
33. Mullings L. Resistance and resilience: the sojourner syndrome and the social context of reproduction in Central Harlem. *Transforming Anthropology* 2005;13(2): 79–91.
34. Vogt D, Bergeron A, Salgado D, Daley J, Ouimette P, Wolfe J. Barriers to Veterans Health Administration care in a nationally representative sample of women veterans. *Journal of General Internal Medicine* 2006;21(S3): S19–S25.
35. Tillman S, Bryant-Davis T, Smith K, Marks A. Shattering silence: exploring barriers to disclosure for African American sexual assault survivors. *Trauma, Violence, & Abuse* 2010;11(2): 59–70.
36. Alvidrez J, Snowden LR, Kaiser DM. Involving consumers in the development of a psychoeducational booklet about stigma for Black mental health clients. *Health Promotion Practice* 2010;11(2): 249–258.
37. Snowden LR. Barriers to effective mental health services for African Americans. *Mental Health Services Research* 2001;3(4): 181–187.
38. Lester K, Artz C, Resick PA, Young-Xu Y. Impact of race on early treatment termination and outcomes in posttraumatic stress disorder treatment. *Journal of Consulting and Clinical Psychology* 2010;78(4): 480.

39. Nicolaidis C, Timmons V, Thomas MJ, et al. "You don't go tell White people nothing": African American women's perspectives on the influence of violence and race on depression and depression care. *Am J Public Health* August 1, 2010;100(8): 1470–1476.
40. Ouimette P, Vogt D, Wade M, et al. Perceived barriers to care among veterans health administration patients with posttraumatic stress disorder. *Psychological Services* 2011;8(3): 212.
41. Edlund MJ, Fortney JC, Reaves CM, Pyne JM, Mittal D. Beliefs about depression and depression treatment among depressed veterans. *Medical Care* 2008;46(6): 581.
42. Sayer NA, Friedemann-Sanchez G, Spoont M, et al. A qualitative study of determinants of PTSD treatment initiation in veterans. *Psychiatry-Interpersonal and Biological Processes* 2009;72(3): 238–255.
43. Spoont MR, Sayer N, Friedemann-Sanchez G, Parker LE, Murdoch M, Chiros C. From trauma to PTSD: beliefs about sensations, symptoms, and mental illness. *Qualitative Health Research* 2009;19(10): 1456–1465.
44. Fontana A, Rosenheck R. Treatment of female veterans with posttraumatic stress disorder: the role of comfort in a predominantly male environment. *Psychiatric Quarterly* 2006;77(1): 55–67.

21 Through a Socio-political Lens

The Relationship of Practice, Education, Research, and Policy to Social Justice

Jill White

In 1995, in an update and critique of Carper's Patterns of Knowing,[1] I introduced a new pattern of knowing called socio-political knowing. This pattern of knowing filled a gap I perceived in Carper's original quartet as it lifted the gaze of the nurse above the nurse-patient dyad and demanded a cognizance of, and engagement with, the environment in which care takes place. It sought to focus the nurses' attention on embedding care within an understanding of the context of the person who is the patient and their social and cultural background, so critical to health status. It demanded the nurse acknowledge him or herself as an influence within the context of care, personally, organizationally, and professionally, and it brought to the attention of the nurse the external perspectives held by health service providers and governments of nursing and nurses, often radically different to nurses perceptions of themselves and their work.

In this chapter I extend the discussion of socio-political knowing to our contemporary circumstances. You will find the words "emancipatory" or "praxis" rarely used in my in discussion of socio-political knowing, even though this knowing clearly furthers our nursing social justice mandate—praxis indeed. In my view socio-political knowing and emancipatory knowing are different. It may be that socio-political knowing is a necessary precursor to emancipatory knowing, but it is also a positioning and practice itself. Socio-political knowing is a broadening of the nurse's gaze to include the "wherein" or context of nursing and those who influence it. Whilst inevitably raising questions of equity and circumstance, of privilege, and of invisibility, socio-political knowing does not necessitate a critical social theory or critical feminist lens. Introduction of the language of emancipation without depth of philosophical understanding can leave people with a shallow veneer of critical social theory or critical feminist theory and a rhetoric of change and emancipation without the knowledge or ability to follow-through with the social challenge inherent in its philosophical stance. Whilst a critical feminist lens is the lens through which I live my life I do not believe it a prerequisite for all who want to contribute as nurses, whereas an understanding of socio-political knowing as a dimension of nursing knowledge is a prerequisite for all.

CONTEMPORARY CONTEXT

We are at a critical time in healthcare where our fascination with high technology and expensive pharmaceuticals has led us to an unsustainable health future and where choices made will influence options for communities to come. In Australia, New Zealand, and the United Kingdom the unaffordability of the health budget is resulting in a focus on cutting costs within existing services, rather than on the development of sustainable, affordable, community-based primary health care initiatives. Nursing's voice in these decisions is critical and socio-political knowing is foundational to inform this voice. In many countries of the world, possibly with the exception of the United States, this lack of nursing voice in policy is, I believe, a result of a fundamental disconnect between practice, education, research, and policy, the very instruments we have to engage with communities and influence those who make social and health policy decisions.

Achieving equity of health outcomes is inherently political—and politics is the ability to guide or influence policy, as policy is the enactment of decisions as they relate to the relative merits of options in the allocation of resources or the regulation of behavior. It has always seemed most strange to me that most nurses do not associate themselves or nursing with politics and don't see it as directly relevant to their professional work. "Justice-making," equitable access to available resources, regulation of behavior for social good, and equity of health outcomes has been at the very heart of nursing from its beginnings. It was the driving force for extraordinary nurses. Florence Nightingale, for example, systematically designed and implemented healthcare services and education systems. She collected data related to health and healthcare practice and developed means of data display in order to make her political point more compelling to policy makers.[2] Nightingale's goal was public policy change for improvements in health, in care of the sick, and in the prevention of illness. Nightingale's body of work provides a lived example of power of conceptualizing practice, education, research, and policy as inseparable for making a difference to health outcomes. However, one must be cautious in eulogizing her successes without understanding her positioning as a well-educated, well-connected, white woman of social position in a particular historical context. The politics of her privilege and actions hold as many lessons as the actions themselves.

The commitment of nursing to the reduction of health disparities as part of our professional social justice mandate through the integration of practice, education, research, and policy has waxed and waned over the intervening 150 years. In 1986 Chopoorian[3] reminded us that "Nursing practitioners continually confront the human responses to underlying social dynamics of poverty, unemployment, undernutrition, isolation and alienation precipitated through structures of society."[(p76)] This human response to such underlying social dynamics was something I saw keenly when nursing in the Emergency Department in a large inner-city hospital in an area of extreme poverty in Sydney. It inspired me to coin the term "socio-political knowing" in order to more fully express the need for a broader and practice focused knowledge base to underpin our daily thoughts and actions.

Since that time there has been an explosion of concern about what has become known as the "social determinants of health." Falk-Rafael[4] is explicit about nursing's responsibilities in this area and she maintains that influencing health policy is our moral obligation. "Nurses, who practice at the intersections of public policy and personal lives, are, therefore, ideally situated and morally obligated to include political advocacy and efforts to influence health public policy in their practice," and she goes on to say that she sees "Justice-making as an expression of caring and compassion."[(p212)]

Given the expanded public discourse about social determinants of health and nursing's central positioning in healthcare provision, one may ask why there is such a disjuncture between the rhetoric of nursing's concern and the lack of evidence of real contribution to the elimination of health inequality.

Clearly we are in vastly different times to those of Nightingale. We have seen enormous gains in women's rights, universal human rights, patient's rights and advocacy, and a rhetoric that has challenged medical dominance, and yet health care services remain focused on cure and heroics. We are, in resource rich and resource poor countries, in a time where our current health systems are progressively financially and environmentally enmeshed in complex economic and structural arrangements, both public and private.

In many countries, including Australia, New Zealand, and the UK, we have seen the disaggregation of influence between practice and education as nursing education has moved from hospital-based apprenticeships into the higher education sector. We have seen a disconnect between research output and the research needed to change models and modes of care, and we have experienced a near absence of nursing voice in public policy debate and influence. We have watched the gains made in nursing influence in the United States with great interest. We have wondered if the key to this was the inextricable and often geographical link between hospitals and universities and questioned whether it was this that provided the glue that prevented the dislocation from practice of the research and education, thus grounding policy input. Since the early days of the Clinton administration and more recently the Obama administration nursing has gained influence. Where the political will has been explicitly for the broader protection of the health of the public, the nursing voice is given room for expression and nurses have been acknowledged as having worthwhile contributions and solutions. This unfortunately has not been replicated elsewhere.

Perhaps in looking at each of our instruments of engagement: practice, education, research, and policy through a socio-political lens, it may be possible to see how, like Nightingale and some of our American colleagues, we may re-integrate them in the interest of stronger political influence and better health outcomes.

PRACTICE

Over many decades there has been an economically driven diminution in public access to primary health care and community nursing services. Outpatient clinics have disappeared from public hospitals, and nurses, once ubiquitous in the community, have largely lost their community connection. What the community expects of a nurse is to be accessible, to help people understand the foreign territory of health care, to attend to their wounds, and to help them heal; to vaccinate their children and identify mystery rashes; someone to talk to of their growing concern about their memory loss or their depression at being diagnosed with a chronic disease; someone who will demystify chemotherapy and make tolerable the extraordinary circumstances in which they may find themselves. The only aspect of nursing that is currently experienced by the public is ill health care during hospitalization.

Out of the public view, nurses have become captives of the business and busyness of the hospital world and the hospital has radically changed the line of sight of the nurse to the connection between health status and public policy. Hospitals are now large intensive care and trauma care units—no longer a site of convalescence, of community clinics for continuity of care, or the site of health teaching, but primarily a site of a "pathophysiological fix." Very often the recipient of treatment is experiencing a form of diminished consciousness, where comfort care becomes secondary to physiological and pharmaceutical monitoring. Hospitals have become environments where families are concerned about the safety of their relatives, as explicated by Claire Fagin in "When care becomes a burden,"[5] where nurses are frustrated at not being able to provide the care they were educated to give and where, out of desperation, unskilled family members are providing what is essentially nursing care.

This situation has been exacerbated by the fact that nurses have failed to educate the public about changed expectations of hospitalization and of care. There is a mismatch between what patients and their families expect of nursing care and what, in times of resource constraint, changed treatment modalities, and minimal length of stay, nurses can be expected to deliver. The consequence of this mismatch is dissatisfaction and confusion for all. In such a circumstance it is hard to imagine what vehicle exists for the nurse to see a connection to a social justice mandate.

The focus of the nurse on the needs of "allocated" patients in a hospital context narrows the nurse's focus from the social political and environmental factors influencing health disparity to one of intensive health care within the confines of an institution. This limits the nurses' exposure to "person knowledge," facilitating only the development of "case knowledge" and "patient knowledge" in Liaschenko and Fisher's[6] trilogy of knowledge used in nursing work. This narrowed view of "person knowledge" is twofold: nurses know little of the person who is the patient because of the acuity and intensity of the illness and the limited interaction due to the brief length of stay. The nurse also learns little of the community from which the person comes and to which they return. The very environment of the hospital prevents the nurse from attending to the person-environment connection made explicit in the classroom.

The commodification of caring[7] has reduced the perception of nurses by hospital management to being replaceable and moveable economic units of organizational cost rather than asset.[7] The result of this ideological shift has been a quest for efficiency and productivity with decreased the ratio of nurses to patients and significant numbers of lesser qualified nurses or health workers, changing both workforce numbers and skill-mix. Nursing's concern for patient safety and concern for the retention of experienced registered nurses within this new environment has resulted in a **workforce** focus to much of the research undertaken by nurses and others.

As an outcome of this workforce focus, nursing job satisfaction indicators were developed through the work of Linda Aiken and her colleagues,[8] the link between levels of registered nurse staffing and patient adverse events has been demonstrated by Cho et al.,[9] and the role of skill mix in patient outcomes quantified by Duffield et al.[10] A further body of workforce research focused on retention of staff through what became known as "Magnet Hospitals" work. This work demonstrated eight dimensions of "magnetism," or the ability of an organization to retain staff. These elements of "magnetism" are now well-known within nursing internationally. The key point here is that the focus of this work is the **hospital** and its organization not the care of the **person** who is the patient.

A second significant body of nursing practice research has been focused on **workplace** environment and the enhancement of team work at a unit or ward level. The Practice Development (PD) movement from the United Kingdom (UK) exemplifies this work. The "Patient Centred Nursing" (PCN) framework of McCormack and McCance[11] has been the strongest influence in this PD area. In Ireland, the UK, Australia, and New Zealand PD has been a positive influence on job satisfaction and climate within the care environment. This in itself is beneficial, however, if one were to look critically at this situation one might see the outcome as being akin to making the inmates happier within the jail, or making the shop floor more pleasant while the factory remains toxic in other ways—feeling better whilst captive within. The PD work remains focused on local solutions to local problems and in a socio-political sense fails to elevate what may be common local problems to researchable and generalizable solutions. The local focus makes a difference at the ward level but it fails to add to the body of international literature and thus influence the practice of other nurses or to influence policy. This, for me, is its greatest weakness. It should not be difficult to include in the PD process a link that would raise up the local problems identified to scalable research in order to add to the literature and nursing's body of knowledge about patient care. A direct link would be forged between the ground floor concerns of practice and patient care, the nursing research agenda, and potentially policy.

Whilst workforce and workplace studies have assisted with retention and skill mix arguments, there have been unintended negative consequences of this preoccupation. Research activity has been diverted away from the practice of nursing, the evidence of its effectiveness and improving health outcomes. A patient, community, employer, or government perspective of this large body of work may be that it is a preoccupation with self-study and an exercise in professional self-interest. Had this time, money and research effort been focused on person/patient care we may have had more substance to offer to policy directions.

EDUCATION

"Health professionals are the service providers who link people to technology, information, and knowledge. They are also caregivers, communicators and educators, team members, managers, leaders, and policy makers"[12(p1924)] Educating for such a complex role is a difficult task for educational institutions, often in tension with the demands of the employers of their graduates. The immediate health system need is for graduates who are able to nurse acutely ill people hospitalized for very short periods of time, often with complex co-morbidities in highly technological environments, and for these new graduates to be "work-ready" on entering the workforce. This hospital-centric need sits in tension with the mission of the education institution to educate the next generation of nurses to be well prepared for both current and future practice, to understand the social determinants of health, to appreciate the complexities of the systems of government and influence that determine health and social policy directions, to understand the vagaries of policy formation and change, and to develop the intellectual habits necessary for life-long learning. This educational goal is described by Frenk et al.[12] as producing graduates who are "educated to mobilize knowledge and to engage in critical reasoning and ethical conduct so that they are competent to participate in patient and population-centred health systems as members of locally responsive and globally connected teams."[(p1924)].

From a patient's perspective the movement away from an apprenticeship model of education within hospitals to the higher education sector has been simultaneous with the decrease in community and hospital nursing staff, the increase in in-patient acuity, and a decreased average length of hospital stay. It is unsurprising then that there is a "muddled perception" in the community consciousness that the unmet expectations of care in hospital and lack of community presence is the fault of baccalaureate education. Patients have little or no line of sight to the changes in skill-mix and staffing levels in hospitals that militate against the nurse being able to provide the care they have been educated to give, inclusive of comfort care. The outcome of this situation is that one hears in general conversation the sentiment that nurses are not being properly "trained" anymore and a community perception, again from general community conversation, that universities are no longer teaching nurses about comfort, care, and compassion. This represents a significant public relations challenge for universities and the nursing profession but one that will only be successful when a consistent message is reinforced by the health services.

Unfortunately, there is a disconnect between the academic world and the world of practice. The university sees its logical role as the provision of a suite of programs representing an educational progression, from undergraduate education to postgraduate specialist education and then potentially to doctoral education, as part of a professional career structure. This natural flow in educational attainment in a career is now a contested one from the perspective of the health system. Staff shortages and lack of funds make study leave provision difficult and the need for specialist graduate education is made less obvious by the decreasing specialization of the medical and surgical wards in our hospitals. The focus within the hospital on "throughput" and "bed management" as a means of enhancing bed utilization has led to an expanding case mix, increasing the diversity of patients in any hospital ward. A consequence of this situation is that nurse "must understand the care requirements, the pharmacology, the treatments, the protocols and preferences of specialist medical staff for an increasingly various patient assignment."[10(p140)] Case mix diversity has the potential to lead to a deskilling of the expert specialist nurse, the rise of the generalist, and presents little incentive for further specialist graduate study for more junior nurses.

There are two unintended consequences for nurses of this system of patient/bed management. The first is an invisible and unaccounted for increase in nursing workload caused by the increased movement of patients within and through the hospital, resulting in what Duffield has identified as "churn."[13] The second unintended consequence is that by decreasing the incentives for nurses to undertake specialist graduate education there is the concomitant loss of the depth and breadth graduate education brings that is beyond the specialist aspects of the curriculum. Lost is the opportunity for in-depth study of multiple and different ideological positioning; the opportunity to study politics, social policy, and political influence, the opportunity to study the moral comportment of nursing, and the opportunity to develop higher order critical thinking skills, to question the "taken for granteds" of privilege and position, and of what constitutes, or could constitute, health and health systems. Lost also is the logical progression for those research-minded scholars to doctoral studies and the development of research expertise.

RESEARCH AND POLICY

Nursing's contribution to evidence-based policy formation has been strained by the demands of government research funding and the "research excellence" exercises that appear to be rapidly spreading around the world, changing only their acronyms en route: RAE (research assessment exercise) in the UK, PBRF (performance based research funding) in NZ, and ERA (Excellence in research for Australia) in Australia. The linking of funding to publication in ranked journals with specific citation ratings and impact factors has a flow-on effect on the style and form of proposals that are developed in order to maximize the chance of competitive funding. It would appear that there is little concern at government levels about the impact of such exercises on the fostering of research that extends from discovery to knowledge translation into clinical practice and outcome evaluation.

What is clear, however, is that knowledge translation into clinical care is enhanced by the physical collocation of the researchers with care delivery. This is a fundamental premise for the development of Academic Health Sciences Centres in the UK; their introduction in Australia and more closely follows the example of university hospitals in the United States that are co-located with educational facilities. However, additionally in the United States, there have been joint clinical-academic appointments for nurse researchers in hospitals since the 1980s. Multidisciplinary evaluation of new modes or models of care, inclusive of measures of patient outcomes, patient and staff satisfaction, and economic evaluation are powerful tools for policy conversations with decision makers at all levels but remain rare in many of our countries.

As we have seen politics is the ability to influence resource allocation and to manipulate other key political levers, such as regulation. Policy is the mechanism by which such decisions are enacted. Policy influence is, there-fore, fundamental to nursing's ability to influence health care priorities and directions, with social justice the desired endpoint of such influence. Why then is nursing so often absent, or far from being seen as a central player, in health care and social policy development? Nurses are always acknowledged as being key policy implementers but rarely as central to policy development and rarely seen as "leading the way" in the health and social policy areas.

In 1996, Cohen and her colleagues[14] developed a four-level framework for exploring stages of political development. These levels were seen as buy-in; self-interest; political sophistication; and leading the way. Cohen and her colleagues selected four dimensions for the analysis of each of these stages: nature of the action; language; coalition building; and nurses as policy shapers. Whilst somewhat dated now it remains a helpful tool for identifying levels of political maturity. When one looks at the common posi-tioning of nursing it is frequently at the "buy-in" or "self-interest" stage, still lacking in sophistication and political savvy. The exception, as indicated earlier, is the United States that, I would suggest, whilst still not "leading the way" is at least at the level of "political sophistication."

Having a framework is, however, far from sufficient and education about and mentoring in the policy process, policy analysis, development, influence, and implementation is essential. Such exposure should be intro-duced in pre-service education as part of socio-political knowing, but the sophistication and complexity of this work can best be developed in graduate studies where these concepts are broadened and deepened and inclusive of emancipatory knowing. Graduate programs enable the building of a cadre of nurses who are well prepared to interact at policy tables. But this too is not sufficient. Being politically successful takes a multipronged strategy including education; research funding for developing the evidence base for policy argument; policy internships or residencies, ideally in nursing policy units to encourage skill development in policy entrepreneurship; but above all, policy leadership and role modeling is required from heads of national nursing organizations, from chief nurses of government, from academics, and from lead clinicians and nurse politicians.

COMING FULL CIRCLE

The current situations in many contexts with the dislocation of nursing practice from education, and from research, and each from the other, together with a general lack of policy savvy and influence could appear potentially depressing to patients, to health professionals, and to governments. We are, however, at an interesting moment in healthcare history, where the focus on acute care is no longer proving to be the most important instrument of health improvement. The successes in the prevention and treatment of acute illnesses have seen them drop from the national and international health priorities. Chronic diseases such as diabetes, heart disease, obesity, mental health, and emerging infectious diseases are now the health priorities.[15] This shift, together with the unaffordability of the continued growth of the acute care system, has brought together a constellation of strange bedfellows. Governments, communities, health professionals, and healthcare businesses are all looking for new directions and there is a growing consensus that this new direction has at its core a greater emphasis on primary health care.[16–20] Despite the lack of progress over several decades of calls for a focus on primary health care, from Alma Ata in 1976, to the Ottawa charter in 1986, and finally to the World Health Organization "Primary Health Care: Now More than Ever" World Report 2008,[15] we are now, in the second decade of the 21st century, beginning to see even conservative governments making tangible movements towards primary health care. Whether this is a philosophical shift from health as individual responsibility to a return to health as social mandate is questionable. Perhaps it is just economic pragmatism. Whatever the rationale, the outcome remains the potential for an improved system of care for people and their communities. Health promotion and disease prevention, chronic disease management in the community, and a public wish for supported dying at home offer nurses a renewed opportunity to reconnect with communities. This shift in service provision opens avenues for nursing involvement in community consultation, coalition building, and action to ameliorate health disparities. Having nurses engaged fully within communities enables the profession to again span both hospital based and community practice working with individuals and populations, to again bear witness to the effects of social policy decisions on the health and well-being of people and to speak, write, and advocate for the amelioration of health disparities—our social justice mandate.

Successful political action does not come easily. If nurses are to maximize political opportunities to make a difference to health outcomes and fulfill the social justice obligation we need to have something to offer at the policy table. Nurses must offer models of care that make a difference, must have the research evidence of the patient and economic benefit of our contribution, must have the ability to be articulate about this contribution, and must have built the coalitions to accomplish political change. If nursing is to make such a contribution, we must do as Nightingale did so long ago—integrate our practice, education, research, and policy endeavors.

It is a time for optimism but this optimism must be tempered with an "eyes wide open" skepticism. Given the complex and changeable socio-political environment in which we all live and in which nursing practice, education, and research take place, it remains a time for the consistent application of a socio-political lens.

REFERENCES

1. White J. Patterns of knowing: review, critique and update. *Adv Nurs Sci* 1995; 17(4): 73–86.
2. Keith J. Florence Nightingale: statistician and consultant epidemiologist. Int Nurs Rev 1988;35(5): 147–150.
3. Chopoorian T. Reconceptualizing the environment. In: Moccia P, ed. *New Approaches in Theory Development*. New York, NY: National League for Nursing; 1986: 39–54.
4. Falk-Rafael A. Speaking truth to power—nursing's legacy and moral imperative. *Adv Nurs Sci* 2005;28(3): 212–223.
5. Fagin C. When care becomes a burden. Milbank Memorial Fund Web site. 2001. http://www.milbank.org/reports/010216fagin.html. Accessed October 24, 2012.
6. Liaschenko J, Fisher A. Theorizing the knowledge that nurses use in the conduct of their work. Scholarly Inquiry for Nursing Practice, 1999;13(1): 29–41.
7. White J. *Commodification of Caring*. Unpublished doctoral thesis. Adelaide, Australia: University of Adelaide; 2004.
8. Aiken L, Clarke S, Sloane D, Sochalski J, Busse R, Clarke H, et al. Nurses' reports on hospital care in five countries. *Health Affairs* 2001;20(3): 43–53.
9. Cho S, Ketefian S. Barkauskas V, Smith D. The effects of nurse staffing on adverse events, morbidity, mortality and medical costs. *Nurs Res* 2003;52(2): 71–79.
10. Duffield C, Roche M, O'Brien-Pallas L, Diers D, Aisbett C, King M, et al. *Glueing It Together: Nurses, Their Work Environment and Patient Safety.* Sydney, Australia: University of Technology, CHSM; 2007. http://www0.health.nsw.gov.au/pubs/2007/nwr_report.html. Accessed October 24, 2012.
11. McCormack B, McCance T. *Person Centred Nursing*. Oxford, UK: Wiley-Blackwell; 2010.

12. Frenk J, Chen L, Bhutta Z, Cohen J, Crisp N, Evans T, et al. Health professionals for a new century: transforming education to strengthen health systems in an independent world. *The Lancet* 2010;376: 1923–1958.

13. Duffield C, Diers D, Aisbett C, Roche M. Churn: patient turnover and case mix. *Nursing Economics* 2009;27(3): 185–191.

14. Cohen S, Mason D, Kovner C, Leavitt J, Pulcini J, Sochalski J. Stages of nursing's political development: where we've been and where we ought to go. *Nurs Outl* 1996;44(6): 259–266.

15. Moussavi S, Chatterji S, Verdes E, Tandon A, Partel V, Uston B. Depression, chronic diseases, and decrements in health: results from the world health surveys. *The Lancet* 2007;370(9590): 851–858.

16. World Health Organization. *The World Health Report 2008—Primary Health Care (Now More Than Ever)*. Geneva, Switzerland: Author, 2009.

17. Australian Government Health and Hospitals Reform Commission. *A Healthier Future for All Australians: National Health and Hospitals Reform Commission—Final Report June 2009*. Canberra, Australia: Commonwealth of Australia, 2009. http://www.yourhealth.gov.au/internet/yourhealth/publishing.nsf/Content/nhhrc-report. Accessed October 22, 2012.

18. Institute of Medicine. The future of nursing: leading change advancing health. October 2010. http://www.iom.edu/Reports/2010/The-Future-of-Nursing-Leading-Change-Advancing-Health.aspx. Accessed October 16, 2012.

19. The Prime Minister's Commission on the Future of Nursing and Midwifery in England. *Frontline Care: The Future of Nursing and Midwifery in England*. London, UK: Author; 2010. http://webarchive.nationalarchives.gov.uk/20100331110400/http://cnm.independent.gov.uk/the-report/. Accessed April 4, 2014.

20. Canadian National Expert Commission. The Health of Our Nation, the Future of Our Health System: A Nursing Call to Action. http://www.cna-aiic.ca/en/on-the-issues/national-expert-commission/. Accessed April 4, 2014.

22 A Passion in Nursing for Justice
Toward Global Health Equity

Afaf I. Meleis and Caroline G. Glickman

INTRODUCTION

Central to nursing's mission is to ensure, to use, and to implement the tenets of social justice as a framework for practice, education, and research. Chapters of this volume are focused on the entire scope of equity inclusive of many of its components of justice. In producing this impressive work, the editors are reclaiming the social mission of nursing and affirming its significance in educating the next generation of nurses, researchers, educators, clinicians, administrators, and leaders in nursing. This is a book that will inspire dialogues about social justice and equity and challenge the readers to think about its meaning, its impact, and the strategies to fully utilize it.

This chapter underpins the importance of the implementation of social justice and equity theoretical models in education, research, and evidence-based practice to advance global health equity. We begin by discussing some of the gross health inequities that pervade all countries (low, mid, and high income), nurses' entrenched commitment to eliminating social injustices and health inequities, and the shortcomings in attaining global health equity as evident in the slow progress of the Millennium Development Goals.[1] Next we expand on the contributions of Justice Theories to advance health equity and how nurses can further contribute to the justice dialogues as well as the vital role they play in advancing health equity through five different components. These components are: notions of health, access to health care, gender issues as front and center in the discipline, maximizing the potential of nurses to practice to their full capacity, and breaking of disciplinary silos. Following this, we discuss the contributions of theories of justice to the discipline of nursing in uncovering inequities and the voices of nurses and their clients. Finally, we underscore the importance of nurses taking pride and embracing their history, as well as the social justice dialogues, to continue to advance knowledge and promote equity for a healthier future for all.

HEALTH INEQUITIES: BARRIERS TO HUMAN PROGRESS AND DEVELOPMENT

Inequality is at the root of injustice in the world and serves as a barrier to human progress and sustainable development. Therefore, we cannot consider social justice and equity without taking a broader view that encompasses a global perspective. Injustice is a major health risk that is not confined to only developing countries. For example the United States outspends all other nations in health care. However, one in five women of reproductive age lack health insurance and therefore cannot afford prenatal care. As a result, maternal mortality in the United States is high for a developed country, ranking 50th among nations with the lowest rates of maternal mortality.[2] Marginalization and discrimination due to race, gender, or socio-economic status perpetuates disempowerment and inequities in health, education, and income in all nations, both rich and poor.

The discipline of nursing has always embraced a profound commitment to social justice, health equity, and empowerment. In reviewing the history of the profession of nursing in many countries, one immediately identifies several common patterns in the health and health care of populations. One such pattern is the crux of the arguments and the narratives provided in this book. Nursing affects people one by one, community by community, and nation by nation. As nurses, we take seriously our moral obligation to make a difference in the health and well-being of individuals and populations, regardless of their socio-economic status. Throughout history, the nursing profession has been built on providing access to health care for vulnerable populations such as the warriors in the Crimean War, the defenders during the Prophet Mohammed era, the poor in New York, and the immigrants in California. Nurses were always there developing systems, processes, or delivering much needed care, both preventive and curative. From these beginnings, nursing as a profession was born, nursing education was developed, nursing theories evolved, and nursing science advanced. Without clearly articulating it or utilizing it, a justice paradigm provided a framework for nursing as a profession and nursing as a discipline. Clinicians, teachers, researchers, and theorists in the discipline of nursing have been dedicated to the global mission of building healthy communities and providing equitable access to health care for all populations as manifested in cursory review of the mission statements of nursing schools. However, perhaps due to structural and political constraints, nurses have neither successfully presented a united front nor a strong voice to change unjust practices or inaccessible health care resources.

MILLENNIUM DEVELOPMENT GOALS: PROMOTING GLOBAL HEALTH EQUITY

There are many indications that we have fallen short in promoting global health equity. A salient indication is the lack of progress made in achieving the Millennium Development Goals (MDGs). The MDGs were endorsed by the United Nations member states in 2001 with the goal to improve the lives of hundreds of millions of people around the world and ensure their basic human rights by 2015. The following are the MDGs:

1. ERADICATE EXTREME POVERTY & HUNGER
   - Reduce by half the proportion of people whose income is less than $1 a day
   - Achieve full and productive employment and decent work for all, including women and young people
   - Reduce by half the proportion of people who suffer from hunger

2. ACHIEVE UNIVERSAL PRIMARY EDUCATION
   - Ensure that all boys and girls complete a full course of primary schooling

3. PROMOTE GENDER EQUALITY AND EMPOWER WOMEN
   - Eliminate gender disparity in primary and secondary education preferably by 2005, and in all levels of education no later than 2015

4. REDUCE CHILD MORTALITY
   - Reduce by two thirds the mortality of children under five

5. IMPROVE MATERNAL HEALTH
   - Reduce maternal mortality by three quarters
   - Achieve universal access to reproductive health

6. COMBAT HIV/AIDS, MALARIA, AND OTHER DISEASES
   - Halt and reverse the spread of HIV/AIDS
   - Achieve, by 2010, universal access to treatment for HIV/AIDS for all those who need it
   - Halt and reverse the incidence of malaria and other major diseases

7. ENSURE ENVIRONMENTAL SUSTAINABILITY
   - Integrate principles of sustainable development into country policies and programs; reverse the loss of environmental resources
   - Reduce biodiversity loss, achieving, by 2010, a significant reduction in the rate of loss
   - Halve the proportion of people without access to safe drinking water and basic sanitation
   - Improve the lives of at least 100 million slum dwellers by 2020

8. DEVELOP A GLOBAL PARTNERSHIP FOR DEVELOPMENT
   - Develop further an open, rule-based, predictable, non-discriminatory trading and financial system
   - Address special needs of the least developed countries, landlocked countries, and small island developing States
   - Deal comprehensively with developing countries' debt

- In cooperation with pharmaceutical companies, provide access to affordable essential drugs in developing countries
- In cooperation with the private sector, make available the benefits of new technologies, especially information and communications technologies.[1]

At the Millennium Development Goals Summit in 2010, it was confirmed that the world is behind in achieving most of these goals. Although significant goals such as decreasing extreme poverty by half and increasing access to safe drinking water have been achieved well before the 2015 target date, much progress remains to be made in order to successfully achieve the rest of the MDGs.[3]

For example, progress remains slow in the reduction of maternal mortality. According to the United Nations, maternal mortality rates in developing regions, such as sub-Saharan Africa and Southern Asia, is still 15 times higher than in developed regions due to a lack of access to skilled health professionals (doctor, nurse, or midwife) to administer interventions that prevent and manage life-threatening conditions resulting from childbirth, such as fistula.[1] Also, despite the progress made in eradicating poverty, hunger continues to pervade many parts of the world. In 2011, the Food and Agriculture Organization of the United Nations estimated that between 2006 and 2008 globally 850 million people, 15.5% of the world's population, suffered from hunger and malnutrition.[1] Worldwide, malnutrition is the cause of one third of all maternal and childhood deaths. Young children who are malnourished are more susceptible to illness and life-threatening health conditions such as diarrhea, malaria, and pneumonia.[4,]

Another indicator is the fight against HIV/AIDS, which started too late with insufficient resources, particularly for heterosexual women who were mistakenly considered not at risk for contracting HIV. This societal mindset disempowered and constrained women from using preventive measures to protect themselves from this life-threatening disease. Today, the worldwide HIV epidemic continues to reveal underlying social injustices, gender inequalities, and violations of girls' and women's human rights. Women in societies and cultures where there are definite gender power imbalances are very vulnerable to HIV even though they do not have multiple partners; in some communities, marriage itself is a risk factor.[5]

The gross injustices faced by the girl-children of the world are a third indication of our failure to effectively advance health equity. In many parts of the world, girl-children are discriminated against starting from birth, through childhood, and into their adulthood. They suffer the most from human trafficking, violence, sexually transmitted diseases, genital mutilation, child labor, bride selling/trading, unwanted pregnancies, "honor killings," and lack of access to education and health care. When the girl-child is born into a culture that does not protect her rights she is most likely to be married before puberty in order to insure protection of her virginity and the honor of her father. Young girls who appear in health care systems as pregnant teens or in surgical units to repair fistulas that they incurred due to pregnancy and delivery-related ruptures are only provided care for the presenting physical conditions rather than the underlying societal inequities that are fundamental to the health or illness condition.

The trafficking and slavery of women from and between developing and developed countries are a fourth major example of failure in translating and implementing a justice paradigm. Girls and women are being transported, willingly or unwillingly, with false promises from Eastern European countries, Latin American countries, and between Asian countries. They are enslaved to work cheaply, to become sex objects, commercial sex workers, or brides for hire. And just as we failed for decades to assess and identify women who are battered in intimate partner relations, and just as there was limited recourse for perpetrators and shelters for protection, there continue to be limited resources and strategies to identify, protect, and shelter the girls and women who are trafficked for either cheap labor, sex enslavement, marriage, or prostitution.

CONTRIBUTIONS OF JUSTICE THEORIES TO ADVANCE HEALTH EQUITY: RAWLS AND SEN

John Rawls' *Theory of Justice*, an important work that helped draw attention to societal injustices, calls for awareness of all constituencies of the presence of injustice, and the need of social cooperation to achieve a just society. Rawls' theory provides general principles and focuses on societies at large and on all institutions within societies.[6] In utilizing this theory, the health system is identified as an institution needing reform in order to insure health equity. Therefore, Rawls' theory[6] posits that health equity cannot be achieved without equity in health care and in economic allocations.[7] Each institution provides a piece in the puzzle of social equity in general. So, what are the pieces of the larger puzzle of equity that may be within the reach and within the mission of nursing as a discipline?

Amartya Sen uses comparative theories of justice and argues that in order for justice to prevail it is necessary to focus on injustices and deal with each one more specifically. By considering justice along a continuum, there is hope that equity can be successfully attained in all societies. He argues against a set of principles developed by Rawls to achieve an impossible goal—an overall "just" society. Sen advocates for focusing on injustices of certain practices or outcomes in which there is major consensus and agreement. In other words, to be effective, nurses can select practices that reflect specific injustices such as disparities in pain management or lack of access to quality care due to gender, race, or class, and develop collective strategies to change these unjust practices. Similarly, nurse scientists may collectively voice concerns about lack of representation of minorities or women in scientific reports.

What could the discipline of nursing contribute to the dialogue about justice and equity and what could the profession offer in operationalizing the theories of justice? The discipline of nursing has a robust history in theoretical development and can continue to further drive the development of coherent justice frameworks to meet the global mission of achieving health equity. Nurses are critical scientific thinkers, innovative champions for justice, and global change agents who operationalize justice theories by creating nursing therapeutics, interventions, and resources tailored to the unique situations and experiences of clients and their families in order to promote equity and improve the health and well-being of all people.

There are five areas from which a dialogue about equity and justice can make a contribution to the overall discourse about equity. The discipline of nursing can affect equity through these components. These are: the notion of health; access to health care; gender issues as front and center in the discipline; maximizing the potential of nurses to practice to their full capacity; and breaking of disciplinary silos.

The Notion of Health

Health, which is one of the central concepts of nursing, is defined by the World Health Organization (WHO) as not merely the absence of disease but the ability of people to experience a sense of well-being. Nurse theorists have complemented the received view of health, empirically based and one dominated by positivism, with a more subjective view that focused on those who experience the health and illness situation. The nursing literature has provided support for the significance of uncovering the lived experience of individuals, and populations as the basis for providing ideas of health as an adaptation.[8,9] Health as defined through awareness, consciousness, space, energy, time, and environment, health as personal empowerment, and health as a process that is dynamic and interactive with community and society presuppose how health could only be understood within an institutional and societal context.[8,9,10] Although each of these models provides the potential to address social justice, none explicitly voice that aspect of the framework. For example, Smith's[9] four models of health and illness, clinical model, role performance model, adaptive model, and eudaemonistic model, offer a progressive expansion of the notion of health but is not grounded in social justice theory. If health is defined by a focus on the quality of life, which is an outcome considered vital for nursing care processes and interventions, then perhaps by insuring the provision of care that promotes equality to all, we may come closer to achieving some level of equity.

Access to Health Care

Although justice for Rawls[6] was articulated brilliantly as a set of principles, i.e., if these broad societal principles are achieved, societies could claim that they operate within an equitable framework, conversely, others argued of the impracticality of this approach. Robert Solomon in his book *A Passion for Justice*, argues from a social norms perspective about ways to achieve equity.[11] He posits that caring and compassion that emerge from having experienced or witnessed indignation, discriminatory resentments, and other negative actions or emotions are front and center in working toward a more equitable and just situation. Nurses often come face to face with discriminatory actions ranging from lack of recognition of suffering to inequity in information dissemination to lack of equity in diagnosis, treatments, and providing preventive measures to rerouting emergency department patients due to lack of insurance or questionable citizenship. Although the ultimate goals of nursing are to provide preventive or therapeutic interventions based on caring, alleviation of suffering, relief from pain, supporting healthy dying, and supporting healthy interactions among other nursing actions, these goals are compromised by inequity and injustices. Many nursing theorists described nursing as a human and caring science that is based on connections and interactions. Questions that could be explored in nursing to further participate in the justice dialogue are: what interactions and connections enhance equity? How does alleviating suffering contribute to a theory of justice? And in what ways do caring and compassion enhance perceived justice and equity in people, communities, and societies? Theories developed in the discipline of nursing should reflect social capital and social impact ideas and concepts. By doing this, differentials in care due to sociocultural or biological factors could become front and center in dialogues within the discipline.

The inequities in resources that lie within the domain of nursing are also manifested in an unequal focus on treatment instead of prevention, on acute illness instead of chronic illnesses, and more on infectious diseases in developing countries and less on neglected diseases in developing and developed countries. Inequitable access to health care is a major global issue and a challenge for which nurses can play a leadership role and have a powerful voice to continue to uncover it.[12]

Models and examples from the field of nursing could enrich theories of justice and equity. Nurses advance social justice through their research by focusing on improving life and health conditions of vulnerable patients and by empowering them to achieve optimum health.[13] For example, some nurse scholars utilize postcolonial feminist and human justice frameworks to uncover gender and structural inequities and oppressive structures. A social justice and equity framework focuses on an analysis of how resources are distributed and the rationale behind the distribution. It also draws attention to how different social groups are compromised through discrimination, stigmatization, and stereotyping.[14]

Postcolonial feminist theory complements a social justice framework. These two theoretical perspectives can work in synergy to advance health equity. Postcolonial feminism sheds light on the historical complexity of gender and ethnic power imbalances within and between systems, respects the agency of all women, and reflects nursing's core values of human dignity, social justice, equity, empowerment, and autonomy. Postcolonial feminism emerged from the feminist philosophy that focuses on the idea that colonialist properties of the past centuries are inextricably bound to the unique gendered realities of non-white and non-Western women.[15] It not only maintains patriarchy as a source of oppression but also examines the impact of how social, political, cultural, and economic inequities serve as underlying influences in health and health care delivery.[16] Postcolonial feminist theory challenges the status quo and dispels myths that tend to stereotype and categorize people, which impede their ability to receive access to equitable health care.[14]

Gender Equity

In the second decade of the 21st century, issues of gender equity are taking a central focus in many dialogues that may range from the global economy to world peace. Although many have described the problems that women and girls face, there has been a realization that girls and women hold the key to improving, if not solving, many of the most in trenchant global issues. Foreign aid, United Nations, the U.S. State Department, and U.S. Foreign Services have all included women and girls front and center in negotiations and in allocation of resources. Nurses have contributed to these gender inequity dialogues through their focus on decreasing infant and maternal mortalities, preparing midwives to enhance healthy parenthood, empowering women through promoting their health, educating health care workers as community extenders, advancing science related to intimate partner violence, developing tools to diagnose skin injuries due to rape, identifying women in violent situations, and providing opportunities for men and women as careerists in the profession of nursing.

Findings from an Institute of Medicine (IOM) report support addressing inequities in the health of women, the social disadvantages on women, and the differences in morbidities, prevalence, and mortalities associated with gender.[17] The inequities start from selective abortion for the girl fetuses resulting from advancement in technology of recognizing the sex of fetuses, to preferential treatment of baby boys through better nutrition and more immediate health care, to under-representation of women in research related to cardiovascular disease (although cardiovascular disease is the number one killer of women). Findings related to longevity demonstrate that in spite of all these inequities women tend to live longer than men. Women's longer lifespans are attributed to their abilities to cope better with stress, worry, resilience, and hard work as well as to their empathetic abilities and focus on nurturing, caring, communication, and connections.[18]

Nurses to Practice Up to Full Capacity

As frontline providers of care, nurses are well-positioned to drive change and advance health equity. However, nurses' potential—the potential of the largest global health care workforce—to play a vital role in improving access to care continues to be squandered by a number of inequities that must be addressed in gender, education, policy, and economic compensation. The marginalization and disempowerment of nurses through limiting their ability to use their education, expertise, and experience hinders them from enhancing access to care and the well-being and quality of life of their clients, thus decelerating progress in meeting the global health care needs and providing accessible quality care.

When supported, nurses are prepared and educated to lead, to practice, to advocate, and to make a difference. Yet they are not provided the policies, the legislative mandates, and the resources that permit them to practice up to their full capacity. A justice framework is needed to uncover oppressive structures and ensure nurses are empowered to practice at their greatest ability under the following conditions:

- Practice to the full extent of their education and training;
- Achieve higher levels of education and training through seamless academic progression;
- Be full partners with physicians and other health care professionals in redesigning health care; and
- Have effective data and information systems.[19]

Breaking of Disciplinary Silos

Breaking down the walls between the different disciplines is a venue that enhances valuation and equity. We need to change educational systems to break down silos and allow for interprofessional education, which would better reflect and contribute to the equity dialogue through providing patient-centered care, improving health outcomes, decreasing costs in developed countries, and improving the quality of care in developing countries. Building interprofessional health care teams and redesigning educational systems is "critical to achieving care that is patient-centered, safer, timelier, and more effective, efficient, and equitable."[20] When health care teams share a common, coherent vision they work more effectively towards achieving their collective goals when providing care. In order to keep pace with the global health issues that coincide with increasing globalization, urbanization, aging, and chronic illness, it is necessary to cultivate a team-based learning environment. A golden moment of great momentum in the transformation of health professional education has been ignited by the *Health Professionals for a New Century: Transforming Education to Strengthen Health Systems in an Interdependent World* report published in 2010 in *The*

Lancet, and the Robert Wood Johnson Foundation and Institute of Medicine (RWJ-IOM) *The Future of Nursing: Leading Change, Advancing Health* report. These ground-breaking reports challenge educators to reshape the education of the future generation of health professionals by integrating the expertise of various disciplines for a future of optimum quality care and a more just and equitable health care system.[19,21] However, key challenges that exist in implementing interprofessional education include a lack of top administrative leadership support for resources to develop an interprofessional element to the curriculum; lack of institutional partners to engage in interprofessional learning; practical issues such as scheduling and finding time to bring students together across disciplines; and training of health professions faculty to effectively teach interprofessional courses.[22] Despite these challenges, many academic institutions in the United States such as Vanderbilt University, The University of Minnesota, Rosalind Franklin University, and Western University of Health Sciences support and implement interprofessional education programs.[22] Internationally, five countries comprising the Asian Network—Vietnam, Thailand, Bangladesh, China, and India—have begun to implement information-sharing initiatives to generate health profession education reform in their own countries and regionally.[23]

Interdisciplinarity and interprofessionalism are the present and the future in educating health care professionals because at the crux of creating safe and quality health care are teams, partnerships, and collaborations. Fostering interprofessional education liberates health care teams from adhering to archaic structures and remaining within their disciplinary silos. As aforementioned, it effectively engages the different professions in both a shared vision and mission, which results in being more effective in managing health care issues and achieving optimum patient health outcomes. Dr. Jordan Cohen, former President and CEO of the Association of American Medical Colleges (AAMC) and 2012–2015 co-chair of the Institute of Medicine Global Forum on Innovation in Health Professional Education stated, "The paradigm of authoritarian captain of the team is shifting toward being an effective and respectful teammate. Well-functioning, interdisciplinary teams of health care professionals are undeniably the key to providing cost-effective, coordinated, high quality care, especially to patients with chronic, unremitting disease. Your generation [new medical school graduates] is in for a profound shift in the time-honored, hierarchical culture of medicine, with doctors on top having unquestioned authority, with nurses having little or no autonomy, and with pharmacists and most other health professionals being slaves to doctors' orders. The new paradigm: non-hierarchical, full participation of all who can help achieve optimal health outcomes."[24]

In 2012, six health professions associations in the United States joined to establish the Interprofessional Education Collaborative (IPEC), a national organization that focuses on reshaping educational programs for nurses, physicians, dentists, pharmacists, public health professionals, and other members of the patient health care team to provide more collaborative and patient-centered care. The founding members include the American Association of Colleges of Nursing, the American Association of Colleges of Osteopathic Medicine, the American Association of Colleges of Pharmacy, the American Dental Education Association, the Association of American Medical Colleges, and the Association of Schools of Public Health. In addition, the Institute of Medicine (IOM) established the Global Forum on Innovation in Health Education as a result of the Lancet Commission and Future of Nursing reports to take the strategic level ideas of these two reports and translate them into action. This multidisciplinary forum provides a platform to dialogue about contemporary issues in health professional education, facilitate sharing of best practices, and create and evaluate new ideas to advance interprofessional education. One of us, (Afaf I. Meleis) has the honor of serving as co-chair of this forum along with Dr. Jordan Cohen, who is mentioned above.

Nurses are vital partners in continuing to generate momentum in interprofessional education as they are uniquely positioned to be a driving force in mobilizing and promoting team work and collaborations in order to provide effective and equitable health care for all populations around the world. Collaboration and partnership between countries and between disciplines to reduce risks for wellness, affirm accountability for wellness, decrease the burden of disease, and build the capacity and sense of responsibility is the framework for the future.[25]

CONTRIBUTIONS OF JUSTICE TO THE PRACTICE OF NURSING

Capacity to Enhance Well-Being

By adopting an equity dialogue, the discipline of nursing can make a difference in nurses' roles, accountability, and their voice in policy changes. The capacity to enhance well-being and enable patients to function up to their full capabilities in spite of suffering acute or chronic illness, handicapping conditions, or debilitating environmental toxins is within the domain of nursing. One of the central goals for nursing care is to provide care that enhances the ability of people to care for themselves and to maximize their sense of well-being. Providing information, although essential, is not sufficient by itself in developing skills of individuals or communities to care for themselves or to prevent further debilitating conditions. Nurses ensure their patients' opportunities for rehearsing, modeling of self-care, and providing equal access to resources until the capabilities of self-care are developed and enhanced.

Personal capabilities and disabilities, immune systems, exposure to toxic and hazardous situations, and climate changes all contribute to inequities in health of individuals and in their capacities to be healthy. Sen[7] proposes that there should be distinctions made between equality in capabilities and equality in resources and distributions. Although members of the discipline may make a contribution to access and resources, there is also a role for the profession that claims that the well-being of human beings is a central goal, to enhance capabilities and capacities.

Finally, social justice theory could contribute to ensuring that patients are making their choices and health care decisions based on equity in the information they receive about all options. Nurses are in the best position to ensure the delivery of all pertinent information.

Voice

Uncovering inequities in health and health care require forming a voice and utilizing that voice. Our example of postcolonial feminism provides a framework for the voice that nurses as theoreticians, clinicians, and scientists can use. As aforesaid, postcolonial feminism provides the lens to recognize and explore oppressions, subordination, and patriarchal, traditional processes and systems that lend to marginalize people and render them more vulnerable to inequalities. These processes and systems that sustain injustice, some taken for granted, some long accepted, are a source for unrelenting inequality. Postcolonial feminism provides the lens to examine how inequalities in the idea of health or health access is located and developed within cultural, social, and historical contexts.

It is a lens that helps in uncovering as well as providing the language to communicate and to be voiced about these inequalities. It is also a lens through which to view how knowledge is developed, how truth is constructed, and how science is viewed. Through this lens, we are given the tools to uncover how students are socialized to devalue the nursing voices and nurses' ways of knowing. Developing an authentic voice in nursing requires acknowledgement and valuation of practice as a source of knowledge as well as support for how nurses tend to uncover the individual and collective voices of their clients.[26] Equity in understanding pain and suffering and the different ways by which it is manifested and in advancing knowledge lie at the crux of utilizing social justice theory as well as informing these theories.

Nurses have always served as a voice for the "voiceless" against injustices and have readily adopted interdisciplinarity and interprofessionalism, proclaiming its value for students and for quality care. Nurses' voices are better heard in affecting policy when others who enjoy greater accepted value and power join in to affirm these principles. In a more just society, and in a more equitable professional environment, nurses' voices of truth and expertise alone should have made the difference. Now that other voices have joined in affirming nurses' vision, these early decades of the 21st century promise to be a turning point. Although the processes to reach these goals reflect inequity, the resultant changes reflect social justice.

A Glimpse from the Past, a Window for the Future

To understand and remember nursing's past is to move forward to the future. The nursing discipline's history serves as a solid foundation to further build nursing science and knowledge and to understand and address current health system problems.[27] A strong connection to nursing history also enables us to understand disenfranchisement, exploitation, and disempowerment, as nurses themselves have experienced these many faces of oppression.[28] Historically, nurses have been seen as handmaidens by physicians and by society rather than as respected peers and science-based health professionals. Nurses have also been marginalized by other nurses due to differences in education (diploma vs. advanced degree) and levels of hierarchy in health care systems. Understanding and embracing nursing's history of oppression, and gender inequities (94% of nurses are women), will stimulate open dialogues and create relationships necessary to overcome obstacles to empowerment.[29] And we must also embrace the history of empowered nurses who have created innovative programs for war victims, for home care, and for global health.[30]

We should have pride in our history, which is full of strong, visionary pioneers who have questioned the status quo and revolutionized many aspects of health care for the betterment of patients and the nursing profession. Maintaining a strong sense of disciplinary identity, acknowledging the significance of nursing's history and theoretical knowledge development, and embracing social justice enhance and make for true equity dialogue. Nurses, in equity dialogue, will continue to have a strong voice, advocate for oppressed groups and for each other, and make a global difference in quality of life and care. Justice and equity dialogues are a means to that end.

REFERENCES

1. United Nations. *The Millennium Development Goals Report 2012*. New York, NY: United Nations Department of Economic and Social Affairs; 2012.
2. WHO, UNICEF, UNFPA, World Bank. *Trends in Maternal Mortality: 1990 to 2010*. Geneva, Switzerland: World Health Organization; 2012.
3. United Nations. *We Can End Poverty 2015—Millennium Development Goals*. http://www.un.org/millenniumgoals/. Accessed on January 7, 2013.
4. World Health Organization. Children: reducing mortality. Fact sheet 178; Sept 2012. http://www.who.int/mediacentre/factsheets/fs178/en/index.html. Accessed on January 7, 2013.
5. UNFPA. *Protecting the Health of Women and Girls*. 2012. http://www.unfpa.org/hiv/women.htm. Accessed on January 7, 2013.
6. Rawls J. *A Theory of Justice*. Cambridge, MA: The Belknap Press of Harvard University Press; 1971.
7. Sen A. Why health equity? *Health Econ* 2002;11(8): 659–666.
8. Roy C. *Introduction to Nursing: An Adaptation Model*. 2nd ed. Englewood Cliffs, NJ: Prentice-Hall; 1984.
9. Smith JA. *The Idea of Health: Implications for the Nursing Professional*. New York, NY: Teachers College, Columbia University; 1983.

10. Jones PS, Meleis AI. Health is empowerment. *Adv Nurs Sci* 1993;15(3): 1–14.
11. Solomon R. *A Passion for Justice: Emotions and the Origins of the Social Contract.* Lanham, MD: Rowman and Littlefield Publishers, Inc; 1995.
12. Racine L, Petrucka P. Enhancing decolonization and knowledge transfer in nursing research with non-western populations: examining the congruence between primary healthcare and postcolonial feminist approaches. *Nurs Inq* 2011;18(1): 12–20.
13. Bathum ME. Global health research to promote social justice: a critical perspective. *Adv Nurs Sci* 2007;30(4): 303–314.
14. Meleis AI, Topaz M. Nursing theory of the future: situation-specific theories. *Pflege* 2011;24(6): 345–347.
15. Mills S. Postcolonial feminist theory. In Jackson S, Jones J eds. *Contemporary Feminist Theories.* Edinburgh, UK: Edinburgh University Press; 1998: 98–112.
16. Racine L. The impact of race, gender, and class in postcolonial feminist fieldwork: a retrospective critique of methodological dilemmas. *Aporia: The Nurs Jour* 2011;3(1): 15–27.
17. Institute of Medicine (IOM). *Clinical Preventive Services for Women: Closing the Gaps.* Washington, DC: The National Academies Press; 2011.
18. Friedman HS, Martin LR. *The Longevity Project: Surprising Discoveries for Health and Long Life from the Landmark Eight-Decade Study.* New York, NY: Penguin; 2012.
19. Institute of Medicine (IOM). *The Future of Nursing: Leading Change, Advancing Health.* Washington, DC: The National Academies Press; 2011.
20. Institute of Medicine (IOM). *Crossing the Quality Chasm: A New Health System for the 21st Century.* Washington, DC: The National Academies Press; 2001.
21. Bhutta ZA, Chen L, Cohen J, Crisp N, Evans T, Fineberg H, et al. Education of health professionals for the 21st century: a global independent commission. *The Lancet* 2010;375(9721): 1137–1138.
22. Interprofessional Education Collaborative Expert Panel. *Core Competencies for Interprofessional Collaborative Practice: Report of an Expert Panel.* Washington, DC: Interprofessional Education Collaborative; 2011.
23. 2011 Health Professionals for a New Century. Asian Network Progress. *News and Views: Follow-Up Action.* http://healthprofessionals21.org. Accessed on March 25, 2013.
24. Cohen J. Are you ready for the paradigm shift? Commencement Speech given at University of California School of Medicine; June 2, 2012 (unpublished). http://www.meded.uci.edu/Cohen_commencement2012.asp. Accessed on December 5, 2012.
25. Gostin L. A framework convention on global health: health for all, justice for all. *JAMA* 2012;307(19): 2087–2092.
26. Georges JM. Linking nursing theory and practice: a critical-feminist approach. *Adv Nurs Sci* 2005;28(1): 50–57.
27. D'Antonio P, Fairman J. Guest editorial: history matters. *Nurs Outlook* 2010;58(2): 113–114.
28. Dong D, Temple B. Oppression: a concept analysis and implications for nurses and nursing. *Nurs Forum* 2011;46(3): 169–176.
29. Fletcher K. Beyond dualism: leading out of oppression. *Nurs Forum* 2006;41(2): 50–59.
30. D'Antonio P. *American Nursing: A History of Knowledge, Authority and the Meaning of Work.* Baltimore, MD: Johns Hopkins University Press, 2010.

Afterword

Paula N. Kagan

When we first imagined putting this book together, I hoped to encourage a broad forum on the topic of emancipatory nursing—broader even than the individual articles published on the topic in academic nursing journals. I wanted to see a variety of views on social justice and nursing collected in one place and, hopefully, opening up to an even wider dialogue on where and how to move the discipline of nursing forward. Thankfully, my partners Peggy Chinn and Marlaine Smith thought so too, and together we moved ahead with the project. We are running out of time. Each new generation of nursing students we produce as novice nurses entering the health care arena *without* an analysis of power and structure, of economics and politics, of the intersection of gender, ethnicity, class, and sexuality (among other domains of life) with health perpetuates the strength of ineffective systems and structures of health care delivery. In addition, this leads to the increased constraints on individual agency and challenges to sustainability that were so eloquently addressed by Joan Anderson in the foreword of this book. Nurses must be, *must live*, within a constant process of critical analysis. This is our charge. Analysis of the social determinants of health and illness, of social justice, and of liberation has historically emerged from nursing and has led to social changes including woman suffrage, professionalization of nursing, sanitation, and providing care where the people are: in their homes and communities. Somehow, along the way, much of this was erased from what many considered "essential" to nursing education. Could this book challenge nurse educators, accreditation organizations, and schools of nursing to make analysis of political, cultural, social, and economic dimensions of health essential and place critical consciousness at the core of every nurse's education?

We are running out of time. A few authors whose works are significantly related to sustainability and the environment had commitments that precluded their participation in this anthology. We are acutely aware of, and regret, their absence in both content and voice. Although we were unable to include a chapter on the human threat to our environment, which mounts moment-by-moment, in turn threatening human, plant, and animal life, this book nonetheless represents a call for more nursing scholarship and political activity relevant to the environment and health. Only a limited number of nurse scholars are today working on questions about human health and the environment, environmental health, sustainability of resources, forensic nursing, and disaster cause, occurrence, outcome, and survival. The greatest threats to human health are environmental; at no other time has a unitary perspective, which poses the inseparability, the indissolubility of humans and environment, been so relevant or so necessary. This is a nursing perspective. Nurses need to commit to the study, the practice, and the political action associated with this dimension of health and illness, in the process, liberating nursing research, education, and practice to go beyond the hospital or sick nursing orientations toward prevention and understanding of humans' integral relationship with the world, its resources, and challenges at the nexus of environmental and human endeavors. The burden of risk, morbidity, and mortality associated with increasing frequency and intensity of so-called weather or natural disasters—read human-made—will disproportionately fall on the poor, disenfranchised, disabled, marginalized, elderly, and women and children. The environment is a social justice issue and a health issue and worthy of emancipatory nursing—worthy of the praxis treated by the authors collected in these pages.

We are running out of time. Putting this book together is a praxiological act of emancipatory nursing. It is a gathering of voices to create an intense rise of volume. Listen. Nurses know many important and unique things about people and communities and their struggles with health and illness. The question addressed in these pages is how, even in light of structural challenges, can nurses best contribute to social justice? How can we best—and sustainably—influence students, faculty, and practitioners regarding the ideas discussed here, such as listening to others, freedom, agency, power, social justice, caring, peace, and the theoretical and practical basis of an imagined emancipatory and critical nursing discipline? Finally, how can we contribute to an effort to let those in other disciplines, who look to nurses for their health expertise and know of the significant scholarship and actions arising from emancipatory nursing?

The answer is, we hope, self-evident in the pages of this anthology. The authors clearly demonstrate that nursing theory, research, education, and practice can be liberated from the constraints of bio-medical models and methods in favor of innovation that takes into consideration persons' and communities' contexts, experiences, social characteristics, and the power dynamics that are integral to their health conditions and outcomes.

The urgency of the effort cannot be over-estimated. However, when I consider the main topics of this anthology—emancipatory nursing, praxis, critical practice, and social justice, I am gratified that we have in the discipline such a significant community of scholars contributing perspectives, standpoints, and methods that are applicable and usable in nursing practice. Practice, as reflected in these chapters and beyond, includes all forms and locations of activities in which nurses engage—from bedside nursing in home and hospital to community nursing to engagement as nurse educators, as administrators, as researchers, as policy makers, as consultants to corporations and organizations, and wherever and however nurses perform the art and science of the discipline. Critical theories that underpin nurses' practice in any of these areas will help to move thinking and doing in nursing from received views based in bio-medical models to a progressive, more humanized, non-routinized focus on care. The health care models incorporating high technology and a focus on cure that is based on an evidence-based protocol of "one size fits all" need to give way to a model of health care that is respectful of difference and the reality of the uniqueness of people and communities. These modes of practice and care are represented by the chapters presented here and are reflectively aimed toward transformation and enhancing social good. In various ways, the authors reflect that basic critique and provide a guide to a unique journey aimed at bettering the outcomes and quality of life of persons and communities.

We are at the point where we can provide a broad set of considerations for new theories that can be developed from critical perspectives and highlight the foundation of emancipatory nursing. Hopefully, many models and theories will be developed in the future to address nursing practice that arises from critical standpoints and frameworks specifically created to take a deep look at social structures, mores, values, habits, rituals, institutions, and behaviors relevant to and occurring during the provision of health care. That these theoretical considerations emerge from the discipline of nursing and have relevance particularly for care offered by nurses does not preclude their relevance for health care providers across disciplines.

So much of the impetus for the initiation of this anthology emerged from my own perspective and those of co-editors Marlaine Smith and Peggy Chinn as nurses who live in the United States at a time when government sponsored single payer health care is still a contentious social and political issue. It may indeed become a reality, *as it should*. The dominance and failure of a mostly white, patriarchal, and wealthy bio-medical establishment to meet the diverse and changing needs of people demands innovation in health care toward goals of inclusion, dignity, and respect regardless of domains or affiliations of color, gender, sexuality, nation, and class. Today, hierarchies of illness are shaped by the prestige of conditions requiring high tech surgical intervention and multiple prohibitively expensive pharmaceuticals down to a level of what most people, most of the time experience and need help with—the everyday realities of influenza, pain, chronic illness, depression, hunger, effects of violence, pregnancy, and childbearing.

The growing desire and considerations for emancipatory theory creates a framework that exists in response to a broken and unrelentingly failing infrastructure in the United States, and perhaps elsewhere, that systematically gears its allocations and resources to the extreme rather than the commonplace. Instead of meeting the public where they are, where they live, and in their contexts and experiential loci, doctor and hospital dominated health care is the most common health care circumstance in which persons find themselves—and that represents the system receiving the greatest economic advantage.

Critical frameworks by which to develop nursing theory, whether arising from the discipline or modified from others, will provide a way for nurses to heighten their awareness of the elements of damaged systems in a manner in which the dynamics of power, influence, and greed that work together to undermine the health of the public, and the arduous work of nurses attempting to care for them, become obvious and recognizable. Moreover, these frameworks may also provide a frame of reference for analysis of health care systems, infrastructures, behaviors, policies, and interpersonal relationships in the health care workplace as well as at its hidden borders and at its unspoken boundaries and margins. Most significantly, it is these frameworks, as analyzed by the works collected in this book, that will inspire nurses to action toward needed social change in nursing and health care, a means for liberation and praxis.

The goal of this anthology was to add significantly to, and push towards, the evolution of nursing—both the discipline and the practice—to unquestioned recognition and acknowledgment as a critical field. Clearly the frameworks, theories, methodologies, and narratives for emancipatory nursing proposed and/or described by the authors in this book go a long way to accomplishing that goal. The authors were concerned always and foremost with social justice and proffered their perspectives and narratives of experiences embedded with conceptualizations of diversity, respect, and dignity; with context, situated knowledges, and participatory problem-solving; and community-based and health promoting. Their collective scholarship is a product of the unique knowledge and expertise of nurses who have developed a critical and feminist theory-based world of scholarship and practice applications. These astonishing scholars liberate through their emancipatory ideas about humans, the environment, health, nursing, caring, power, and change. Emancipatory nursing is no longer underrepresented in the literature.

One final note: along with my co-editors, I recognize that we may have inadvertently neglected to invite others whose works deserve to be recognized in this field. The authors of the works collected here reflect the social and political contexts of western, Euro-centric nursing; they are by vast majority women and with few exceptions white and from English-speaking nations such as the United States, Canada (English and Quebecois), New Zealand, and Australia. We are well aware that there are many topics and authors relevant to the concept of emancipatory nursing whose ideas are not reflected here—but we see this not as a limitation but a challenge to continue the work of broadening the horizons and meanings of critical analysis and praxis that we have begun. Indeed, we have come full circle to envisioning a second volume that will focus on enhancing the emancipatory diversity of critical nursing consciousness—broadening the dialogue and pushing the emancipatory possibilities of nursing praxis even further beyond the limits of the present.

Paula N. Kagan, PhD, RN
November 2013

Contributors

Joan M. Anderson, PhD (Sociology), MSN, RN, Professor Emerita, University of British Columbia School of Nursing, has conducted extensive research in the areas of culture, gender, migration, health, and inequities in health and health care through the lens of postcolonial feminist inquiry and, more recently, critical humanism. With colleagues in academic and clinical settings, she has engaged in knowledge translation research with health professionals at the point of care, administrators, and policy makers. Dr. Anderson's active scholarship includes writing, consultation, serving on advisory committees, knowledge translation, and other forms of dissemination of her research.

JoAnne Banks, RN, PhD is the Bertha L. Shelton Professor of Research at Winston-Salem State University. "I am deeply interested in the multitude of life that surrounds me. Building connections within/across groups and species of life is essential to honoring my reason for being on the planet. I stand on the shoulders of a rich and diverse group of ancestors. My academic life is centered on the development of culturally and contextually consistent strategies to promote the health and well-being of Black women. I have been particularly interested in storytelling as an intervention strategy and data collection method. For the past 15 years, I have had the pleasure of working with Black women to develop storytelling and other strategies that assist in achieving and sustaining physically active lifestyles. Currently, I am extending this work to include Latina women."

Helene Berman, RN, PhD, is a professor and the Associate Dean (Research) in the Faculty of Health Sciences at Western University, and Research Scholar, Centre for Research and Education on Violence against Women and Children. Her research interests include the intersections of gender, race, and class in the context of interpersonal and structural violence. She has led two national studies on violence in the lives of girls and young women, and is currently the Principal Investigator on a Canadian Institutes of Health Research (CIHR) Team Grant, "Promoting Health through Collaborative Engagement with Youth: Overcoming, Resisting and Preventing Structural Violence." Other current research includes an examination of the transition to motherhood among women who have experienced past trauma. Helene is a past president of the Nursing Network on Violence against Women International.

Doris M. Boutain, PhD, RN is an associate professor in the Department of Psychosocial and Community Health, University of Washington School of Nursing. She is a community health researcher, nurse, and educator committed to using social justice as a framework to promote and protect health among underserved populations and communities. Her chronic disease prevention research is anchored in understanding how health disparities are created and can be addressed from working collaboratively across multiple sectors. Her work advocates for system change to promote population and community health for those most at risk of poor health outcomes. Dr. Boutain earned a degree in nursing from Southern University and MN and PhD degrees from the University of Washington School of Nursing.

Annette J. Browne, PhD, RN is a professor in the School of Nursing at the University of British Columbia in Vancouver, British Columbia, Canada. Her research focuses on strategies for fostering greater health equity and mitigating the negative effects of health inequities. Examples of her current research are focused on: promoting health equity for vulnerable populations in primary health care clinics; improving health care for Indigenous women experiencing violence; addressing the health effects of structural inequities and structural violence; and the relevance of cultural safety for health services. Her work is aimed at promoting health equity through improvements in nursing practice, health care delivery, and health policy.

Mary K. Canales, PhD, RN is a professor in the Department of Nursing at the University of Wisconsin-Eau Claire. She received her master's degree from Georgetown University in Washington, DC, and her PhD from the University of Wisconsin-Madison. Her scholarly interests include food insecurity and poverty, social justice, and health, particularly related to health inequities and the theoretical concept of othering. At the University of Wisconsin-Eau Claire she teaches undergraduate community and mental health and health policy and research at the graduate level. She serves as the Equity, Diversity, and Inclusivity (EDI) Fellow for the university.

C. Susana Caxaj, PhD, RN is a registered nurse and doctoral candidate at Western University, Canada. She is a recipient of the Canadian Vanier Scholarship (2011–2013) and has a clinical background in mental health psychiatric nursing. Her research has focused on refugee and immigrant youth well-being and more recently, on the relationship between community mental health and mining mega-projects among diverse indigenous populations. In 2012, Susana was a key organizer in the Peoples International Health Tribunal, the first tribunal of this nature focused on health, in where affected communities throughout Mesoamerica put Goldcorp on a moral trial for harms to health, human rights, and the environment. Goldcorp was found guilty by an international panel of judges.

Loryle (Laurie) M. Cender, RN, MSN is a doctoral student in the School of Nursing at the University of British Columbia. Laurie's clinical work as a clinical nurse specialist in pediatric cardiology and cardiac surgery has shaped her research interests. Her doctoral research focuses on promoting equity in parental antenatal decision-making support.

Peggy L. Chinn, RN, PhD, FAAN is the Founding Editor of *Advances in Nursing Science*, which since 1978 has been a premier journal publishing cutting-edge scholarship in nursing. She authors books and journal articles on nursing theory, feminism and nursing, the art of nursing, and nursing education. She was a co-founder of the group "Cassandra: Radical Feminist Nurses Network" that existed throughout the 1980s and of the current web-based "NurseManifest" project. She and Maeona Kramer, co-authors of the book *Knowledge Development in Nursing*, developed a conceptual approach to emancipatory knowing as integral to the essence and foundation of nursing.

Kierrynn Davis, RN, PhD is an adjunct fellow, School of Health and Human Sciences, Southern Cross University, Lismore, NSW, Australia. Her main research interests are violence against women and children and surviving relationship trauma. She has conducted sole and collaborative emancipatory research projects for the last two decades. Her research findings have been published in books and journals.

Gweneth Hartrick Doane, RN, PhD has an interdisciplinary background (nursing/psychology) and is a professor of Nursing at the University of Victoria, Canada. Her scholarly work focuses on relational inquiry with a particular emphasis on the integration of relational ontology, knowledge, and responsive action. She has translated this work within the areas of relational practice, family nursing, ethics, end-of-life care, and teaching and learning.

Denise J. Drevdahl, PhD, RN is a professor in the Nursing Program at the University of Washington–Tacoma. She received her master's degree from the University of Colorado Health Sciences Center and her PhD from the University of Washington. Her research interests include social justice and public health nursing, race/ethnicity and the delivery of health care, clinical trial decision making, and RN decision making with respect to pain medication administration in the Emergency Department. At the University of Washington Tacoma she has taught graduate and under-graduate courses in diversity, ethics, community/public health, health and human rights, and global health.

Robin A. Evans-Agnew, PhD, RN is an assistant professor, University of Washington–Tacoma Nursing and Healthcare Leadership program. Robin joined the faculty at the University of Washington in 2012. His major interests are in participatory research and environmental justice; with a focus on the critical examination of intersections between health care, chronic disease management (including asthma), and policy change. He received his PhD (2011) and MN (1989) from the University of Washington and his BSN (1994) from Johns Hopkins University.

Marilou Gagnon, RN, ACRN, PhD is an associate professor at the School of Nursing, Faculty of Health Sciences, University of Ottawa and Director of the Unit for Critical Research in Health. Her work is underpinned by critical and sociopolitical approaches. Her fields of study include questions related to the body and technology, power and discourse, and social justice. As a member of the University of Ottawa Research Chair in Forensic Nursing, she is working on a number of projects on HIV criminalization, HIV-related stigma and discrimination in health care settings, and human rights.

Jane M. Georges, PhD, RN is a professor at the Hahn School of Nursing and Health Science at the University of San Diego since 1996. She received her PhD in Nursing Science from the University of Washington and her MS in Nursing from the University of California, San Francisco. She teaches Philosophy of Science and Nursing Theory in the PhD program in Nursing Science at the University of San Diego. Her principal scholarly interests include power relations, suffering, and compassion, and she has published widely on these topics during the past decade.

Nel Glass, RN, PhD, FACN is a research professor of Nursing at Australian Catholic University, Melbourne, Victoria, Australia. Her main research interests are resilience, optimism, well-being, and healing. She has been involved in conducting sole and collaborative emancipatory research projects since the 1990s. Her research findings have been disseminated in books, journals, and art exhibitions.

Caroline G. Glickman, MIM is the associate director of the Office of the Dean at the University of Pennsylvania School of Nursing where she manages and implements a broad range of special projects and initiatives to advance the school's strategic international and national priorities, primarily in support of women's health and interprofessional education initiatives. She has co-authored with Dr. Afaf Meleis an article titled, "Empowering Expatriate Nurses: Challenges and Opportunities—a Commentary." Caroline holds a master's degree in international marketing and a bachelor's degree in Spanish and marketing from Saint Joseph's University in Philadelphia, Pennsylvania.

Pamela Grace, PhD, RN, FAAN is an associate professor of Nursing and Ethics at Boston College. She is an experienced nurse who has completed graduate degrees in both nursing and philosophy. Her research and scholarly interests are in exploring the foundations and boundaries of professional responsibilities for individual and social good. She has written and presented extensively on these and related ethical nursing issues.

Paula N. Kagan, PhD, RN is an associate professor at the School of Nursing DePaul University, Chicago, where she teaches graduate courses in theory, ethics, policy, and research underpinned with intersectional, critical feminist, and unitary frameworks. Dr. Kagan received the Illinois Board of Higher Education Nurse Educator Fellowship Award and the DePaul University Humanities Center Fellowship for her analysis of documentary filmmaking as nursing praxis. She has authored articles on listening, nursing philosophy, innovations in research, and health policy. Dr. Kagan is an OpEd Project—Public Voices through Leadership Fellow.

Peninnah M. Kako, PhD, RN, FNP-BC, APNP is an associate professor at the University of Wisconsin–Milwaukee, College of Nursing. Dr. Kako's research focuses on improving health care access for women living with HIV in sub-Saharan Africa. She has led a community health study abroad program to Kenya and also teaches in the DNP program. She maintains her clinical practice as a nurse practitioner providing primary health care for incarcerated populations.

Ursula A. Kelly, PhD, RN, ANP-BC, PMHNP-BC has served as the nurse scientist at the Atlanta VAMC for over three years. She is principal investigator of a study examining PTSD treatment barriers and facilitators for female veterans who experienced military sexual trauma and co-investigator of a VA PTSD/MST Treatment Program Evaluation study. Kelly maintains clinical practices as an adult and psychiatric/mental health nurse practitioner and has received numerous awards for her work with female veterans with PTSD. Her research and clinical expertise are the impact of interpersonal violence on women's mental and physical health. The central foci of her research have been posttraumatic stress disorder (PTSD) and depression in women who experienced intimate partner violence and military sexual trauma (MST), particularly exploring barriers to care and developing and evaluating innovative treatment models.

Terri LaCoursiere-Zucchero, PhD, RN, FNP-BC is a Post-doctoral Nurse Research Fellow at the Bedford VA Medical Center and Assistant Professor in the Graduate School of Nursing at the University of Massachusetts, Worcester. Her interest in social justice stems from her clinical experience as a Family Nurse Practitioner working with homeless and other vulnerable populations. Terri's scholarly work focuses on the complex care needs of homeless and unstably housed individuals and families who have co-morbid medical, psychiatric, and substance use disorders. She believes *housing is health care* and that nursing has a responsibility to address this critical issue. She maintains a clinical practice at Boston Health Care for the Homeless Program where she enjoys growing and learning together with her patients, colleagues, and students.

Beverly Malone, PhD, RN, FAAN is the chief executive officer of the National League for Nursing. Dr. Malone's tenure at the NLN has been marked by a retooling of the league's mission to reflect the core values of caring, diversity, integrity, and excellence and an ongoing focus on advancing the nation's health. Her distinguished career has mixed policy, education, administration, and clinical practice. In 1996, she was elected to two terms as president of the American Nurses Association (ANA) before becoming the deputy assistant secretary for health within the U.S. Department of Health and Human Services in 2000. Just prior to joining the NLN, Dr. Malone was general secretary of the Royal College of Nursing (RCN), the United Kingdom's largest professional union of nurses. In 2010, she was ranked #29 among the 100 Most Powerful People in Healthcare by *Modern Healthcare* magazine. Dr. Malone is a member of the Institute of Medicine.

Afaf I. Meleis, PhD, DrPS(Hons), FAAN is the Margaret Bond Simon Dean of Nursing at the University of Pennsylvania School of Nursing, Professor of Nursing and Sociology, and director of the school's WHO Collaborating Center for Nursing and Midwifery Leadership. Prior to coming to Penn, she was a professor at the University of California Los Angeles and the University of California San Francisco for 34 years. Dr. Meleis' research focuses on global health, immigrant health, women's health, and on the theoretical development of the nursing discipline. Dr. Meleis completed her Bachelor of Science in Nursing degree at the University of Alexandria, Egypt, a master's in nursing, a master's in sociology, and a PhD in medical and social psychology at the University of California, Los Angeles.

Lucy Mkandawire-Valhmu, RN, PhD is an associate professor in the College of Nursing at University of Wisconsin–Milwaukee (UWM). Her research focuses on the intersections of HIV and gender based violence in the lives of East African women. She leads the College of Nursing study abroad program to Malawi at UWM where students have the opportunity to participate in research and service while also learning about community health nursing.

Selina A. Mohammed, PhD, MPH, RN is an associate professor in Nursing and Health Studies at the University of Washington Bothell. Her research interests include examining the impact of racialized discrimination and other structural disadvantages on health and using critical research methodologies to explore how historical, sociocultural, political, and economic contexts contribute to health inequities, particularly for American Indians. Dr. Mohammed holds a master of science in nursing from the University of Michigan, master of public health from the University of Washington, and doctor of philosophy in nursing science from the University of Washington.

Carol Pillsbury Pavlish, PhD, RN, FAAN is currently an associate professor in the School of Nursing at the University of California Los Angeles and Professor Emeritus at St. Catherine University. She currently works with a research team investigating early indicators and interventions for ethical conflicts at end of life. Carol also researches women's health and human rights. She has partnered with the American Refugee Committee and worked with displaced populations in the post-conflict settings of Rwanda, Sudan, and Uganda since 2000. Based on those experiences she co-authored a nursing research textbook with Dr. Margaret Dexheimer Pharris, *Community-Based Collaborative Action Research: A Nursing Approach*, which was honored with an AJN Book of the Year Award for 2011.

Amélie Perron, RN, PhD is an associate professor at the School of Nursing, Faculty of Health Sciences, University of Ottawa, and a member of the University of Ottawa Research Chair in Forensic Nursing and of the Unit for Critical Research in Health. Her interests include nursing care provided to captive and marginalized populations, forensic and psychiatric nursing, power relationships, as well as issues of discourse, risk, gender, and ethics. She also writes on topics relating to the state of nursing knowledge and epistemology. She has published extensively in peer-reviewed journals and is an editor for *Aporia*, an open access peer-reviewed nursing journal (http://www.aporiajournal.com).

Donna J. Perry, PhD, RN is an assistant professor at the University of Massachusetts Graduate School of Nursing in Worcester, MA. She is also a nurse scientist at Massachusetts General Hospital. Dr. Perry is active in community service on issues of peace and social justice. She is Vice Chair of the Center for Nonviolent Solutions' Board of Directors. Dr. Perry's program of research focuses on human decision making around contemporary issues of social transformation that impact health related to peace, justice, and human rights. The research is conducted within an emerging theory developed by Dr. Perry called transcendent pluralism, which is a theory about the evolution of human dignity. She has lectured both nationally and internationally on topics ranging from health care to environmental justice. She had worked on global health projects in Abu Dhabi, Cuba, Guatemala, India, Israel, and Palestine. Dr. Perry has published a number of journal articles, book chapters, and two books. Her most recent book, entitled: *The Israeli-Palestinian Peace Movement: Combatants for Peace* provides the results of a research study with members of an Israeli-Palestinian peace group working nonviolently for peace and justice.

Margaret Dexheimer Pharris, PhD, RN, FAAN is the Associate Dean for Nursing at St. Catherine University in St. Paul and Minneapolis, Minnesota. As the Associate Dean, she oversees the education of over 800 nursing students from Associate Degree to DNP and actively collaborates on inter-professional education with the directors of the 30+ health programs within St. Catherine's Henrietta Schmoll School of Health. Dr. Pharris received her MS in Nursing, MPH, and PhD from the University of Minnesota, where she also completed a two-year interdisciplinary fellowship in Adolescent Health. In 2001, Dr. Pharris co-authored an Office of Women's Health grant that established a National Community Center of Excellence in Women's Health at NorthPoint Health & Wellness Center in North Minneapolis. To fulfill grant requirements, Dr. Pharris worked with women in multiethnic North Minneapolis to initiate a process of community-based collaborative action research within a unitary-participatory theoretical framework inspired by Dr. Margaret Newman's theory of health as expanding consciousness. Dr. Pharris has lectured widely on community-based collaborative action research and creating equitable, inclusive nursing education, and practice environments.

Debby A. Phillips, PhD, PMHCNS is a clinician, scholar, and educator who works to prevent human violence. Dr. Phillips is a psychiatric mental health Clinical Nurse Specialist and a Post-Traumatic Stress Disorder expert working with people of all ages who have survived diverse forms of violence. Dr. Phillips' scholarship likewise focuses on human violence. Grounded in a strong belief that humans are not innately programmed to act violently, her research moves away from examining individuals and their commonly assumed underlying biological pathology and examines society and how it produces the embodied possibility of acting violently, as well as the violence enacted though society's discourses.

Sheryl Reimer-Kirkham, PhD, RN is a professor and the Director of the Graduate program in the School of Nursing at Trinity Western University in Langley, British Columbia, Canada. Her research is in the area of plurality and equity in health care, focusing on the intersections of religion, spirituality, race, class, and gender, and is demonstrating how religion and spirituality are negotiated for social inclusion or exclusion in post-secular health care settings and how religion and spirituality may form social pathways to health and illness. Another arm of her scholarship focuses on knowledge translation for a palliative approach. She is the Co-Director of Trinity Western University's Centre for Equity and Global Engagement (http://www.twu.ca/cege) and co-edited the book, *Religion, Religious Ethics, and Nursing* (Fowler, Reimer-Kirkham, Sawatzky, and Johnston Taylor, Springer, 2012).

Trudy Rudge RN, BA(Hons), PhD is in the unique position of having an appointment as a chair in nursing with a focus in the humanities and social sciences at the Sydney Nursing School, the University of Sydney. This appointment is centered in the dual recognition of her ongoing research program analyzing nurses and their work using philosophy, anthropology, and contemporary social analyses and the centrality of social and philosophical knowledge to enabling sound nursing practice and disciplinary development. She has published with Dave Holmes (2010) *Abjectly Boundless: Bodies, Boundaries and Health Work* and with Dave Holmes and Amélie Perron (2012) *(Re)thinking Violence in Health Care Settings: A Critical Approach*, both published by Ashgate, Farnham, UK. She is advisory editor to *Nursing Inquiry* and on many editorial boards of journals in nursing and the social sciences.

Marie-Anne Sanon, PhD, RN is currently a post-doctoral fellow at the University of Michigan, School of Nursing. She earned her PhD with a specialty focus on occupational health as a Centers for Disease Control (CDC)–National Institute for Occupational Safety and Health (NIOSH)–Education Research Center (ERC) Fellow from the University of Washington, Seattle. Dr. Sanon completed her master's degree in communities, populations, and health at the University of Washington, Tacoma, School of Nursing. Her program of research focuses on optimizing the health of workers in the United States, specifically immigrant workers in service industries.

Marlaine C. Smith, RN, PhD, FAAN is Dean and Helen K. Persson Eminent Scholar at the Christine E. Lynn College of Nursing at Florida Atlantic University. She is the co-editor of the third edition of *Nursing Theories and Nursing Practice* and *Caring in Nursing Classics*, and has authored articles related to nursing philosophy, caring as a philosophy, theory and ethic, and issues of discrimination, equality, and social justice. Her theoretical work has focused on caring within a unitary worldview, and her research is related to healing outcomes of touch for those with life-threatening illnesses.

Patricia E. Stevens, PhD, RN, FAAN is a professor at the University of Wisconsin–Milwaukee. She is a feminist scholar who has done extensive research in the area of HIV/AIDS and women's health and is an expert in qualitative research methods and community based participatory research. She has published more than 100 peer reviewed articles in professional journals.

Sally Thorne, RN, PhD, FAAN, FCAHS is a professor and the former Director at the University of British Columbia School of Nursing in Vancouver, Canada. Her scholarly contributions span the fields of nursing theory and philosophy, applied qualitative methodology, and the substantive areas of chronic illness and cancer patient experience. Her work reveals sustained fascination for the manner in which health system structure and ideology shape inequities in health experience. She serves on several national boards, playing an active role in advancing professional nursing perspectives at policy tables. She also currently serves as Editor-in-Chief of *Nursing Inquiry*.

Colleen Varcoe, RN, PhD is a professor in the School of Nursing at the University of British Columbia. Her research focuses on women's health with emphasis on violence and inequity and the culture of health care with an emphasis on ethics. Completed research includes studies of the interacting risks of violence and HIV infection for rural and Aboriginal women, rural maternity care for Aboriginal women, ethics and health policy, and the health effects of violence. Current research includes studies to promote equity in primary health care and studies of a health intervention for women who have experienced violence.

Jean Watson, PhD, AHN-BC, FAAN is Distinguished Professor and Dean Emerita, University of Colorado Denver, College of Nursing Anschutz Medical Center campus, where she held the nation's first endowed Chair in Caring Science for 16 years. She is founder of the original Center for Human Caring in Colorado; past President of the National League for Nursing; and founding member of International Association in Human Caring and International Caritas Consortium. Her latest activities include Founder and Director of the non-profit foundation: Watson Caring Science Institute (http://www.watsoncaringscience.org). Dr. Watson has earned undergraduate and graduate degrees in nursing and psychiatric-mental health nursing and holds her PhD in educational psychology and counseling. She was designated a Living Legend in 2013 by the American Academy of Nursing.

Jill White, AM, RN, RM, MEd, PhD is currently the Dean of the Sydney Nursing School at the University of Sydney, Australia's oldest and one of its most prestigious universities. Prior to taking up this appointment in 2008 Jill was Dean at the University of Technology, Sydney, and Chair of the Nursing and Midwifery Department at Victoria University in Wellington, New Zealand. From the earliest days in her nursing career Jill has been interested in social justice issues, however, this interest was deepened to a strong commitment during her very formative and privileged time in New Zealand. Jill is Immediate Past Chair of the Australian Nursing and Midwifery Accreditation Council (ANMAC).

Danny G. Willis, DNS, RN, PMHCNS is an associate professor and department chair at Boston College, William F. Connell School of Nursing. His research, practice, and publications focus on the phenomenon and meanings of healing for boys and men who have lived through marginalizing and traumatic violence as well as nursing philosophy and nursing's theoretical development. The National Institute of Nursing Research (NINR) has funded his research focused on men's lived experiences of healing from child maltreatment.

Index